D1557770

Catheter Based Valve and Aortic Surgery

Gorav Ailawadi • Irving L. Kron
Editors

Catheter Based Valve and Aortic Surgery

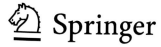 Springer

Editors
Gorav Ailawadi, MD
Chief, Section of Adult Cardiac Surgery
Surgical Director
Advanced Cardiac Valve Center
University of Virginia
Department of Surgery
Charlottesville, VA, USA

Irving L. Kron, MD
Hurt Watts Professor and Chairman
University of Virginia Hospital
Department of Surgery
Charlottesville, VA, USA

ISBN 978-1-4939-3430-0   ISBN 978-1-4939-3432-4   (eBook)
DOI 10.1007/978-1-4939-3432-4

Library of Congress Control Number: 2016933482

Springer New York Heidelberg Dordrecht London
© Springer Science+Business Media New York 2016

Printed on acid-free paper

Springer Science+Business Media LLC New York is part of Springer Science+Business Media (www.springer.com)

Preface

The treatment of cardiac diseases has had several breakthroughs in the last 70 years, starting with the development of the cardiopulmonary bypass machine, as well as artificial valves and ventricular assist devices. The treatment of coronary artery disease dramatically changed when Andreas Gruentzig presented an early experience with catheter-based angioplasty in 1977. Roughly 10 years later, angioplasty was more common than coronary artery bypass grafting.

For the last 60+ years, significant valve disease has been primarily treated with surgical repair or replacement. In 2002, Alan Cribier performed the world's first transcatheter aortic valve replacement, dramatically changing the course of catheter-based valve therapies. Over the last 10 years, multiple studies investigating catheter-based aortic valve replacement, including the PARTNER and CoreValve Pivotal Trials, have led to approval for these devices in high-risk and inoperable patients with severe aortic stenosis. Trials with the MitraClip device have also led to approval in patients with primary mitral pathology at prohibitive risk for surgery.

Recently, there have been multiple new catheter-based technologies targeting structural diseases of the heart that are challenging traditional open surgery as well as increasing the patient population who are able to be treated. As such, the purpose of this book is to provide the readers an up-to-date reference for catheter-based valve technology.

The first section of this book focuses on aortic valve disease with an emphasis on the technique of transfemoral and alternative access TAVR as well as valves on the horizon and valve-in-valve TAVR. The next section evaluates mitral valve therapies which are rapidly evolving including MitraClip and Annular methods of repair with the final chapters evaluating transcatheter mitral valve replacement. Next, the pulmonary valve is evaluated in depth along with percutaneous and alternative approaches to transcatheter pulmonary valve replacement. The final section considers the "forgotten" tricuspid valve as a major area of growth with new annular repair techniques on the horizon.

In summary, the cardiac surgeon and cardiologist must be aware of these new therapies. It is not unlikely that over the next 5–10 years, many of the diseases traditionally treated with valve surgery will be treated with the evolving and novel catheter-based options for repair and replacement discussed in this text.

Charlottesville, VA   Gorav Ailawadi
                                                                         Irving L. Kron

Contents

Contributors

Gorav Ailawadi, MD Section of Adult Cardiac Surgery, Department of Surgery, Advanced Cardiac Valve Center, University of Virginia, Charlottesville, VA, USA

Rizwan Attia, BMedSci, MBChB, MRCS, PhD Department of Cardiothoracic Surgery, Guys and St. Thomas' Hospital, London, UK

Waqar Aziz, MB, BCh, BAO, MSc, MRCPI, MRCP Department of Cardiology, Guys and St. Thomas' Hospital, London, UK

Vinnie (Vinayak) Bapat, MBBS, MS, FCRS, FRCSCTh Department of Cardiothoracic Surgery, Guys and St. Thomas' Hospital, London, UK

Anson Cheung, MD Division of Cardiac Surgery, St. Paul's Hospital, Vancouver, BC, Canada

Juan A. Crestanello, MD Division of Cardiac Surgery, Department of Surgery, Wexner Medical Center, The Ohio State University, Columbus, OH, USA

Stephen W. Davies, MD, MPH Department of Surgery, University of Virginia Medical Center, Charlottesville, VA, USA

Abhay A. Divekar, MBBS, MD Division of Pediatric Cardiology, University of Iowa Children's Hospital, Iowa City, IA, USA

Emily Downs, MD Department of Surgery, Thoracic Surgery Resident, University of Virginia, Charlottesville, VA, USA

Ted Feldman, MD, FSCAI, FACC, FESC Cardiac Catheterization Laboratory, Cardiology Division, Evanston Hospital, NorthShore University HealthSystem, Evanston, IL, USA

James J. Gangemi, MD Department of Surgery, University of Virginia Medical Center, Charlottesville, VA, USA

Nadim Geloo, MD Department of Cardiology, Sentara Rockingham Memorial Hospital, Harrisonburg, VA, USA

Barry George, BE, MD, FACC, FACI, FACP Division of Cardiovascular Medicine, Department of Medicine, Wexner Medical Center, The Ohio State University, Columbus, OH, USA

Timothy J. George, MD Division of Thoracic and Cardiovascular Surgery, Department of Surgery, The University of Virginia Hospital Medical Center, Charlottesville, VA, USA

Ravi K. Ghanta, MD Division of Thoracic Cardiovascular Surgery, University of Virginia, Charlottesville, VA, USA

Matthew J. Gillespie, MD Division of Cardiology, Department of Pediatrics, The Children's Hospital of Philadelphia, Perelman School of Medicine, University of Pennsylvania, Philadelphia, PA, USA

Paul A. Grayburn, MD Department of Cardiology, Baylor University Medical Center, Baylor Heart and Vascular Institute, Dallas, TX, USA

Christoph Hammersting, MD Department of Cardiology, Pulmonology, Angiology, and Internal Intensive Care, University Hospital, University of Bonn, NRW, Bonn, Germany

Matthew C. Henn, MD Division of Cardiothoracic Surgery, Department of Surgery, Barnes-Jewish Hospita, Washington University School of Medicine, St. Louis, MO, USA

Phillip A. Horwitz, MD Department of Internal Medicine, University of Iowa Carver College of Medicine, Iowa City, IA, USA

Hanna A. Jensen, MD, PhD Joseph B. Whitehead Department of Surgery, Emory University School of Medicine, Atlantic, GA, USA

Department of Cardiothoracic Surgery, Structural Heart and Valve Center, Emory University Hospital Midtown, Atlantic, GA, USA

Samir R. Kapadia, MD, FACC Department of Cardiovascular Medicine, Cleveland Clinic Hospital, Cleveland, OH, USA

Susheel Kodali, MD Department of Interventional Cardiology, Columbia University Medical Center, New York, NY, USA

Kevin Lichtenstein, BM, BS Division of Cardiac Surgery, University of British Columbia, Vancouver, BC, Canada

Francesco Maisano, MD Department of Cardiovascular Surgery, University Hospital of Zurich, Zurich, Switzerland

S. Chris Malaisrie, MD Division of Cardiac Surgery, Bluhm Cardiovascular Institute, Northwestern University/Northwestern Memorial Hospital, Chicago, IL, USA

Hersh S. Maniar, MD Division of Cardiothoracic Surgery, Department of Surgery, Barnes-Jewish Hospital, Washington University School of Medicine, St. Louis, MO, USA

Arul Furtado, MD Joseph B. Whitehead Department of Surgery, Emory University School of Medicine, Atlantic, GA, USA

Department of Cardiothoracic Surgery, Structural Heart and Valve Center, Emory University Hospital Midtown, Atlantic, GA, USA

Rick Meece, ACS, RDCS, RCIS, FASE Department of Cardiology, St. Thomas Hospital, Nashville, TN, USA

M. Andrew Morse, MD Department of Cardiology, St. Thomas Hospital, Nashville, TN, USA

Jared E. Murdock, MD Joseph B. Whitehead Department of Surgery, Emory University School of Medicine, Atlantic, GA, USA

Department of Cardiothoracic Surgery, Structural Heart and Valve Center, Emory University Hospital Midtown, Atlantic, GA, USA

Georg Nickenig, MD Department of Cardiology, Pulmonology, Angiology, and Internal Intensive Care, University Hospital, University of Bonn, NRW, Bonn, Germany

Michael L. O'Byrne, MD, MSCE Division of Cardiology, Department of Pediatrics, The Children's Hospital of Philadelphia, Perelman School of Medicine, University of Pennsylvania, Philadelphia, PA, USA

Puja B. Parikh, MD, MPH Department of Medicine, Stony Brook University Medical Center, South Setauket, NY, USA

Francesco Prione, MD St. Thomas Hospital, London, UK

Rahee Radia Department of Cardiology, Guys and St. Thomas' Hospital, Rickmansworth, Herts, UK

Michael Ragosta, MD Cardiovascular Division, Cardiac Catheterization Laboratory, University of Virginia Health System, Charlottesville, VA, USA

Mohammad Qasim Raza, MD Department of Cardiovascular Medicine, Cleveland Clinic Hospital, Cleveland, OH, USA

Jeffrey B. Rich, MD Virginia Cardiac Surgery, Quality Initiative, Virginia Beach, VA, USA

Evelio Rodriguez, MD Department of Cardiology, St. Thomas Hospital, Nashville, TN, USA

Mohammad Sarraf, MD Cardiac Catheterization Laboratory, Cardiology Division, Evanston Hospital, NorthShore University HealthSystem, Evanston, IL, USA

Sarah A. Schubert, MD Division of Thoracic Cardiovascular Surgery, University of Virginia, Charlottesville, VA, USA

Robert Schueler, MD Department of Cardiology, Pulmonology, Angiology, and Internal Intensive Care, University Hospital, University of Bonn, NRW, Bonn, Germany

Matthew L. Stone, MD Department of Surgery, University of Virginia Medical Center, Charlottesville, VA, USA

Amjadullah Syed, MD Joseph B. Whitehead Department of Surgery, Emory University School of Medicine, Atlantic, GA, USA

Department of Cardiothoracic Surgery, Structural Heart and Valve Center, Emory University Hospital Midtown, Atlantic, GA, USA

Deepak Talreja, MD, FACC Department of Cardiology, Sentara Heart Program, Eastern Virginia Medical School, Virginia Beach, VA, USA

Maurizio Taramasso, MD Department of Cardiovascular Surgery, University Hospital of Zurich, Zurich, Switzerland

Vinod H. Thourani, MD Joseph B. Whitehead Department of Surgery, Emory University School of Medicine, Atlantic, GA, USA

Department of Cardiothoracic Surgery, Structural Heart and Valve Center, Emory University Hospital Midtown, Atlantic, GA, USA

Joseph W. Turek, MD, PhD Division of Pediatric Cardiac Surgery, University of Iowa Children's Hospital, Iowa City, IA, USA

Michael H. Yamashita, MDCM, MPH Division of Cardiac Surgery, Bluhm Cardiovascular Institute, Northwestern University/Northwestern Memorial Hospital, Chicago, IL, USA

Leora T. Yarboro, MD Department of Surgery, University of Virginia, Charlottesville, VA, USA

Firas Zahr, MD Department of Internal Medicine, University of Iowa Carver College of Medicine, Iowa City, IA, USA

Alan Zajarias, MD Division of Cardiovascular Diseases, Department of Medicine, Barnes-Jewish Hospital, Washington University School of Medicine, St. Louis, MO, USA

Chapter 1
Aortic Valve Anatomy: Implications for Transcatheter Aortic Valve Replacement

Sarah A. Schubert and Ravi K. Ghanta

The aortic valve is a semilunar valve positioned between the left ventricle (LV) and the aorta. Proper functioning of the valve with unobstructed opening during systole and hermetic closure during diastole is critical for cardiac output and function. Transcatheter intervention on the aortic valve requires a comprehensive understanding of aortic valve anatomy, including the structure of the aortic root, position of the aortic valve annulus, and valve leaflets, including surrounding anatomic relationships with the coronary ostia, membranous septum, mitral valve, and outflow tract.

Anatomy

The aortic valve is the most centrally located cardiac valve, sitting just posterior and medial to the pulmonary valve and anterior to the tricuspid and mitral valves (Fig. 1.1) [1]. Aortic valve structure and function is intimately related to the surrounding aortic root—a structure that extends from basal attachments of the aortic valve leaflets in the LV to the superior attachment at the sinotubular junction (STJ) (Fig. 1.2). Two thirds of the aortic root is attached to the muscular ventricular septum, while one third is attached to the fibrous aorto-mitral continuity and fibrous trigones. Important structures contained within the aortic root include the sinuses of Valsalva, the coronary ostia, the aortic valve leaflets, and the interleaflet triangles (Fig. 1.3).

The STJ is a distinct ridge of circular tissue that delineates the start of the ascending aorta. The aortic valve leaflets are parabolically attached to the aortic root, with their attachments extending from the LV to the STJ. Due to this relationship,

S.A. Schubert, MD • R.K. Ghanta, MD (✉)
Division of Thoracic Cardiovascular Surgery, University of Virginia, 1215 Lee Street,
PO Box 800679, Charlottesville, VA 22908, USA
e-mail: ss9kw@virginia.edu; rkg3y@virginia.edu

© Springer Science+Business Media New York 2016
G. Ailawadi, I.L. Kron (eds.), *Catheter Based Valve and Aortic Surgery*,
DOI 10.1007/978-1-4939-3432-4_1

1

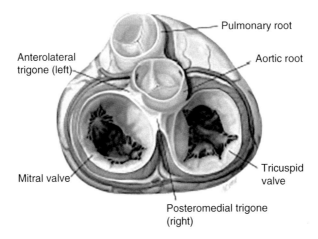

Fig. 1.1 Aortic valve seated within the heart, anchored between the pulmonary valve and atrioventricular valves and in continuity with the fibrous skeleton of the heart. (Source: Carpentier A, Adams DH, Filsoufi F. Surgical Anatomy and Physiology. In: Carpentier's Reconstructive Valve Surgery: From Valve Analysis to Valve Reconstruction. Maryland Heights, MO: Saunders Elsevier; 2010:209–216.)

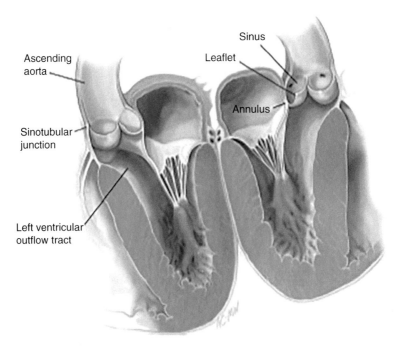

Fig. 1.2 Left atrium, left ventricle, and aortic root opened longitudinally. The left ventricular outflow tract serves as the proximal delineation of the aortic root and the sinotubular junction is the distal boundary. (Source: Carpentier A, Adams DH, Filsoufi F. Surgical Anatomy and Physiology. In: Carpentier's Reconstructive Valve Surgery: From Valve Analysis to Valve Reconstruction. Maryland Heights, MO: Saunders Elsevier; 2010:209–216.)

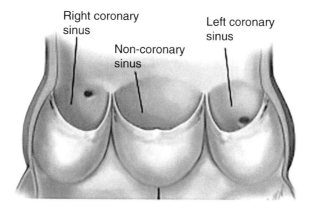

Fig. 1.3 Opened aortic valve demonstrating coronary ostia within the sinuses of Valsalva. (Source: Carpentier A, Adams DH, Filsoufi F. Surgical Anatomy and Physiology. In: Carpentier's Reconstructive Valve Surgery: From Valve Analysis to Valve Reconstruction. Maryland Heights, MO: Saunders Elsevier; 2010:209–216.)

widening of the STJ, as seen with an ascending aortic aneurysm, frequently leads to aortic insufficiency. The normal diameter of the STJ ranges from 29 to 33 mm in average adults without aortic valve pathology [2]. In patients with aortic stenosis, the diameter at the STJ is often significantly wider—a fact that must be taken into consideration when sizing and positioning transcatheter aortic valves within the root [3].

Inferior to the STJ, the aortic root widens to almost twice the radius of the aorta, forming the sinuses of Valsalva [4]. These sinuses give rise to the coronary ostia and physiologically function to augment coronary perfusion and valve closure. During diastole, the sinuses support a reservoir of blood to perfuse the coronary arteries. During systole, the sinuses prevent the valve leaflets from occluding the coronary ostia and allow formation of eddy currents within the sinus to exert pressure on the valve leaflets to close at end-systole [5].

The aortic valve most commonly consists of three leaflets, each named according to their position relative to the coronary arteries: right coronary leaflet, left coronary leaflet, and noncoronary (or posterior) leaflet. Each leaflet consists of a hinge, belly, and coapting edge (Fig. 1.4). The hinge is the semilunar attachment of the leaflet to the wall of the proximal aorta, forming the scalloped hemodynamic border between the LV and the aorta. The belly is the main body of the leaflet extending medially from the hinge, forming the inferior aspect of each corresponding sinus of Valsalva. In a competent aortic valve, each free leaflet edge coapts with the adjacent leaflet edge for a distance of several millimeters. These coapting edges are thin, fibrous structures termed lunulae. At the midpoint of each lunulae is a small fibrous nodule known as the nodule of Arantius; these complete valve coaptation and ensure valve competency [6]. Each leaflet is composed primarily of connective tissue contained within three distinct histologic layers (Fig. 1.5). The fibrosa lies on the aortic side of the leaflet and is comprised primarily of collagen fibers, while the ventriculosa lies on the ventricular side of the leaflet and is comprised primarily of radially oriented

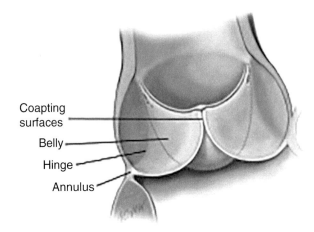

Fig. 1.4 Each leaflet is comprised of a belly, hinge, and the coapting edge. (Source: Carpentier A, Adams DH, Filsoufi F. Surgical Anatomy and Physiology. In: Carpentier's Reconstructive Valve Surgery: From Valve Analysis to Valve Reconstruction. Maryland Heights, MO: Saunders Elsevier; 2010:209–216.)

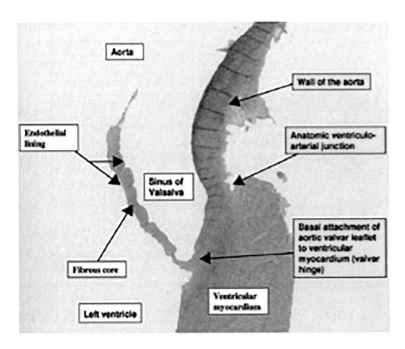

Fig. 1.5 Histologic layers of the aortic valve leaflets from ventricular side to aortic side: ventriculosa, spongiosa, and fibrosa. Also demonstrated is the anatomic ventriculo-arterial junction (Source: Piazza et al. [7])

elastic fibers, all of which given strength to the valve leaflets. The spongiosa layer lies between the ventriculosa and fibrosa and is made of mucopolysaccharide ground substance, imparting a certain amount of flexibility within each leaflet [1].

Only rarely are the valve leaflets of equal size. A study of 200 normal hearts found considerable variation between the average widths of the leaflets; average width of the right coronary, noncoronary, and left coronary leaflets was 25.9, 25.5, and 25.0 mm, respectively. Variation also exists within the height of each coronary cusp, although the mean height from the center of the leaflet to the free edge was 14.1 mm [8]. Such variability in leaflet sizes must be considered during transcatheter prosthetic valve sizing, as it can confound measurements of the aortic annulus and contribute to inaccurate prosthesis sizing.

The aortic valve leaflet is a scalloped structure with a nadir in the LV and a superior edge in the aorta at the level of the STJ, and the leaflets serve to define the hemodynamic border. The hemodynamic border is crown-like in shape, following the parabolic attachments of the aortic valve leaflets (Fig. 1.6). In contrast, the anatomic ventriculo-arterial border is a circular border, lying just superior to the nadir of the leaflet cusps. The anatomic border is a histologically defined boundary, with myocardium proximally and aortic tissue distally [4].

The term aortic annulus is frequently utilized in describing the aortic valve and is critical in sizing for aortic valve replacement. Although there is continued debate about the existence of a true aortic annulus, during surgical aortic valve replacements, the suture line is generally located just at the anatomic junction of the ventricle and aorta [4].

The commissure of each leaflet is the peripheral point of coaptation of adjacent leaflets to the wall of the aorta; thus, in a normal trileaflet aortic valve, there are three commissures. The commissure formed by the right and left coronary leaflets lies anterior and leftwards within the aorta, adjacent to the pulmonary artery. The

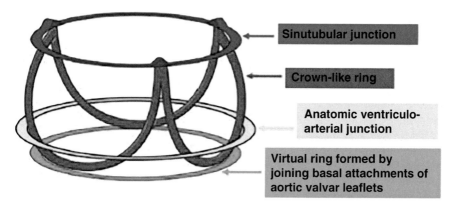

Fig. 1.6 Three-dimensional arrangement of the aortic root, demonstrating the crown-like suspension of the leaflets within the root and the corresponding circular anatomic landmarks (Source: Piazza et al. [7])

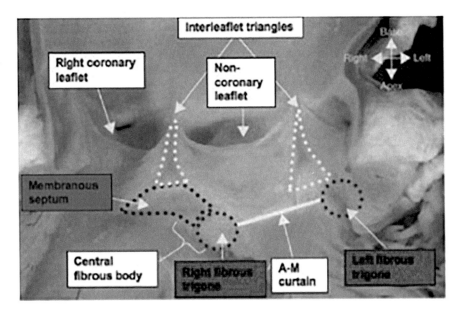

Fig. 1.7 Opened aortic root demonstrating the leaflets and interleaflet triangles and their continuity with the fibrous trigones, membranous septum, and aorto-mitral continuity (Source: Piazza et al. [7])

left and noncoronary commissure lies posterior and rightward. The right and non-coronary commissure lies anterior and rightward, adjacent to the right atrium.

Each commissure forms the apices of the interleaflet triangles—the areas under the inferior borders between each scalloped leaflet (Fig. 1.7). The base of each inter-leaflet triangle is formed by an imaginary line connecting the nadir of each leaflet hinge. The interleaflet triangle between the right and left coronary leaflets is con-tiguous with the potential space between the anterior aortic wall and the posterior portion of the pulmonary trunk of pulmonary infundibulum. Moving clockwise within the aortic root, the right and noncoronary interleaflet triangle is in continuity with the membranous ventricular septum, thus placing it in close proximity to the right atrium and the septal leaflet of the tricuspid valve (Fig. 1.7). The tricuspid septal leaflet divides the membranous septum into its ventricular and atrioventricu-lar portions and forms one side of the triangle of Koch. Of note, the apex of this anatomic triangle contains the atrioventricular (AV) node, placing it in close prox-imity to the subvalvar regions of the aortic valve, thus making the AV node vulner-able during traditional or transcatheter aortic valve replacement. The bundle of His also typically travels out from within this subcommissural space of the right and noncoronary interleaflet triangle, so it is also at risk for injury during aortic valve replacement. The third interleaflet triangle is that between the left and noncoronary leaflets, which extends proximally as the aorto-mitral continuity and ultimately forms the anterior leaflet of the mitral valve [7, 9].

Common Anatomic Variants

Bicuspid aortic valves are a common anatomic variant, occurring in 1–2 % of the population [10]. Most commonly in bicuspid aortic valves, the right and left coronary leaflets are fused, thus forming anterior and posterior leaflets with right and left true commissures; however, right and left leaflets with anterior and posterior commissures can also be formed. The right and noncoronary leaflets can also be fused, which occurs in approximately 15–30 % of cases [11]. Most significantly, in the context of aortic valve replacement, bicuspid aortic valves are widely known to be associated with a greater incidence of both infective endocarditis and aortic stenosis. It has been estimated that 50 % of adults with aortic stenosis have a bicuspid aortic valve, and approximately 25 % of cases of infective endocarditis develop on a bicuspid valve [12]. Bicuspid aortic valves were previously considered a contraindication to transcatheter valve placement because of the risk of aortic dissection with valve deployment and because of incorrect valve placement and deployment because of the elliptical valve orifice, but there have been reports of successful transcatheter aortic valve replacements in patients with bicuspid aortic valves [13].

Anomalous coronary arteries are a relatively rare, albeit important, anatomic abnormality affecting the aortic valve and root that must be considered when planning transcatheter aortic valve replacement. Normally positioned coronary arteries arise from their respective ostia positioned within the sinuses of Valsalva; that is, the right coronary artery ostium lies within the rightward facing sinus and the left coronary artery ostium arises from the leftward facing sinus, with both sinuses adjacent to the pulmonary trunk. Although most ostia lie within the central portion of the sinus, they can also lie at the sinus periphery and as much as 1 cm distal to the STJ. Broadly, clinically significant anomalous coronary artery origins can be dichotomized into those coronary arteries arising from the wrong sinus of Valsalva and those coronary arteries arising from the pulmonary artery. The incidence of anomalous coronary arteries has been estimated at 0.3 % in autopsy studies [14]. Coronary arteries with aberrant origins in the wrong sinus are much more common than those taking off from the pulmonary artery, with the most common abnormality being a left circumflex artery arising from the right sinus of Valsalva. Coronary arteries arising from the main pulmonary artery or its branches are a much less common anomalous configuration, especially in adults. Anomalous left coronary artery from the pulmonary artery (ALCAPA) and anomalous right coronary artery from the pulmonary artery are relatively rare congenital malformations, and these patients typically present early in life with symptoms of myocardial ischemia and heart failure, primarily due to coronary steal phenomenon. Even less common abnormalities include coronary artery fistulae in which the coronary ostia communicate directly with the cardiac chambers and coronaries with anomalous origins from more distal aortic branches [15, 16]. Although there are myriad anomalous configurations of coronary arteries and their ostia, the positions and courses of the coronaries should be considered prior to transcatheter valve placement to avoid coronary injury and ensure adequate coronary perfusion following valve deployment.

Imaging of the Aortic Root and Valve

Transcatheter aortic valve prostheses sit within the aortic root, and intimate knowl-edge of the entire aortic root anatomy is critical. Each patient's specific anatomy should be fully queried prior to transcatheter valve placement; most importantly, the STJ diameter, the aortic annulus diameter, the location and height of the coronary artery ostia, and the presence of septal hypertrophy should be determined. Transthoracic echocardiography (TTE) is the standard initial imaging modality for characterization of valvular morphology. TTE is invaluable for the definition of individual aortic valve anatomy (Fig. 1.8), and it also allows for the determination of the severity of aortic stenosis, diameter of aortic valve annulus, ejection fraction, left ventricular hypertrophy, concomitant valvular disease, and any wall motion abnormalities indicative of ischemic or infarcted myocardium.

Additional imaging with multi-slice computed tomography (CT) or cardiac mag-netic resonance imaging (CMRI) is also necessary for complete evaluation of the aortic valve (Figs. 1.9 and 1.10). Both types of imaging allow measurement of the annular diameter, dimensions within the root, and, most importantly, the measurement of the height of the coronary ostia relative to the aortic annulus. CT has several advan-tages over CMRI, including its speed and greater patient tolerance. Most importantly, however, CT allows visualization of calcification, which is not visible on CMRI. Calcification of the aortic valve leaflets, aortic root, and aortic arch must be considered prior to transcatheter valve placement. Bulky calcification of the leaflets

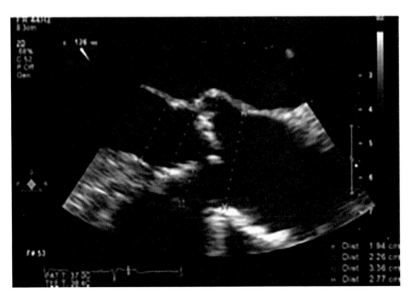

Fig. 1.8 Measurement of the diameters of the aortic annulus, sinotubular junction, and ascending aorta on transthoracic echocardiography is essential for correct selection and positioning of the implanted transcatheter aortic valve. (Courtesy of the University of Virginia Department of Radiology and Cardiovascular Imaging)

Fig. 1.9 (**a**) Axial and (**b**) coronal multi-slice CT imaging of the aortic root allows assessment of calcification, coronary anatomy, and dimensions of the root and native aortic valve (Source: Zamorano et al. [17])

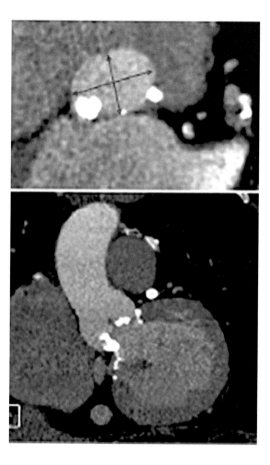

Fig. 1.10 MRI imaging of the aortic root allows assessment of coronary anatomy and dimensions of the root and native aortic valve. (Courtesy of the University of Virginia Department of Radiology and Cardiovascular Imaging)

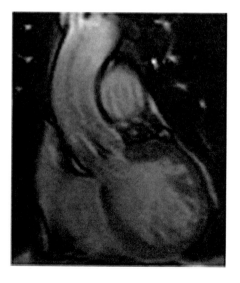

and within the root increases the risk of paravalvular leaks, as the outer surface of the prosthesis does not fit snugly within the native aortic valve. Leaflet calcification also increases the risk of coronary occlusion, as the native leaflets are displaced against the aortic wall and possibly overlying the coronary ostia. Excessive calcification within the annulus and root may also cause asymmetric valve deployment, increasing the risk of coronary ostial compression and improper seating of the valve within the root [17].

Conclusion

Knowledge of the aortic valve and root anatomy is essential to transcatheter replacement of the valve, and an understanding of the functional anatomy can minimize the risks of coronary ischemia, paravalvular leaks and regurgitation, and patient-prosthesis mismatch with transcatheter aortic valve replacement.

References

1. Gross L, Kugel MA. Topographic anatomy and histology of the valves in the human heart. Am J Pathol. 1931;7:445–74.
2. Reid K. The anatomy of the sinus of Valsalva. Thorax. 1970;25:79–85.
3. Crawford MH, Roldan CA. Prevalence of aortic root dilatation and small aortic roots in valvular aortic stenosis. Am J Cardiol. 2001;87:1311–3.
4. Sutton JP, Ho SY, Anderson RH. The forgotten interleaflet triangles: a review of the surgical anatomy of the aortic valve. Ann Thorac Surg. 1995;59:419–27.
5. Gatzoulis MA. Heart and mediastinum. In: Standring S, editor. Gray's anatomy: the anatomic basis of clinical practice. 40th ed. Spain: Elsevier; 2008. p. 960–82.
6. Mercer JL, Benedicty M, Bahnson HT. The geometry and construction of the aortic leaflet. J Thorac Cardiovasc Surg. 1973;65:511–8.
7. Piazza N, de Jaegere P, Schultz C, et al. Anatomy of the aortic valvar complex and its implications for transcatheter implantation of the aortic valve. Circ Cardiovasc Interv. 2008;1:74–81.
8. Vollebergh FE, Becker AE. Minor congenital variations of cusp size in tricuspid aortic valves: possible link with isolated aortic stenosis. Br Heart J. 1977;39:1006–11.
9. Anderson RH. Clinical anatomy of the aortic root. Heart. 2000;84:670–3.
10. Lewis T, Grant RT. Observations related to subacute infective endocarditis. Heart. 1923;4:21–99.
11. Roberts W. The congenitally bicuspid aortic valve: a study of 85 autopsy cases. Am J Cardiol. 1970;26:72–83.
12. Ward C. Clinical significance of the bicuspid aortic valve. Heart. 2000;83:81–5.
13. Himbert D, Pontnau F, Messika-Zeitoun D, Descoutures F, et al. Feasibility and outcomes of transcatheter aortic valve implantation in high-risk patients with stenotic bicuspid aortic valves. Am J Cardiol. 2012;110:877–83.
14. Alexander RW, Griffith GC. Anomalies of the coronary arteries and their clinical significance. Circulation. 1956;14:800–5.
15. Angelini P, Velasco JA, Flamm S. Coronary anomalies: incidence, pathophysiology, and clinical relevance. Circulation. 2002;105:2449–54.
16. Loukas M, Groat C, Khangura R, Owens DG, Anderson RH. The normal and abnormal anatomy of the coronary arteries. Clin Anat. 2009;22:114–28.
17. Zamorano JL, Goncalves A, Lang R. Imaging to select and guide transcatheter aortic valve implantation. Eur Heart J. 2014;35:1578–87.

Chapter 2
Transfemoral TAVR: Balloon-Expandable Valves

Puja B. Parikh and Susheel Kodali

Introduction

Following the first-in-man implantation of a transcatheter heart valve (THV) in 2002, transcatheter aortic valve replacement (TAVR) procedures have significantly increased over the past decade with more than 100,000 deployed THVs worldwide to date [1–4]. TAVR has been demonstrated to be a viable treatment option for patients with symptomatic severe aortic stenosis (AS) who are high risk for standard surgical aortic valve replacement (SAVR) [5–8] as well as for those considered to be inoperable [9–14]. In 2014, the American College of Cardiology in conjunction with the American Heart Association recommended the utilization of TAVR for patients with severe AS who were deemed inoperable (Class I) and/or at high risk for surgical AVR (Class IIa) [15] (Table 2.1).

The early TAVR experiences were performed with a balloon-expandable THV system, involving a bioprosthetic tissue valve sewn inside an expandable stent frame, crimped onto a balloon, and subsequently deployed with balloon inflation. Rapid progress has resulted in accelerated clinical development of new balloon-expandable devices and clinical studies (in the setting of a multidisciplinary heart team) over the past decade. This chapter will review the main characteristics of the balloon-expandable THV systems used for TAVR, the mechanisms of implantation,

P.B. Parikh, MD, MPH (✉)
Department of Medicine, Stony Brook University Medical Center, 101 Nicolls Road, Health Sciences Center T16-080, Stony Brook, NY 11794, USA
e-mail: pujaparikhmd@gmail.com

S. Kodali, MD
Department of Interventional Cardiology, Columbia University Medical Center, 177 Fort Washington Avenue, 5-501C, New York, NY 10032, USA
e-mail: sk2427@cumc.columbia.edu

© Springer Science+Business Media New York 2016
G. Ailawadi, I.L. Kron (eds.), *Catheter Based Valve and Aortic Surgery*,
DOI 10.1007/978-1-4939-3432-4_2

Table 2.1 Balloon-expandable transcatheter heart valves commercially available in the United States and/or Europe

Company	Device name	TF delivery sheath	THV size	FDA approval	First CE mark approval
Edwards Lifesciences	SAPIEN	RetroFlex3 (22/24Fr)	23 and 26 mm	November 2011	September 2007
Edwards Lifesciences	SAPIEN XT	NovaFlex+ (16/18/20Fr)	23, 26, and 29 mm	June 2014	March 2010
Edwards Lifesciences	SAPIEN 3	Commander (14/16Fr)	20, 23, 26, and 29 mm	–	January 2014

TF transfemoral, *THV* transcatheter heart valve, *FDA* Food and Drug Administration, *CE* European Commission

and the short- and long-term outcomes, valve hemodynamics, and durability associated with such systems in patients with severe AS undergoing TAVR via transfemoral (TF) approach.

Balloon-Expandable THVs

All balloon-expandable TAVR systems are composed of three integrated components: a metallic support frame, a bioprosthetic trileaflet valve, and a delivery catheter. The THV is crimped directly onto a delivery catheter before insertion into the patient and is delivered by inflation of the balloon once the prosthesis is in the correct position. The first iteration of the balloon-expandable valve consisted of equine pericardial tissue sewn inside of a stainless steel stent frame, which was crimped onto a commercially available balloon valvuloplasty catheter. Many of the initial cases including the first-in-man case in April 2002 were performed via an antegrade transfemoral transvenous transseptal approach due to the large size of the delivery catheter. This device, which became known as the Cribier-Edwards valve, was used in the initial feasibility trials in both Europe and the United States. The transvenous transseptal approach proved to be technically challenging and resulted in many intra-procedural complications even in the most experienced hands [1, 16]. The balloon-expandable TAVR system evolved quickly, and new THVs with different delivery approaches were developed as noted below. However, many features have remained constant, including the tubular-slotted metallic frame, pericardial bioprosthetic valve leaflets sewn to the frame, and a fabric "skirt" covering the bottom of the frame to provide a seal at the annulus and reduce paravalvular regurgitation.

SAPIEN THV

The SAPIEN THV (Edwards Lifesciences, Irvine, CA) valve like its predecessor still consisted of a balloon-expandable THV with a stainless steel frame and a polyethylene terephthalate fabric skirt. However, the leaflet material was changed from equine to bovine pericardial tissue, which allowed for tissue processing comparable to surgical valves including anti-calcification treatments [17–20] (Fig. 2.1a). The SAPIEN valve was the first THV to be commercially available in Europe (for TF and transapical (TA) approach) as well as in the United States (TF only) [3, 21–23]. The valve was available in 23- and 26-mm sizes, requiring 22- and 24-French (Fr) RetroFlex 3 delivery catheter systems, respectively (Fig. 2.2a), for implantation via the TF approach. In patients where the peripheral vasculature was prohibitive for the delivery catheter, there was a transapical delivery system that allowed for implantation of the THV via a lateral thoracotomy. The SAPIEN valve was evaluated extensively in multicenter registries as well as the PARTNER I trial [6–11, 14]. It received CE mark approval in 2007 and was approved by the FDA in November 2011 for commercial use in the United States in patients with severe AS deemed inoperable for SAVR (as deemed by a multidisciplinary heart team). The indications were expanded to include patients at high risk for SAVR, and the transapical approach was approved in October 2012.

SAPIEN XT THV

Further design modifications of the SAPIEN THV led to the development of the SAPIEN XT THV (Edwards Lifesciences, Irvine, CA) which began clinical evaluation in 2010. This device which was initially developed in 23-, 26-, and 29-mm sizes represented a more radical design change with the goal of creating a lower-profile system. The SAPIEN XT consists of a trileaflet pericardial bovine valve mounted onto a unique cobalt-chromium tubular stent frame (Fig. 2.1b). Its stent frame design permits thinner struts, allowing for a lower crimped profile (and smaller sheath diameter), without compromising structural integrity or radial force and stiffness [24, 25]. The inflow of the frame is covered with fabric for provision of an annular seal, and the geometry of this valve allows for a partially closed

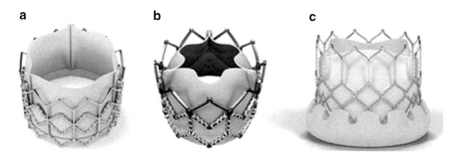

Fig. 2.1 Edwards balloon-expandable TAVR systems: (**a**) balloon-expandable SAPIEN, (**b**) balloon-expandable SAPIEN XT, and (**c**) balloon-expandable SAPIEN 3 (Edwards Life Sciences, Irvine, CA)

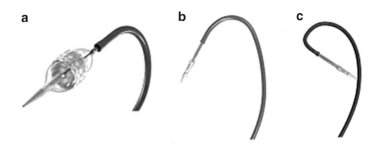

Delivery System	RetroFlex3 Sheath	NovaFlex+ eSheath	Commander eSheath
Valve Type	SAPIEN	SAPIEN XT	SAPIEN 3
Sheath ID unexpanded	22Fr (23mm valve) 24Fr (26mm valve)	16Fr (23mm valve) 18Fr (26mm valve) 20Fr (29mm valve)	14Fr (20-, 23-, and 26mm valves) 16Fr (29mm valve)
Indicated vessel size	≥7mm	6mm (16Fr) 6.5mm (18Fr) 7mm (20Fr)	5.5mm (14Fr) 6mm (16Fr)

Fig. 2.2 Edwards transfemoral sheaths: (**a**) RetroFlex3, (**b**) NovaFlex+, and (**c**) Commander (Edwards Life Sciences, Irvine, CA)

configuration. Further reduction in system profile was enabled due to an endovascular docking maneuver, such that the valve was crimped onto the catheter shaft for arterial entry, and in the descending aorta, the valve was loaded onto the balloon by pulling back the balloon delivery catheter. The SAPIEN XT THV received FDA approval in June 2014 and is the device commercially available in the United States. The NovaFlex + delivery system, utilized for SAPIEN XT implantation via a TF approach, utilizes 16-Fr (23-mm valve), 18-Fr (26-mm valve), and 20-Fr (29-mm valve) expandable sheaths (e-sheath, Edwards Lifesciences, Irvine, CA) (Fig. 2.2b).

The SAPIEN XT's ease of use and reduced vascular complications (compared to the older-generation SAPIEN THV) in patients with severe symptomatic AS were confirmed in PARTNER IIB, a randomized multicentered trial comparing the SAPIEN THV to the SAPIEN XT THV in patients with severe symptomatic AS deemed inoperable [12]. In PARTNER IIB, 560 patients with severe symptomatic AS deemed inoperable were randomized to transfemoral TAVR with SAPIEN THV versus the SAPIEN XT THV. Designed as a noninferiority study, the primary endpoint was a nonhierarchical composite of all-cause mortality, disabling stroke, and rehospitalization for AS symptoms and/or procedural complications at 1 year. At 30 days, while rates of all-cause (5.1 % vs. 3.5 %) and cardiovascular mortality (3.3 % vs. 1.8 %), disabling stroke (3.0 % vs. 3.2 %), rehospitalization (10.2 % vs. 11.6 %), myocardial infarction (0.7 % vs. 1.8 %), and need for permanent pacemaker (5.9 % vs. 6.4 %) were similar between the SAPIEN THV and SAPIEN XT THV arms, respectively (p=NS for all), the rate of major vascular complications was significantly higher in the SAPIEN THV arm (15.5 % vs. 9.6 %, $p = 0.04$), driven by higher rates of perforation (4.8 % vs. 0.4 %, $p = 0.003$) and dissection (9.2 % vs. 4.3 %, $p = 0.03$). At 1 year, no significant difference was noted in the primary composite endpoint (34.7 % (SAPIEN) vs. 33.9 % (SAPIEN XT); noninferiority $p = 0.0034$), and rates of all-cause mortality (23.7 % vs. 22.5 %), disabling stroke (4.6 % vs. 4.5 %), and rehospitalization (19.0 % vs. 17.4 %) were similar in both arms ($p = NS$ for all) [12].

SAPIEN 3 THV

The SAPIEN 3 THV (Edwards Lifesciences, Irvine, CA) is the latest version of the balloon-expandable platform. It consists of a trileaflet pericardial bovine valve mounted in a cobalt-chromium stent with an additional external polyethylene terephthalate skirt or "cuff" to further reduce PVR (Fig. 2.1c). The frame geometry has also been modified with larger cells distally to allow for unimpeded access to the coronaries. The SAPIEN 3 Commander delivery system provides precise positioning features for more coaxial and optimal position as well as a lower-profile delivery system [26–31]. The SAPIEN 3 is available in 20-, 23-, 26-, and 29-mm sizes, and all but the 29-mm valve are delivered through a 14-Fr e-sheath (Edwards Lifesciences, Irvine, CA) (Fig. 2.2c). The SAPIEN 3 THV became CE mark approved in January 2014 and is commercially available in Europe.

First-in-man studies demonstrated excellent short-term outcomes with the SAPIEN 3 THV [28]. Comparison to the second-generation SAPIEN XT has demonstrated reduced rates of PVR and less frequent postdilatation. In a case-matched study with echo core laboratory analysis, a total of 27 patients who underwent TAVR with the SAPIEN 3 were matched for prosthesis size (26 mm), aortic annulus area, and mean diameter measured by computed tomography as well as left ventricular ejection fraction (LVEF), body surface area, and body mass index with 50 patients treated with the SAPIEN XT [29]. Prosthesis size was determined by oversizing of 1–15 % of the annulus area. The need for postdilatation was higher in the SAPIEN XT group (20 % vs. 4 %, $p = 0.047$), while the mean residual gradient and effective orifice area were similar in both groups. The incidence of at least mild PVR was greater with the SAPIEN XT (42 % vs. 7 %, $p = 0.002$) than with the SAPIEN 3, as was at least moderate PVR (8 % vs. 0 %). SAPIEN 3 implantation was the only factor associated with trace or no paravalvular leak after TAVR ($p = 0.007$) [29].

One recent prospective multicentered study involving 150 patients with severe symptomatic AS of intermediate or high risk who underwent TAVR (64 % TF approach) with the SAPIEN 3 THV demonstrated low rates of significant PVR (moderate PVR 3.5 %, severe PVR 0 %) at 30 days [32]. TF approach was associated with low mortality (2.1 %), no disabling stroke (0 %), and fully percutaneous access and closure in 95.8 %. Non-TF alternative access was associated with higher rates of mortality (11.6 %) and stroke (5.6 %).

Other Balloon-Expandable THVs

The Innovare balloon-expandable system (Braile Biomedica, Sao Jose do Rio Preto, Brazil), a trileaflet bovine pericardial valve mounted in a cobalt-chromium frame, is designed initially to be implanted via transapical approach [33]. One unique feature of this device is that it is available in multiple sizes from 20- to 28-mm in 2-mm increments. The delivery catheter ranges from 20-Fr (20-, 22-, and 24-mm valves) to 22-Fr (26- and 28-mm valves). Early studies demonstrated procedural success rates of 91 % with 30-day and 1-year mortality rates of 18.2 % and 39.5 %, respectively, in patients with severe symptomatic AS [33]. Peak and mean gradients at 1-year follow-up were 21.3 ± 12.4 mmHg and 10.5 ± 6.9 mmHg, respectively.

The Colibri balloon-expandable system (Colibri Heart Valve, Broomfield, CO, USA) is a low-profile (14-Fr), pre-mounted, prepackaged TAVR system [34]. It is comprised of porcine pericardial leaflets (constructed via a unique folding method) sewn into a stainless steel frame. The first implant was performed in November 2012. Feasibility studies are currently in progress.

TAVR: Implantation and Procedural Considerations

Transfemoral (TF) Approach

With device modifications resulting in smaller delivery catheters, the TF approach has become the predominant access choice in the majority of TAVR-performing centers [35]. However, careful evaluation of the vascular anatomy is critical to reduce vascular complications, which have been shown to impact late mortality [36]. In general, a comprehensive evaluation of bilateral iliofemoral anatomy using computed tomography is required before TAVR. Several factors have been shown to impact the risk of vascular complications including vessel size, tortuosity, and calcification [36–41]. Earlier studies demonstrated that a sheath to femoral artery ratio of greater than 1.05 is predictive of a vascular complication [37]. However, with newer expandable sheaths that enter the artery at a smaller diameter, this ratio may be different. Although femoral arterial access was initially obtained via surgical cutdown, the majority of procedures are currently performed via a fully percutaneous approach utilizing closure devices [38, 42]. Recommended femoral diameters for the balloon-expandable THVs are noted in Fig. 2.2.

Key elements of optimal fluoroscopic guidance when obtaining femoral access should include identification of the mid-third of the femoral head and angiographic confirmation of the level of arterial entry using contrast [43]. Location of needle entry may be altered based upon CT findings of high bifurcation of the common femoral artery and/or significant calcium precluding optimal preprocedural deployment of suture-based vascular closure devices. The crossover balloon technique [44] is also frequently utilized by most institutions in which the femoral artery that will not be used for large sheath delivery is accessed first (using fluoroscopic and/or ultrasound guidance); a catheter (i.e., an internal mammary artery catheter) is utilized to identify the aortoiliac bifurcation; and an extra support guidewire is inserted under direct fluoroscopic visualization to the contralateral distal superficial femoral artery to serve as a "safety wire" in the setting of an ileofemoral injury on the side of the large delivery sheath. While access of the femoral artery intended for large sheath placement can be achieved using an angiogram from the contralateral side, so that the site of needle entry can be directly assessed, comprehensive preprocedural CT evaluation can avoid administration of this additional contrast.

Alternative Access Approaches

In patients with prohibitive peripheral arterial disease or tortuosity of vessels, TAVR can be performed through a transapical or transaortic approach. The initial studies with alternative access were performed using the SAPIEN device via the transapical (TA) approach [21, 23]. TA-TAVR is performed by creating a left anterolateral intercostal incision to expose the left ventricular apex. Direct needle puncture of the apex after placement of pledgeted purse-string sutures allows introduction of a hemostatic sheath into the left ventricle. Valve position and deployment are performed in a manner similar to transfemoral approach as described below. After valve deployment, the sheath is removed from the apex, and hemostasis is achieved by tightening of the previously placed purse-string sutures. Outcomes from the TA approach have been variable, and a recent propensity-matched analysis demonstrated higher mortality and length of stay with this approach when compared with transfemoral [45]. However, these comparisons are inherently difficult as the populations for transapical and transfemoral are different. Another commonly used alternative access approach is the transaortic (TAo) approach [46, 47]. With this approach, the ascending aorta is exposed via either a hemisternotomy or a right upper thoracotomy. After exposure, purse-string sutures are placed, and the delivery sheath is introduced directly into the aorta. Valve delivery and deployment is similar to the other approaches. Some operators have suggested that the transaortic approach has some advantages over transapical such as less pain and faster recovery. However, these approaches have never been compared directly. Beyond transapical and transaortic, a limited number of cases have been performed via either the carotid or subclavian arteries with acceptable results [48–50].

Valve Sizing

Appropriate valve sizing is crucial to getting a successful result with minimal paravalvular regurgitation. Oversizing the prosthesis results in better annular seal but must be balanced with the risk of annular rupture. The term "cover index" is used to quantify the degree of oversizing and is calculated by the following formula: (prosthesis size—annulus size)/prosthesis size. The initial studies using cover index were performed with 2D measurements and demonstrated that oversizing by at least 8 % resulted in less regurgitation [51, 52]. However, it became clear that 2D measurements were not adequate since the annulus was a 3D structure. Currently, aortic annular area assessments are determined with 3D assessments derived from gated computed tomography angiography (CTA) or transesophageal echocardiogram (TEE). Several studies have demonstrated that valve sizing using multislice computed tomography angiography (MSCT)-derived annular areas results in less AR than sizing performed with either 2D or 3D transesophageal echocardiogram (TEE) [53, 54]. However, a more recent study utilizing novel method for making 3D measurements on TEE showed no difference between MSCT and TEE [55]. The feasibility and safety of balloon aortic valvuloplasty (BAV) to size the aortic annulus has been demonstrated and may also be an important adjunct to TEE when selecting valve size, as implantation of the minimal valve greater than the BAV annulus size has been shown to be safe and results in no adverse events [56].

Predilatation and Valve Deployment

Balloon aortic valvuloplasty (BAV) is routinely performed in order to predilate the stenosed aortic valve prior to balloon-expandable TAVR. Although predilatation is considered to be essential for the preparation of the valve landing zone, there is no clear evidence to support its clinical value and has been linked to several complications. Some studies have supported the feasibility and safety of TAVR without predilatation [57]. The ongoing, prospective, two-armed, multicenter EASE-IT registry has been designed to obtain essential data concerning procedural success rates, adverse events, and mortality in a large cohort of patients undergoing transapical TAVR using the Edwards SAPIEN 3 balloon-expandable valves with and without pre-ballooning [58]. Some literature has noted difficulty in device crossing and implantation without predilatation [59].

Following BAV, the THV is subsequently positioned using fluoroscopy, angiography, and transesophageal echocardiography guidance. A coplanar view with the nadirs of all three cusps in the same plane is essential to ensure proper deployment of the valve. Optimal fluoroscopic angles for valve deployment can also be ascertained via various imaging systems [60]. Transesophageal echocardiography can be helpful in positioning the valve, especially in cases with renal dysfunction where minimizing contrast use is important [61, 62]. Valve expansion is then achieved via balloon inflation under rapid pacing (180–220 beats per minute) so as to minimize cardiac output and avoid valve embolization during deployment. A slow balloon inflation technique has been reported to help minimize the risk of THV malpositioning and may allow for partial repositioning of the THV during deployment [63]. Pre-, intra-, and postprocedural deployment of a SAPIEN 3 valve via TF approach are demonstrated in Fig. 2.3.

A simplified percutaneous approach using local anesthesia has become increasingly popular in Europe and the United States given the multiple advantages it offers in the elderly and frail populations. One single-center study prospectively evaluated

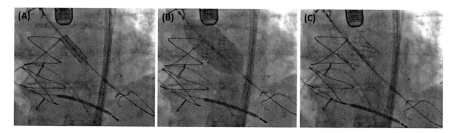

Fig. 2.3 Deployment of a 26-mm SAPIEN 3 valve via transfemoral approach: (**a**) pre-valve deployment, (**b**) during valve deployment, and (**c**) post-valve deployment

151 patients who underwent TAVR with SAPIEN/SAPIEN XT valves using only local anesthesia and fluoroscopic guidance (i.e., no TEE guidance) and demonstrated a greater than 95 % procedural success rate and a low rate of complications [64].

Postdilatation

Postdilatation (PD) is performed in ~10–40 % of transfemoral TAVR cases [52, 65]. Patients undergoing PD tend to have a larger aortic annulus and lower cover index. They usually have larger areas of PVR immediately after deployment with significant reduction in PVR area attributable to PD. While a nonsignificant greater rate of cerebrovascular events have been noted in patients undergoing PD, no significant differences in major aortic injury and/or permanent pacemaker implantation rates have been noted in comparison to patients not undergoing PD [52].

A technique of intentionally underexpanding the balloon-expandable valve by underfilling the deployment balloon with subsequent PD as needed has been described [66]. No adverse effect in clinical outcomes, THV gradients, or THV areas was noted with this technique, which may potentially reduce the risk of annular injury and PVR in selected patients.

Clinical Outcomes

The PARTNER Trials

PARTNER I

The PARTNER I trial involved two cohorts of patients with severe symptomatic AS—a high-risk cohort and an inoperable cohort. The high-risk cohort was studied in PARTNER IA, a noninferiority study which randomized 699 patients with severe symptomatic AS deemed high risk to TAVR with the SAPIEN THV versus SAVR [6].

TAVR and SAVR were associated with similar rates of all-cause mortality (24 % vs. 27 %), cardiovascular mortality (14 % vs. 13 %), and readmission at 1 year ($p=$NS for all). Patients undergoing TAVR had significantly higher rates of stroke (30 days: 5.5 % vs. 2.4 %, $p=0.04$; 1 year: 8.3 % vs. 4.3 %, $p=0.04$) and vascular complications (30 days: 17 % vs. 4 %, $p<0.001$; 1 year: 18 % vs. 5 %, $p<0.001$) at both 30 days and 1 year [6]. Two-year data demonstrated no significant differences in all-cause (34 % vs. 35 %) or cardiovascular mortality (21 % vs. 21 %) between the TAVR and SAVR arms, respectively ($p=$NS for both), and a trend toward higher rates of stroke in the TAVR arm (11.2 % vs. 6.5 %, $p=0.05$) [7]. Five-year data demonstrated similar rates of death (67.8 % vs. 62.4 %, $p=0.76$) in the TAVR and SAVR arms, respectively. Rates of significant aortic regurgitation were higher in the TAVR group (14 % vs. 1 %, $p<0.0001$) and were associated with increased 5-year risk of mortality in the TAVR group [8].

The inoperable cohort was studied in PARTNER IB, which randomized 358 patients with severe symptomatic AS deemed inoperable (defined as having an estimated risk of death or serious irreversible morbidity exceeding 50 %) to TF TAVR with the SAPIEN THV versus medical therapy (included balloon aortic valvuloplasty) [9]. At 1 year, the TAVR arm was associated with significantly lower rates of all-cause mortality (30.7 % vs. 50.7 %, $p<0.001$) and cardiovascular mortality (20 % vs. 42 %, $p<0.001$) and lower readmission rates for AS or procedure-related complications (22 % vs. 44 %, $p<0.001$). The rate of the composite endpoint of all-cause mortality or repeat hospitalization was significantly lower in the TAVR arm (42.5 % vs. 71.6 %, $p<0.001$). At 1 year, the rate of NYHA Class III or IV symptoms was significantly lower in the TAVR arm (25.2 % vs. 58.0 %, $p<0.001$). TAVR was associated with increased stroke rates at 30 days (6.7 % vs. 1.7 %, $p=0.03$) and at 1 year (10.6 % vs. 4.5 %, $p=0.04$) and more frequent major vascular complications at both 30 days (31 % vs. 5 %, $p<0.001$) and 1 year (32 % vs. 7 %, $p<0.001$) compared to patients receiving standard medical therapy [9]. Two-year and three-year data demonstrated continued improved all-cause (2 years, 43 % vs. 68 %, $p<0.001$; 3 years, 54 % vs. 81 %, $p<0.001$) and cardiovascular mortality (2 years, 31 % vs. 62 %, $p<0.001$; 3 years, 41 % vs. 75 %, $p<0.001$) in the TAVR arm and higher rates of stroke in the TAVR arm compared to standard medical therapy (2 years, 13.8 % vs. 5.5 %, $p=0.01$; 3 years, 15.7 % vs. 5.5 %, $p=0.012$) [10, 11]. Recent data on 5-year outcomes of PARTNER IB demonstrated significantly lower rates of all-cause (72 % vs. 94 %, $p<0.0001$) and cardiovascular mortality (57 % vs. 86 %, $p<0.0001$) in patients undergoing TAVR compared to standard medical therapy [14].

The PARTNER IA and IB studies demonstrated no deterioration in functioning of the SAPIEN THV (as assessed by absence of increase in transvalvular gradient, attrition of valve area, or significant total or paravalvular regurgitation) at up to 5 years [6–11, 14].

PARTNER II

The PARTNER II trial, which commenced in 2011, involved cohorts of varying surgical risk. The inoperable cohort was studied in PARTNER IIB, a noninferiority study which randomized 560 patients with severe symptomatic AS deemed inoperable (defined as having an estimated risk of death or serious irreversible morbidity exceeding 50 %) to TF TAVR with the SAPIEN THV versus the SAPIEN XT THV [12]. The primary endpoint was a nonhierarchical composite endpoint of all-cause mortality, disabling stroke, or rehospitalization for treatment of severe AS or procedural-related complications at 1 year. During the procedure, the SAPIEN XT was associated with reduced anesthesia time and a trend toward less frequent requirement for intra-aortic balloon pump and/or more than one THV and less frequent risk of an aborted procedure. At 30 days, no significant risk in all-cause (5.1 % vs. 3.5 %) or cardiovascular mortality (3.3 % vs. 1.8 %), disabling stroke (3.0 % vs. 3.2 %), rehospitalization (10.2 % vs. 11.6 %), myocardial infarction (0.7 % vs. 1.8 %), new pacemaker implantation (5.9 % vs. 6.4 %), or major bleeding (16.4 % vs. 15.7 %) was noted between the SAPIEN and SAPIEN XT arms, respectively ($p=$NS for all); however, the SAPIEN XT arm was associated with reduced vascular complications (15.5 % vs. 9.6 %, $p=0.04$), driven by reduced rates of dissections (9.2 % vs. 4.3 %, $p=0.03$) and perforations (4.0 % vs. 0.4 %, $p=0.003$). At 1 year, no significant difference was noted in the primary composite endpoint (34.7 % vs. 33.9 %, noninferiority $p=0.0034$), and rates of all-cause mortality (23.7 % vs. 22.5 %), disabling stroke (4.6 % vs. 4.5 %), and rehospitalization (19.0 % vs. 17.4 %) were similar between the SAPIEN and SAPIEN XT arms, respectively. Secondary endpoints, including NYHA Class, total aortic regurgitation, PVR, and aortic valve area, were also similar between both arms [12]. However, the rate of moderate or severe PVR (20.9 % for SAPIEN, 29.2 % for SAPIEN XT) was higher than reported in previous studies. This difference may be due to a difference in core lab methodology as this study placed an emphasis on circumferential extent in determining PVR severity. An analysis by a core lab consortium has subsequently demonstrated that with this method, moderate PVL may be overestimated in ~15 % of cases [67].

The PARTNER IIA study randomized intermediate-risk patients (STS calculated risk of 4–8 %) with severe symptomatic AS to TAVR with a SAPIEN XT THV versus SAVR [12]. The primary endpoint of the study is all-cause mortality or disabling stroke at 2 years. PARTNER IIA has completed enrollment, and its 2-year results are eagerly anticipated.

In the PARTNER IIB valve-in-valve registry [nested registry 7 (NR7)], 99 patients with failed aortic surgical bioprostheses who were deemed inoperable were enrolled and underwent a valve-in-valve TAVR with a SAPIEN XT THV [68]. One-year data demonstrated a 19.9 % and 15.9 % rate of all-cause and cardiovascular mortality, respectively, a 3.2 % risk of stroke, and 1.1 % risk of new pacemaker implantation. No significant difference in clinical outcomes was noted with TF versus transapical approach in patients undergoing valve-in-valve TAVR (Table 2.2).

The PARTNER II study also consisted of multiple nested registries involving the SAPIEN 3 THV. The PARTNER II SAPIEN 3 (S3) high-risk/inoperable registry and intermediate-risk registry completed enrollment in 2014. Thirty-day rates of adverse events in both registries were low. All-cause and cardiovascular mortality rates were 2.2 % and 1.4 % for the high-risk/inoperable registry and 1.1 % and 0.9 % for the intermediate-risk registry, respectively. Rates of any stroke and disabling stroke were 1.5 % and 0.9 % for the high-risk/inoperable registry and 2.6 %

Table 2.2 Long-term clinical outcomes in PARTNER I

		PARTNER I Cohort A			PARTNER I Cohort B		
		TAVR	SAVR	p value	TAVR	BAV/ Med Rx	p value
1 Year [6, 9]	All-cause death	24 %	27 %	0.45	31 %	50 %	<0.001
	CV death	14 %	13 %	0.63	20 %	42 %	<0.001
	Stroke	8.7 %	4.3 %	0.03	10.6 %	4.5 %	0.04
2 Year [7, 10]	All-cause death	34 %	35 %	0.78	43 %	68 %	<0.001
	CV death	21 %	21 %	0.80	31 %	62 %	<0.001
	Stroke	11.2 %	6.5 %	0.05	13.8 %	5.5 %	0.01
5 Year [8, 14]	All-cause death	68 %	62 %	0.76	72 %	94 %	<0.0001
	CV death	–	–	–	57 %	86 %	<0.0001
	Stroke	15.9 %	14.7 %	0.35	16 %	18 %	<0.05

BAV balloon aortic valvuloplasty, *Med Rx* medical therapy, *CV* cardiovascular

and 1.0 % for the intermediate-risk registry. Rates of moderate or severe PVR were 2.9 % and 4.2 % in the high-risk/inoperable and intermediate-risk registries, respectively [69]. The PARTNER II S3 NR7 (20-mm valve registry) is currently enrolling patients.

Balloon-Expandable Versus Self-Expanding THVs

The multicentered, German CHOICE study is the only randomized trial comparing balloon-expandable THVs to self-expanding THVs in high-risk patients with severe AS scheduled to undergo TAVR. CHOICE randomized 240 high-risk patients with severe symptomatic AS and an anatomy suitable for the transfemoral TAVR to receive the SAPIEN XT versus the CoreValve (Medtronic Inc, Minneapolis, MN) [70]. The primary endpoint was device success, a composite endpoint of successful vascular access and deployment of the device and retrieval of the delivery system, correct position of the device, intended performance of the heart valve without moderate or severe regurgitation, and only one valve implanted in the proper anatomical location. Device success was higher in the balloon-expandable valve group (95.9 % vs. 77.5 %, $p < 0.001$) compared to the self-expandable valve group, primarily driven by a significantly lower frequency of residual more-than-mild aortic regurgitation (4.1 % vs. 18.3 %; $p < 0.001$) and less frequent need for implanting more than 1 valve (0.8 % vs. 5.8 %, $p = 0.03$) in the balloon-expandable valve group. While cardiovascular mortality at 30 days was similar in both groups (4.1 % vs. 4.3 %, $p = 0.99$), placement of a new permanent pacemaker was less frequent in the balloon-expandable valve group (17.3 % vs. 37.6 %, $p = 0.001$) [70].

Pooled prospective data from two German centers of 394 patients (276 treated with Medtronic CoreValve and 118 with Edwards SAPIEN XT) demonstrated significantly higher rates of more-than-mild AR with the CoreValve than with the SAPIEN XT in unadjusted analyses (12.7 % vs. 2.6 %, $p=0.002$) and following propensity adjustment (adjusted OR 4.59, 95 % CI 1.03–20.44) [71]. The occurrence of any degree of AR was also higher with the CoreValve (71.6 % vs. 56.9 %, $p=0.004$). One-year survival was comparable between both valve types (83.8 % CoreValve vs. 88.2 % SAPIEN XT, $p=0.42$) but was significantly worse in patients with more-than-mild AR (69.8 % vs. 87.4 %, $p=0.004$). Short-term mortality rates have also been noted to be similar in both transcatheter valve groups [72].

A propensity-matched analysis from the PRAGMATIC Plus Initiative, pooled data obtained from four European centers, demonstrated no differences in 30-day outcomes between the Edwards SAPIEN valves (SAPIEN/SAPIEN XT) ($n=204$) and the Medtronic CoreValve ($n=204$) (all-cause mortality (MCV, 8.8 % vs. ESV, 6.4 %; $p=0.352$), cardiovascular mortality (MCV, 6.9 % vs. ESV, 6.4 %; $p=0.842$), myocardial infarction (MCV, 0.5 % vs. ESV, 1.5 %; $p=0.339$), stroke (MCV, 2.9 % vs. ESV, 1.0 %; $p=0.174$), or device success (MCV, 95.6 % vs. ESV, 96.6 %; $p=0.611$)) [73]. There were also no differences in major vascular complications (MCV, 9.3 % vs. ESV, 12.3 %; $p=0.340$) or life-threatening bleeding (MCV, 13.7 % vs. ESV, 8.8 %; $p=0.120$). MCV was associated with more permanent pacemakers (22.5 % vs. 5.9 %; $p<0.001$). At 1 year, there were no differences in all-cause (MCV, 16.2 % vs. ESV, 12.3 %; $p=0.266$) or cardiovascular (MCV, 8.3 % vs. ESV, 7.4 %; $p=0.713$) mortality [73].

Complications

Complications associated with TAVR include vascular complications, valve malpositioning, regurgitation, embolization, coronary compromise, conduction abnormalities, stroke/transient ischemic attack, acute kidney injury, cardiac tamponade, and hemodynamic collapse [74]. A thorough understanding of the procedure and early identification and management of complications are necessary for procedural success.

Paravalvular Regurgitation (PVR)

Multiple studies have demonstrated that PVR after TAVR is associated with poor survival after balloon-expandable TAVR [7, 75, 76]. With the first-generation SAPIEN valve, the rate of moderate or severe PVL is ~10 % and mild ~40 % [76, 77]. Recent studies of the SAPIEN XT have demonstrated slightly lower rates of both mild PVR (40 %) and more-than-mild PVR (2–8 %) [29, 70, 71]. However, this may be due to differences in ascertainment or may represent decreases in PVR with incorporation of CT sizing algorithms. External adaptive skirts on newer-generation THVs have led to further reduction in rates of PVR. The SAPIEN 3 has been associated with a very low rate of moderate or severe PVR (3.5 %) [32] and reduced need for balloon postdilatation—much lower than that observed with the SAPIEN XT [29].

Conduction Disturbances

Cardiac conduction disturbances requiring PPM are a frequent complication of TAVR. Low transcatheter valve implantation has been associated with new left bundle branch block, complete heart block, and need for permanent pacemaker implantation [25]. In the PARTNER trial and its continued access registry, a new PPM was required in 8.8 % of individuals undergoing TAVR (with a SAPIEN THV) without a preexisting pacemaker [78]. By multivariable analysis, predictors of permanent pacemaker implantation included right bundle branch block (odds ratio (OR), 7.03, 95 %; confidence interval (CI), 4.92–10.06), prosthesis diameter/left ventricular (LV) outflow tract diameter (for each 0.1 increment, OR, 1.29, 95 %; CI, 1.10–1.51), LV end-diastolic diameter (for each 1 cm, OR, 0.68, 95 %; CI, 0.53–0.87, $p=0.003$), and treatment in the continued access registry (OR, 1.77, 95 %; CI, 1.08–2.92). At 1 year, new pacemaker implantation was associated with a significantly higher rate of mortality or rehospitalization (42.0 % vs. 32.6 %, $p=0.007$), driven by a trend toward higher rates of rehospitalization (23.9 % vs. 18.2 %, $p=0.05$), but no change in LV ejection fraction [78].

Electrophysiological study performed in the catheterization room immediately before the initial balloon valvuloplasty and immediately after Edwards SAPIEN prosthesis implantation demonstrated several important findings including significantly prolonged His-ventricle interval (56 vs. 47 ms, $p<0.001$) and antegrade Wenckebach point (354 vs. 334 ms, $p=0.001$) postprocedure compared to preprocedure [79]. The effect of Edwards SAPIEN on the conduction system was mostly infranodal and temporary.

Malpositioning

Malposition of current balloon-expandable aortic valves can vary and is a largely preventable complication. An early study noted a rate of 5.3 % in 170 patients receiving a balloon-expandable valve, with the majority of malpositioning occurring supravalvular and all cases demonstrated embolization of the transcatheter valve to the ascending aorta within a few cardiac cycles following deployment (i.e., no late embolization was observed) [80]. In most cases, the prosthesis was uneventfully repositioned in the more distal aorta. However, this represented early operator experience as well as a first-generation device, which was known to move cranially during inflation. Subvalvular positioning can result in severe aortic regurgitation due to lack of seal at the annulus with the skirt of the prosthesis. Rates of implantation of a second transcatheter valve are now typically around 1 % [70, 80]. An improved understanding of the procedure will likely minimize this possibility and mitigate the consequences should malposition occur.

Aortic Root/Annular Rupture

Aortic root rupture is a major life-threatening concern with balloon-expandable TAVR. LVOT calcification (nearly 11-fold higher risk of rupture), aggressive ≥ 20 % annular area oversizing (8–9-fold higher risk of rupture), and postdilatation (PD) have been associated with an increased risk of aortic root rupture during TAVR with balloon-expandable prostheses [81, 82]. Multislice computed tomography-based assessment of aortic annulus dimension in conjunction with adapted sizing guidelines may reduce the incidence of severe oversizing. In cases where there is excessive oversizing of the valve, underfilling and underexpansion has been proposed as a strategy to reduce the risk of annular injury [81]. The authors propose reducing the inflation volume by ~10 % which roughly correlates to 1 cm^3 for 23-mm valve, 2 cm^3 for 26-mm valve, and 3 cm^3 for the 29-mm valve. In this study, authors noted no difference in THV performance with the strategy of underdeployment (Table 2.3).

Bleeding and Vascular Complications

Bleeding after TAVR can be as high as approximately 30 % (any bleeding) and is independently associated with a nearly threefold higher risk of 1-year mortality (HR 2.54, 95 % CI 1.3–4.9, $p=0.002$) [83]. Earlier studies involving the SAPIEN THV

Table 2.3 Complications associated with balloon-expandable TAVR

Complications associated with balloon-expandable TAVR [74]
• Paravalvular regurgitation (PVR)
• Conduction abnormalities (e.g., new left bundle branch block (LBBB), atrioventricular block, need for new pacemaker implantation)
• Annular rupture
• Aortic injury
• Malpositioning
• Valve embolization
• Injury to mitral valve apparatus
• Coronary obstruction
• Stroke/transient ischemic attack
• Vascular complications (e.g., hematoma, dissection, perforation)
• Bleeding
• Acute kidney injury

demonstrated an approximate 20 % rate of vascular complications, including perforations/rupture (requiring surgical bypass) and dissection (necessitating stenting) [39]; however, lower rates were noted over time as operator experience heightened and delivery catheter sheath sizes were significantly reduced [12]. With current-generation SAPIEN XT and SAPIEN 3 systems, the vascular complication rates are ~5 % [32, 69].

Stroke

Prior randomized studies had raised major safety concerns because of increased stroke/transient ischemic attack (TIA) rates with TAVR compared to medical treatment and surgical aortic valve replacement (SAVR). A recent meta-analysis of over 10,000 patients undergoing TF, transapical or trans-subclavian TAVR for native severe AS demonstrated an overall 30-day stroke/TIA of 3.3 % (range 0–6 %), with the majority being major strokes (2.9 %) [84]. During the first year after TAVR, stroke/TIA increased up to 5.2 %. Differences in stroke rates were associated with different approaches and valve prostheses used, with the lowest stroke rates after transapical TAVR with the SAPIEN THV (2.7 %). Thirty-day mortality was nearly fourfold higher in patients with stroke compared to those without stroke (25.5 % vs. 6.9 %). Data recently presented utilizing the SAPIEN 3 device in over 1500 patients demonstrated significantly lower stroke rates in high- and intermediate-risk patients (any stroke ~2.5 %, major stroke ~1 %). These rates are with careful neurologic oversight, which has been shown to increase stroke reporting. A recent publication demonstrated that stroke rates following surgical AVR are underestimated if a neurologist does not evaluate the patient (7 % vs. 17 %) [85]. In addition to clinical stroke, studies have noted a nearly 70–80 % incidence of new ischemic lesions on diffuse-weighted magnetic resonance imaging (DW-MRI) following TAVR [86]. While reduction in the number of new lesions has been demonstrated with cerebral embolic protection filters [87], larger studies are currently in progress to assess the impact of cerebral embolic protection filters on neuroimaging and neurological symptoms [88].

Conclusions

Since the first-in-man transcatheter heart valve implantation in 2002, balloon-expandable THVs have played a major role in the development of TAVR in the last decade. TAVR is currently the standard of care for patients with severe symptomatic AS who are considered inoperable and is considered a viable treatment option to SAVR in those patients considered at high risk. Further refinements in THV and delivery catheter technology and the demonstration of the efficacy of TAVR (compared to SAVR) in lower-risk patients will lead to a significant increase in TAVR implementation in the near future.

References

1. Cribier A, Eltchaninoff H, Bash A, et al. Percutaneous transcatheter implantation of an aortic valve prosthesis for calcific aortic stenosis: first human case description. Circulation. 2002;106:3006–8.
2. Bande M, Michev I, Sharp AS, Chieffo A, Colombo A. Percutaneous transcatheter aortic valve implantation: past accomplishments, present achievements and applications, future perspectives. Cardiol Rev. 2010;18:111–24.
3. Chodor P, Wilczek K, Przybylski R, et al. Immediate and 6-month outcomes of transapical and transfemoral Edwards-Sapien prosthesis implantation in patients with aortic stenosis. Kardiol Pol. 2010;68:1124–31.
4. Varadarajan P, Kapoor N, Bansal RC, Pai RG. Clinical profile and natural history of 453 non-surgically managed patients with severe aortic stenosis. Ann Thorac Surg. 2006;82:2111–5.
5. Adams DH, Popma JJ, Reardon MJ, et al. Transcatheter aortic-valve replacement with a self-expanding prosthesis. N Engl J Med. 2014;370:1790–8.
6. Smith CR, Leon MB, Mack MJ, et al. Transcatheter versus surgical aortic-valve replacement in high-risk patients. N Engl J Med. 2011;364:2187–98.
7. Kodali SK, Williams MR, Smith CR, et al. Two-year outcomes after transcatheter or surgical aortic-valve replacement. N Engl J Med. 2012;366:1686–95.
8. Mack MJ, Leon MB, Smith CR, et al. 5-year outcomes of transcatheter aortic valve replacement or surgical aortic valve replacement for high surgical risk patients with aortic stenosis (PARTNER 1): a randomised controlled trial. Lancet. 2015;385:2477–84.
9. Leon MB, Smith CR, Mack M, et al. Transcatheter aortic-valve implantation for aortic stenosis in patients who cannot undergo surgery. N Engl J Med. 2010;363:1597–607.
10. Makkar RR, Fontana GP, Jilaihawi H, et al. Transcatheter aortic-valve replacement for inoperable severe aortic stenosis. N Engl J Med. 2012;366:1696–704.
11. Kapadia SR, Tuzcu EM, Makkar RR, et al. Long-term outcomes of inoperable patients with aortic stenosis randomly assigned to transcatheter aortic valve replacement or standard therapy. Circulation. 2014;130:1483–92.
12. Leon M. A randomized evaluation of the SAPIEN XT transcatheter valve system in patients with aortic stenosis who are not candidates for surgery: PARTNER II, Inoperable cohort. American College of Cardiology Scientific Sessions, 2013.
13. Popma JJ, Adams DH, Reardon MJ, et al. Transcatheter aortic valve replacement using a self-expanding bioprosthesis in patients with severe aortic stenosis at extreme risk for surgery. J Am Coll Cardiol. 2014;63:1972–81.
14. Kapadia SR, Leon MB, Makkar RR, et al. 5-year outcomes of transcatheter aortic valve replacement compared with standard treatment for patients with inoperable aortic stenosis (PARTNER 1): a randomised controlled trial. Lancet. 2015;385:2485–91.
15. Nishimura RA, Otto CM, Bonow RO, et al. 2014 AHA/ACC guideline for the management of patients with valvular heart disease: a report of the American College of Cardiology/American Heart Association Task Force on Practice Guidelines. J Thorac Cardiovasc Surg. 2014;148:e1–132.
16. Cribier A, Eltchaninoff H, Tron C, et al. Early experience with percutaneous transcatheter implantation of heart valve prosthesis for the treatment of end-stage inoperable patients with calcific aortic stenosis. J Am Coll Cardiol. 2004;43:698–703.

17. Cribier A, Litzler PY, Eltchaninoff H, et al. Technique of transcatheter aortic valve implantation with the Edwards-Sapien heart valve using the transfemoral approach. Herz. 2009;34:347–56.
18. Maisano F, Michev I, Denti P, Alfieri O, Colombo A. Transfemoral transcatheter aortic valve implantation using the balloon expandable SAPIEN transcatheter heart valve device. Multimedia manual of cardiothoracic surgery: MMCTS/European Association for Cardio-Thoracic Surgery 2008; 2008: mmcts 2007 003087.
19. Thielmann M, Eggebrecht H, Wendt D, et al. New techniques for the treatment of valvular aortic stenosis--transcatheter aortic valve implantation with the SAPIEN heart valve. Minim Invasive Ther Allied Technol. 2009;18:131–41.
20. Holoshitz N, Kavinsky CJ, Hijazi ZM. The Edwards SAPIEN transcatheter heart valve for calcific aortic stenosis: a review of the valve, procedure, and current literature. Cardiol Ther. 2012;1:6.
21. Walther T, Simon P, Dewey T, et al. Transapical minimally invasive aortic valve implantation: multicenter experience. Circulation. 2007;116:I240–5.
22. Thomas M, Schymik G, Walther T, et al. Thirty-day results of the SAPIEN aortic Bioprosthesis European Outcome (SOURCE) Registry: A European registry of transcatheter aortic valve implantation using the Edwards SAPIEN valve. Circulation. 2010;122:62–9.
23. Kempfert J, Rastan A, Holzhey D, et al. Transapical aortic valve implantation: analysis of risk factors and learning experience in 299 patients. Circulation. 2011;124:S124–9.
24. Freeman M, Webb JG. Edwards SAPIEN and Edwards SAPIEN XT transcatheter heart valves for the treatment of severe aortic stenosis. Expert Rev Med Devices. 2012;9:563–9.
25. Binder RK, Webb JG, Toggweiler S, et al. Impact of post-implant SAPIEN XT geometry and position on conduction disturbances, hemodynamic performance, and paravalvular regurgitation. J Am Coll Cardiol Intv. 2013;6:462–8.
26. Binder RK, Rodes-Cabau J, Wood DA, Webb JG. Edwards SAPIEN 3 valve. EuroIntervention. 2012;8(Suppl Q):Q83–7.
27. Binder RK, Schafer U, Kuck KH, et al. Transcatheter aortic valve replacement with a new self-expanding transcatheter heart valve and motorized delivery system. J Am Coll Cardiol Intv. 2013;6:301–7.
28. Binder RK, Rodes-Cabau J, Wood DA, et al. Transcatheter aortic valve replacement with the SAPIEN 3: a new balloon-expandable transcatheter heart valve. J Am Coll Cardiol Intv. 2013;6:293–300.
29. Amat-Santos IJ, Dahou A, Webb J, et al. Comparison of hemodynamic performance of the balloon-expandable SAPIEN 3 versus SAPIEN XT transcatheter valve. Am J Cardiol. 2014;114(7):1075–82.
30. Minha S, Waksman R. Evaluation of the Edwards Lifesciences SAPIEN transcatheter heart valve. Expert Rev Med Devices 2014;11(6):553–62
31. Ribeiro HB, Doyle D, Nombela-Franco L, et al. Transapical implantation of the SAPIEN 3 valve. J Card Surg. 2013;28:506–9.
32. Webb J, Gerosa G, Lefevre T, et al. Multicenter evaluation of a next-generation balloon-expandable transcatheter aortic valve. J Am Coll Cardiol. 2014;64:2235–43.
33. Gaia DF, Palma JH, Ferreira CB, et al. Transapical aortic valve implantation: results of a Brazilian prosthesis. Rev Bras Cir Cardiovasc. 2010;25:293–302.
34. Fish RD, Paniagua D, Urena P, Chevalier B. The Colibri heart valve: theory and practice in the achievement of a low-profile, pre-mounted, pre-packaged TAVI valve. EuroIntervention. 2013;9(Suppl):S111–4.
35. Webb JG, Chandavimol M, Thompson CR, et al. Percutaneous aortic valve implantation retrograde from the femoral artery. Circulation. 2006;113:842–50.
36. Genereux P, Webb JG, Svensson LG, et al. Vascular complications after transcatheter aortic valve replacement: insights from the PARTNER (Placement of AoRTic TraNscathetER Valve) trial. J Am Coll Cardiol. 2012;60:1043–52.

37. Hayashida K, Lefevre T, Chevalier B, et al. Transfemoral aortic valve implantation new criteria to predict vascular complications. J Am Coll Cardiol Intv. 2011;4:851–8.
38. Hayashida K, Lefevre T, Chevalier B, et al. True percutaneous approach for transfemoral aortic valve implantation using the Prostar XL device: impact of learning curve on vascular complications. J Am Coll Cardiol Intv. 2012;5:207–14.
39. Ducrocq G, Francis F, Serfaty JM, et al. Vascular complications of transfemoral aortic valve implantation with the Edwards SAPIEN prosthesis: incidence and impact on outcome. EuroIntervention. 2010;5:666–72.
40. Kadakia MB, Herrmann HC, Desai ND, et al. Factors associated with vascular complications in patients undergoing balloon-expandable transfemoral transcatheter aortic valve replacement via open versus percutaneous approaches. Cir Cardiovasc Interv. 2014;7:570–6.
41. Van Mieghem NM, Nuis RJ, Piazza N, et al. Vascular complications with transcatheter aortic valve implantation using the 18 Fr Medtronic CoreValve System: the Rotterdam experience. EuroIntervention. 2010;5:673–9.
42. Toggweiler S, Gurvitch R, Leipsic J, et al. Percutaneous aortic valve replacement: vascular outcomes with a fully percutaneous procedure. J Am Coll Cardiol. 2012;59:113–8.
43. Cilingiroglu M, Feldman T, Salinger MH, Levisay J, Turi ZG. Fluoroscopically-guided micropuncture femoral artery access for large-caliber sheath insertion. J Invasive Cardiol. 2011;23:157–61.
44. Genereux P, Kodali S, Leon MB, et al. Clinical outcomes using a new crossover balloon occlusion technique for percutaneous closure after transfemoral aortic valve implantation. J Am Coll Cardiol Intv. 2011;4:861–7.
45. Blackstone EH, Suri RM, Rajeswaran J, et al. Propensity-matched comparisons of clinical outcomes after transapical or transfemoral transcatheter aortic valve replacement: a placement of aortic transcatheter valves (PARTNER)-I trial substudy. Circulation. 2015;131:1989–2000.
46. Bapat VV, Attia R. Transaortic transcatheter aortic valve implantation using the Edwards Sapien valve. Multimedia manual of cardiothoracic surgery: MMCTS/European Association for Cardio-Thoracic Surgery 2012; 2012: mms017.
47. Bapat V, Khawaja MZ, Attia R, et al. Transaortic transcatheter aortic valve implantation using Edwards Sapien valve: a novel approach. Catheter Cardiovasc Interv. 2012;79:733–40.
48. Rajagopal R, More RS, Roberts DH. Transcatheter aortic valve implantation through a trans-carotid approach under local anesthesia. Catheter Cardiovasc Interv. 2014;84:903–7.
49. Huber C, Praz F, O'Sullivan CJ, et al. Transcarotid aortic valve-in-valve implantation for degenerated stentless aortic root conduits with severe regurgitation: a case series. Interact Cardiovasc Thorac Surg. 2015;20:694–700.
50. Reardon MJ, Adams DH, Coselli JS, et al. Self-expanding transcatheter aortic valve replacement using alternative access sites in symptomatic patients with severe aortic stenosis deemed extreme risk of surgery. J Thorac Cardiovasc Surg. 2014;148(6):2869–76.e1–7.
51. Samim M, Stella PR, Agostoni P, et al. A prospective "oversizing" strategy of the Edwards SAPIEN bioprosthesis: results and impact on aortic regurgitation. J Thorac Cardiovasc Surg. 2013;145:398–405.
52. Daneault B, Koss E, Hahn RT, et al. Efficacy and safety of postdilatation to reduce paravalvular regurgitation during balloon-expandable transcatheter aortic valve replacement. Cir Cardiovasc Interv. 2013;6:85–91.
53. Jilaihawi H, Kashif M, Fontana G, et al. Cross-sectional computed tomographic assessment improves accuracy of aortic annular sizing for transcatheter aortic valve replacement and reduces the incidence of paravalvular aortic regurgitation. J Am Coll Cardiol. 2012;59:1275–86.
54. Jilaihawi H, Doctor N, Kashif M, et al. Aortic annular sizing for transcatheter aortic valve replacement using cross-sectional 3-dimensional transesophageal echocardiography. J Am Coll Cardiol. 2013;61:908–16.
55. Khalique OK, Kodali SK, Paradis JM, et al. Aortic annular sizing using a novel 3-dimensional echocardiographic method: use and comparison with cardiac computed tomography. Circ Cardiovasc imaging. 2014;7:155–63.

56. Babaliaros VC, Junagadhwalla Z, Lerakis S, et al. Use of balloon aortic valvuloplasty to size the aortic annulus before implantation of a balloon-expandable transcatheter heart valve. J Am Coll Cardiol Intv. 2010;3:114–8.
57. Davies WR, Bapat VN, Hancock JE, Young CP, Redwood SR, Thomas MR. Direct TAVI using a balloon-expandable system: a novel technique to eliminate pre-deployment balloon aortic valvuloplasty. EuroIntervention. 2014;10:248–52.
58. Bramlage P, Strauch J, Schrofel H. Balloon expandable transcatheter aortic valve implantation with or without pre-dilation of the aortic valve - rationale and design of a multicenter registry (EASE-IT). BMC Cardiovasc Disord. 2014;14:160.
59. Chan PH, Mario CD, Moat N. Transcatheter aortic valve implantation without balloon predilatation: not always feasible. Catheter Cardiovasc Interv. 2013;82:328–32.
60. Blumenstein JM, Van Linden A, Moellmann H, et al. DynaCT-guided anatomical rotation of the SAPIEN XT valve during transapical aortic valve implantation: proof of concept. Thorac Cardiovasc Surg. 2013;61:409–13.
61. Hahn RT, Abraham T, Adams MS, et al. Guidelines for performing a comprehensive transesophageal echocardiographic examination: recommendations from the American Society of Echocardiography and the Society of Cardiovascular Anesthesiologists. J Am Soc Echocardiogr. 2013;26:921–64.
62. Hahn RT, Little SH, Monaghan MJ, et al. Recommendations for comprehensive intraprocedural echocardiographic imaging during TAVR. J Am Coll Cardiol Img. 2015;8:261–87.
63. Mok M, Dumont E, Doyle D, Rodes-Cabau J. Transcatheter aortic valve implantation using the slow balloon inflation technique: making balloon-expandable valves partially repositionable. J Card Surg. 2012;27:546–8.
64. Durand E, Borz B, Godin M, et al. Transfemoral aortic valve replacement with the Edwards SAPIEN and Edwards SAPIEN XT prosthesis using exclusively local anesthesia and fluoroscopic guidance: feasibility and 30-day outcomes. J Am Coll Cardiol Intv. 2012;5:461–7.
65. Hahn RT, Pibarot P, Webb J, et al. Outcomes with post-dilation following transcatheter aortic valve replacement: the PARTNER I trial (placement of aortic transcatheter valve). J Am Coll Cardiol Intv. 2014;7:781–9.
66. Barbanti M, Leipsic J, Binder R, et al. Underexpansion and ad hoc post-dilation in selected patients undergoing balloon-expandable transcatheter aortic valve replacement. J Am Coll Cardiol. 2014;63:976–81.
67. Hahn RT, Pibarot P, Weissman NJ, Rodriguez L, Jaber WA. Assessment of paravalvular aortic regurgitation after transcatheter aortic valve replacement: intra-core laboratory variability. J Am Soc Echocardiogr. 2015;28:415–22.
68. Suri RMWJ, Mack M. Transcatheter aortic valve replacement for failed surgical bioprostheses: one year update – PARTNER II valve-in-valve registry. Washington, DC: Transcatheter Cardiovascular Therapeutics; 2014.
69. Kodali S. Clinical and echocardiographic outcomes at 30 days with the Sapien 3 TAVR system in inoperable, high-risk, and intermediate-risk AS patients. San Diego, CA: American College of Cardiology; 2015.
70. Abdel-Wahab M, Mehilli J, Frerker C, et al. Comparison of balloon-expandable vs self-expandable valves in patients undergoing transcatheter aortic valve replacement: the CHOICE randomized clinical trial. JAMA. 2014;311:1503–14.
71. Abdel-Wahab M, Comberg T, Buttner HJ, et al. Aortic regurgitation after transcatheter aortic valve implantation with balloon- and self-expandable prostheses: a pooled analysis from a 2-center experience. J Am Coll Cardiol Intv. 2014;7:284–92.
72. Bosmans JM, Kefer J, De Bruyne B, et al. Procedural, 30-day and one year outcome following CoreValve or Edwards transcatheter aortic valve implantation: results of the Belgian national registry. Interact Cardiovasc Thorac Surg. 2011;12:762–7.
73. Chieffo A, Buchanan GL, Van Mieghem NM, et al. Transcatheter aortic valve implantation with the Edwards SAPIEN versus the Medtronic CoreValve Revalving system devices: a multicenter collaborative study: the PRAGMATIC Plus Initiative (Pooled-RotterdAm-Milano-Toulouse In Collaboration). J Am Coll Cardiol. 2013;61:830–6.

74. Chakravarty T, Jilaihawi H, Doctor N et al. Complications after transfemoral transcatheter aortic valve replacement with a balloon-expandable prosthesis: The importance of preventative measures and contingency planning. Catheter Cardiovasc Interv. 2013 Feb 21. [Epub ahead of print].
75. Athappan G, Patvardhan E, Tuzcu EM, et al. Incidence, predictors, and outcomes of aortic regurgitation after transcatheter aortic valve replacement: meta-analysis and systematic review of literature. J Am Coll Cardiol. 2013;61:1585–95.
76. Kodali S, Pibarot P, Douglas PS, et al. Paravalvular Regurgitation after Transcatheter Aortic Valve Replacement with the Edwards Sapien Valve in the PARTNER trial: characterizing patients and impact on outcomes. Eur Heart J. 2015;36(7):449–56.
77. Hahn RT, Pibarot P, Stewart WJ, et al. Comparison of transcatheter and surgical aortic valve replacement in severe aortic stenosis: a longitudinal study of echocardiography parameters in cohort A of the PARTNER trial (placement of aortic transcatheter valves). J Am Coll Cardiol. 2013;61:2514–21.
78. Nazif TM, Dizon JM, Hahn RT, et al. Predictors and clinical outcomes of permanent pacemaker implantation after transcatheter aortic valve replacement: the PARTNER (Placement of AoRtic TraNscathetER Valves) trial and registry. J Am Coll Cardiol Intv. 2015;8:60–9.
79. Eksik A, Gul M, Uyarel H, et al. Electrophysiological evaluation of atrioventricular conduction disturbances in transcatheter aortic valve implantation with Edwards SAPIEN prosthesis. J Invasive cardiol. 2013;25:305–9.
80. Al Ali AM, Altwegg L, Horlick EM, et al. Prevention and management of transcatheter balloon-expandable aortic valve malposition. Catheter Cardiovasc Interv. 2008;72:573–8.
81. Barbanti M, Yang TH, Rodes Cabau J, et al. Anatomical and procedural features associated with aortic root rupture during balloon-expandable transcatheter aortic valve replacement. Circulation. 2013;128:244–53.
82. Blanke P, Reinohl J, Schlensak C, et al. Prosthesis oversizing in balloon-expandable transcatheter aortic valve implantation is associated with contained rupture of the aortic root. Cir Cardiovasc Interv. 2012;5:540–8.
83. Borz B, Durand E, Godin M, et al. Incidence, predictors and impact of bleeding after transcatheter aortic valve implantation using the balloon-expandable Edwards prosthesis. Heart. 2013;99:860–5.
84. Eggebrecht H, Schmermund A, Voigtlander T, Kahlert P, Erbel R, Mehta RH. Risk of stroke after transcatheter aortic valve implantation (TAVI): a meta-analysis of 10,037 published patients. EuroIntervention. 2012;8:129–38.
85. Messe SR, Acker MA, Kasner SE, et al. Stroke after aortic valve surgery: results from a prospective cohort. Circulation. 2014;129:2253–61.
86. Daneault B, Kirtane AJ, Kodali SK, et al. Stroke associated with surgical and transcatheter treatment of aortic stenosis: a comprehensive review. J Am Coll Cardiol. 2011;58:2143–50.
87. Linke A. Technology Overview and Perspectives From the CLEAN-TAVI Randomized Trial. Chicago, IL: Transcatheter Valve Therapeutics; 2015.
88. Kodali S. Updates From the US FDA–Approved Sentinel TAVR Safety and Efficacy Study. Chicago, IL: Transcatheter Valve Therapeutics; 2015.

Chapter 3
TAVR with CoreValve via Transfemoral Approach

Juan A. Crestanello and Barry George

Introduction and Device Description

The CoreValve (Medtronic Inc., Minneapolis, MN) is a self-expanding transcatheter valve approved by the FDA for commercial use in the USA for patients at high or at extreme risk for surgery after the completion of the US CoreValve Pivotal trial [1, 2]. The CoreValve can be delivered via a transfemoral, axillary, or direct aortic approach [1, 2]. In this chapter, we will discuss the transfemoral approach.

The CoreValve transcatheter system consists of three components: the valve, the delivery catheter, and the loading system. The CoreValve comes in four sizes (23, 26, 29, and 31 mm). The CoreValve is a porcine pericardial valve mounted on a self-expanding nitinol frame. The nitinol frame has three portions: an inflow, a constrain, and an outflow portion (Fig. 3.1). The **inflow portion** anchors the valve to the annulus. A pericardial skirt covers the first 12 mm of the stent sealing the valve to the aortic annulus to prevent paravalvular leak [1, 2]. The high radial force of the inflow portion is partially responsible for compressing the conduction system and for the need for permanent pacemaker. The **constrain portion** (Fig. 3.1) contains the pericardial valve leaflets and is responsible for valve competency. This narrow portion of the stent that sits at the sinuses of Valsalva is designed to avoid the coronary ostia. The **outflow portion** sits in the ascending aorta to orient and stabilize the stent. The commissures of the valve leaflets are also attached at this level.

J.A. Crestanello, MD (✉)
Division of Cardiac Surgery, Department of Surgery, Wexner Medical Center,
The Ohio State University, N-825 Doan Hall, 410 West 10th Avenue, Columbus, OH, USA
e-mail: juan.crestanello@osumc.edu

B. George, BE, MD, FACC, FACI, FACP
Division of Cardiovascular Medicine, Department of Medicine,
Wexner Medical Center, The Ohio State University, 473 West 12th Avenue,
Suite 200 DHLRI, Columbus, OH 43210, USA
e-mail: barry.george@osumc.edu

© Springer Science+Business Media New York 2016
G. Ailawadi, I.L. Kron (eds.), *Catheter Based Valve and Aortic Surgery*,
DOI 10.1007/978-1-4939-3432-4_3

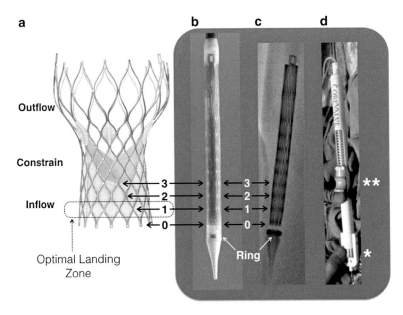

Fig. 3.1 (**a**) CoreValve bioprosthesis with the inflow, constrain, and outflow portion. (**b**) Valve loaded in the capsule of the delivery system. (**c**) Fluoroscopic appearance of the valve loaded in the capsule of the delivery system. When the valve is loaded in the capsule, the superimposition of the nodes creates bands. These bands are used for guidance during deployment. The distance between nodes is 4 mm. The numbers (0–3 name the nodes). The ring is the radiopaque marker at the end of the capsule. Note that the first 12 mm (node 0–3) of the inflow portion is covered by a pericardial skirt. The optimal landing zone to assure sealing between the skirt and the aortic annulus is between 2 and 6 mm (within 2 mm of node 1). That means that the native annular plane is at that level. The nadir of the prosthetic leaflets is also at 12 mm. If the native annulus is above this point, the skirt won't seal. D. Shows the handle of the delivery catheter with the micro (*asterisk*) and macro (*double asterisk*) knobs

The **delivery system** is 18F in diameter. The valve is loaded inside a capsule (Fig. 3.1b, c). The valve is deployed by turning the handle micro-knob that withdraws the capsule allowing the valve to expand [1, 2].

Patient Evaluation and Procedure Planning

Anatomic Evaluation

Echocardiography

Echocardiography is used for functional assessment and to determine the number of leaflets of the aortic valve. Prosthesis size selection based on echocardiography is no longer used since it is associated with an increased rate of paravalvular leak [3].

Table 3.1 CoreValve prosthesis dimensions and multidetector computed tomography (MDCT) angiogram-derived aortic root and iliofemoral access dimensions for each CoreValve size

	CoreValve dimensions			
CoreValve size	**23 mm**	**26 mm**	**29 mm**	**31 mm**
CoreValve stent inflow diameter (mm)	23	26	29	31
CoreValve stent constrain diameter (mm)	20	22	24	24
CoreValve stent outflow diameter (mm)	34	40	43	43
CoreValve stent height (mm)	48.8	55.5	53.4	52.4
	MDCT-derived aortic root dimensions			
Annulus mean diameter (mm)	18–20	20–23	23–26	26–29
Annulus perimeter (mm)	56.5–62.8	62.8–72.3	72.3–81.6	81.6–91.1
Sinus of Valsalva diameter (mm)	≥25	≥27	≥29	≥29
Sinus of Valsalva height (mm)	≥15	≥15	≥15	≥15
Ascending aorta max diameter (mm)	≤34[a]	≤40[b]	≤43[b]	≤43[b]
	Iliofemoral access dimensions			
Minimum arterial diameter (mm)	6	6	6	6
Delivery catheter diameter (F)	18	18	18	18

CoreValve size selection is based on these dimensions. CoreValve can accommodate aortic valve annulus with mean diameters from 18 to 29 mm and mean perimeters from 56.5 to 91.1 mm. The CoreValve sizes (23, 26, 29, and 31 mm) reflect the diameter of the inflow portion. In order to minimize paravalvular leak, the recommended CoreValve/annulus oversizing is 15 % of the aortic annulus perimeter determined by MDCT. Ascending aorta diameter at 3 cm ([a]) and at 4 cm ([b]) from annulus

Multidetector Computed Tomography Angiogram

Multidetector computed tomography (MDCT) angiogram is the primary imaging modality to select valve size and access route [4, 5]. The aortic root, the entire aorta, and the iliofemoral vessels are evaluated. Table 3.1 shows the MDCT-derived measurements required for each valve size [4].

Aortic root evaluation: Images are acquired during end systole (20–50 % phase of the cardiac cycle) due to the larger annular size during systole. Images are post processed and reconstructed to obtain the best image of the aortic root.

Annular measurements (Fig. 3.2): The aortic annulus is the landing target. Two measurements are obtained from the annulus: (a) annulus diameter (major and minor diameters are measured and the mean diameter is calculated) and (b) annulus perimeter which is measured by tracing the circumference of the annulus. The aortic valve number of cusps, degree and extension of leaflet, and annular calcification are also assessed. Asymmetric, focal, or excessive calcification may prevent the expansion of the stent and lead to increased risk of paravalvular regurgitation, coronary obstruction, annular rupture, and need for post-deployment valvuloplasty.

The sinuses of Valsalva (SOV) diameter and height and the distance from the aortic annulus to the coronary artery ostium are evaluated to prevent coronary obstruction by the displaced native leaflets (Table 3.1, Fig. 3.2). The combination of a large annulus, small sinuses, and a low-lying coronary ostium can lead to coronary

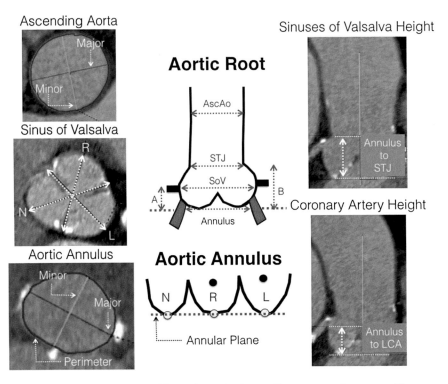

Fig. 3.2 MDCT of the aortic root. The aortic annulus is not a discrete anatomic structure. The annular plane (aortic annulus) is the plane that intersects the nadir of all three aortic valve cusps. Reconstructions of the aortic root are performed and dimensions are obtained from the left ventricular outflow tract, the aortic annulus (Annulus) (major, minor, and mean diameter and perimeter), each sinus of Valsalva diameter (SoV), sino-tubular junction (STJ) diameter (minor, major, and mean), and ascending aorta diameter (minor, major, and mean) at 4 cm from the annular plane (AscAo). The distances from the annular plane to each coronary artery ostium (coronary artery height, A) and to the sino-tubular junction for each sinus (sinus of Valsalva height, B) are also measured. N, noncoronary sinus; L, left coronary sinus; R, right coronary sinus. *LCA* left coronary artery

obstruction. The chances of coronary obstruction are low if the distance from the aortic annulus to the ostium is greater than 10–14 mm. In the presence of patent coronary artery bypass grafts, the anatomic consideration for compromise of the coronary arteries is more relative. The outflow portion of the stent lies in the ascending aorta and should make contact with the aortic wall (Table 3.1). The LVOT is assessed for size, basal septal hypertrophy, and calcifications that may compromise the expansion of the stent and risk paravalvular leak and or pop-out of the valve. The aortic root angulation is also assessed (Fig. 3.3).

Valve size selection: The size of the annulus is the main determinant to select the size of the valve (Table 3.1). The mean diameter and the perimeter are considered. The recommended CoreValve/annulus oversizing is 15 % of the aortic annulus perimeter [1, 2]. For example, for annulus dimensions between 18 and 20 mm (perimeter 56.5 to 62.8 mm), a 23 mm CoreValve should be used. For annulus dimensions between 20 and 23 (perimeter between 62.8 and 72.3), a 26 mm

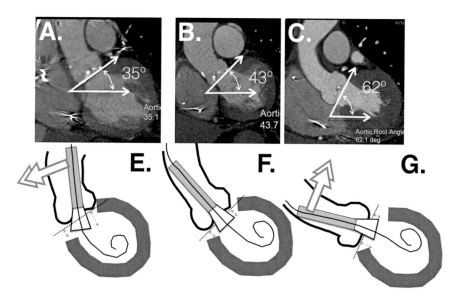

Fig. 3.3 MDCT determination of the aortic root angulation. The aortic root angulation is the angle between the plane of the aortic valve and the horizontal plane. It should be less than 70°. The ideal anatomy is when the aortic root angulation is such that the valve is completely coaxial to the aorta and perpendicular to the plane of the annulus (**b, f**). Vertical aortas (angle <45° angle, **a, e**) or horizontal aortas (angle >45° **c, g**) prevent the CoreValve to be coaxial to the plane of the aortic annulus and may lead to uneven deployment with one side too deep and the other too shallow (*red arrows*). This may be corrected by adjusting the position of the guidewire to the lesser or greater curvature of the aorta (*gray arrows*)

CoreValve is selected (Table 3.1). The size of the SOV should also be considered to avoid compromising the coronary ostia. The height of the SOV should be ≥15 mm, and there should be a 5 mm clearance between the constrain portion and the sinus of Valsalva (Table 3.1, Fig. 3.2). For example, in a 29 mm valve, the constrain portion is 24 mm; therefore, the sinuses of Valsalva should be at least 29 mm. When the annulus dimensions (diameter and perimeter) are in the intermediate range, other criteria should be considered. They are the diameter and height of the sinuses of Valsalva, the distance of the coronary arteries to the annulus, and the size of the sino-tubular junction (STJ). For example, with an annulus diameter and circumference of 23 and 72.3 mm either a 26 or a 29 mm CoreValve can be used. If the SOV diameter is less than 29 mm, then a 26 mm valve should be selected. If the distance of the coronary ostia to the annulus or the diameter at the STJ is also on the small side, the smaller valve should be used. The calcification of the annulus is also important to consider in these intermediate circumstances. A heavy calcified, symmetric annulus is more likely to accept and seal the smaller valve. If there is very little or asymmetric calcification, a larger valve will likely seal better.

The aorta, iliac, and common femoral arteries are assessed through non-gated acquisition (Fig. 3.4) [4, 5]. The femoral and iliac vessels should be at least 6 mm in diameter to accept an 18F delivery sheath.

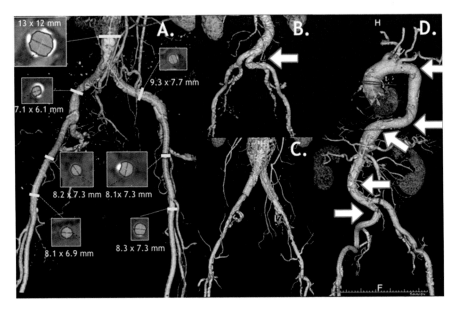

Fig. 3.4 Iliofemoral artery evaluation: The femoral and iliac arteries are evaluated for size (**a**, minor and major diameter), calcification and its extension (severity, focal, circumferential), tortuosity (**d**), acute angulation (**b**, **d** *arrows*), focal dissection, aneurysm (**c**), mural thrombosis, atherosclerotic plaque, previous surgery, or endografts (**c**). The combination of a borderline size artery with heavy calcification and tortuosity is a contraindication for femoral access. However, a relatively small, straight artery with no significant calcification can be used even if the diameter is borderline

Preprocedure Evaluation

Preprocedure evaluation should be performed to asses for comorbidities, frailty, dementia, and other risk factors that may limit the possibilities of clinical improvement after the aortic stenosis is relieved. Coronary anatomy, cardiac function, and other valvular abnormalities should be assessed preoperatively. Prophylactic antibiotics and dual antiplatelet therapy with aspirin (325 mg) and clopidogrel (300 mg) are administered before the procedure [1, 2]. An active fixation temporary pacemaker lead is placed in the right ventricle for pacing during the procedure.

Although traditionally most TAVR procedures are performed under general anesthesia, there is a trend to perform them under monitored anesthesia care (MAC). MAC may be associated with less hemodynamic compromise, lower rate of pneumonia, and decreased length of hospital stay [6].

CoreValve Deployment

The steps in the deployment of the CoreValve are (1) vascular access, (2) crossing the aortic valve and hemodynamic assessment of the aortic stenosis, (3) aortic valvuloplasty, (4) valve deployment, (5) post-deployment valve assessment, and (6) vascular access repair.

Vascular Access

Both common femoral arteries are accessed percutaneously. The patient is then heparinized to an ACT > 300 s. The side of the delivery sheath is pre-closed (Perclose ProGlide, Abbott Vascular, Abbott Park, Illinois). Then, an Amplatz Super Stiff Guidewire (Boston Scientific, Natick, MA) is inserted into the descending thoracic aortic. The iliofemoral arteries are progressively dilated with 12, 14, and 18F dilators and the delivery sheath is inserted. We routinely use the Gore Dryseal Sheath (W. L. Gore & Ass., Inc. Newark, DE). The SoloPath balloon-expandable sheath (Terumo Interventional Systems, Somerset, NJ) has a smaller insertion profile that is useful in patients with borderline access because of size or concentric calcifications. We use a longer sheath (40 or 65 cm 18F, Check-Flo, Cook Medical, Bloomington, IN) for severe tortuosity of the abdominal or thoracic aorta, aortic aneurysm, localized dissection in the aorta, large plaque, or mural thrombus. This avoids dragging the delivery catheter through the area of concern and may avoid that area if valve retrieval is necessary. A femoral artery cut down is rarely done.

A reference pigtail is placed through the contralateral femoral artery into the noncoronary cusp of the aortic valve to be used for angiography and as a landmark during deployment. The implantation projection is selected next (Fig. 3.5).

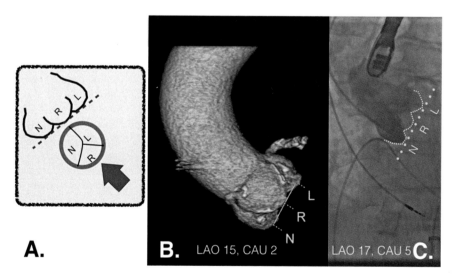

Fig. 3.5 The deployment projection is the projection where the nadirs of the 3 cusps of the aortic valve are aligned in a single plane (**a**). MDCT usually provides valuable information about this projection and minimizes contrast injection during the TAVR procedure (**b**). During the procedure, a root angiogram is obtained with the reference pigtail placed in the noncoronary sinus of Valsalva (**c**). For most patients, the deployment projection is close to 10–15° LAO and 5–10° caudal. N, noncoronary sinus of Valsalva; R, right coronary sinus of Valsalva; L, left coronary sinus of Valsalva. *LAO* left anterior oblique projection

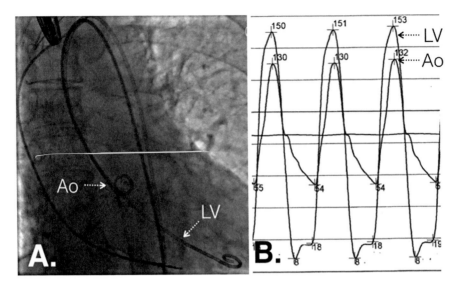

Fig. 3.6 (**a**) The aortic valve is crossed and pigtails are placed in the ascending aorta (Ao) and left ventricle (LV). (**b**) Simultaneous aortic and left ventricular pressures are measured. Aortic systolic and diastolic pressures, left ventricular systolic and end-diastolic pressures, and peak to peak and mean aortic gradients are recorded

Crossing the Aortic Valve and Baseline Hemodynamic Assessment

The aortic valve is crossed using a straight tip guidewire. Once the aortic valve is crossed, the projection is changed to RAO. This opens up the left ventricle and prevents the inadvertent perforation of the ventricle during the placement of the stiff guidewire. Simultaneous pressures in the left ventricle and aorta are measured (Fig. 3.6). Then, in the RAO projection, an Amplatz Super Stiff Guidewire is placed in the left ventricular apex. This is a straight guidewire with a 1 cm flexible tip previously shaped to a pigtail configuration (Boston Scientific, Natick, MA).

Aortic Valvuloplasty

Aortic valvuloplasty is not routinely performed except in patients with heavily calcified aortic valve or bicuspid valves. Although implantation success rate with and without valvuloplasty is the same, preimplantation valvuloplasty is associated with a higher rate of stroke and permanent pacemaker [7]. Preimplantation valvuloplasty is performed with a 5 or 6 cm long NuMED Z-MED II balloon (B. Braun Medical Inc., Bethlehem, PA). The size of the balloon is selected not to exceed the smaller transverse diameter of the aortic annulus by MDCT. During valvuloplasty the heart is paced at 160 to 180 bpm to decrease stroke volume.

Valve Deployment

The CoreValve is advanced across the aortic valve and the parallax of the ring at the lower end of the capsule is removed. The ideal deployment projection is when the valve is completely coaxial to the aorta and perpendicular to the plane of the annulus (Fig. 3.3b, f). However, given the angulation of the ascending aorta and the ventricle, that situation is rare (Fig. 3.3a, c) and guidewire adjustment is necessary to make the valve more coaxial. The optimal deployment depth is when the annular plane is within 2 mm from node 1 (2–6 mm depth) of the CoreValve using the pigtail in the noncoronary cusp as a landmark for the annular plane (Figs. 3.1 and 3.5). Valve deployment is performed by 2 operators. Operator number one is located closer to the delivery sheath and controls the shaft of the delivery catheter. Operator number one advances and withdraws the catheter to make adjustment in the valve position. Operator number 2 controls the catheter handle, the micro-knob, and the guidewire. As the micro-knob is turned, the capsule withdraws and the valve expands. Adjustments in the valve position are made by moving the shaft of the catheter by operator number one or by adjusting the guidewire by operator number 2 (Fig. 3.7). The valve is deployed by slowly withdrawing the capsule (Fig. 3.8). By withdrawing the capsule, the inflow portion of the valve starts to expands. It usually makes contact with the annulus when the capsule is around node 3 (Fig. 3.8c). This part of the deployment should be done slowly with frequent angiograms to assess the depth of the prosthesis. After annular contact, the valve position can only be adjusted by pulling on the delivery catheter and it cannot be advanced into a lower position. At this point, the valve is fully occlusive of the LVOT and the blood pressure starts to fall. Rapid ventricular pacing (120 bpm) is started and the valve is quickly released up to the 2/3 deployment point (Fig. 3.8d). At this point the

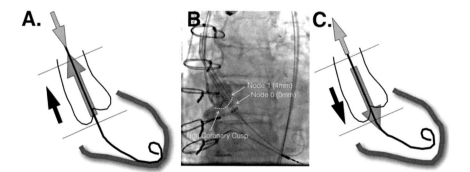

Fig. 3.7 Adjustments in the CoreValve position during deployment can be made by operator number one by pulling or pushing on the catheter shaft. Movements of the guidewire move the valve in the opposite direction than the guidewire movement. Pushing on the guidewire brings the valve toward the aorta (**a**) while pulling on the guidewire has the opposite effect (valve moves toward the ventricle, **c**). (**b**) CoreValve across the aortic valve. Note the nadir of the right coronary cusp (annular plane) is between node 0 and 1 of the CoreValve. Thus, the depth of the CoreValve is approximately 2 mm

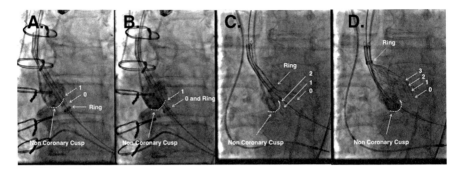

Fig. 3.8 CoreValve deployment starts with the valve node 1 aligned with the nadir of the noncoronary cusp (**a**). Then the ring (radiopaque marker at the end of the capsule and as such the ring reflects the movement of the capsule) is moved to node 0 (**b**). As the capsule withdraws, the inflow portion of the valve starts to expand. It usually makes contact with the annulus when the end of the capsule (ring) is around node 3 (**c**). Note that the depth of the valve is maintained fairly constant with node 1 aligned with the nadir of the noncoronary cusp. At this point, rapid ventricular pacing is started and the capsule is rapidly withdrawn to the 2/3 deployment point (**d**)

bioprosthesis leaflets are fully functioning. The position, height, and expansion of the inflow portion are assessed by TEE and angiography. If the valve is too deep (low in the ventricle), adjustments can be made by carefully pulling on the delivery catheter to withdraw the valve to a more superficial level. If the prosthesis is too superficial (high, toward the aorta), the valve can still be completely retrieved by withdrawing the delivery catheter and re-sheathing the valve into the delivery sheath. Then the valve can be removed from the patient. When satisfactory position is achieved, the reference pigtail catheter is withdrawn into the ascending aorta, the valve is released by dialing the micro-knob until the valve is fully released from the delivery catheter, and the valve frame loops are disengaged.

Post-deployment Valve Assessment

Post-deployment valve assessment is accomplished by hemodynamics, aortography (Fig. 3.9), and TEE. Hemodynamic assessment is performed by simultaneously measuring aortic and left ventricular pressure with pigtail catheters (Fig. 3.10) [8]. TEE is performed to asses height of implantation, stent expansion, left ventricular function, presence of pericardial effusion, and degree or aortic insufficiency both transvalvular and paravalvular. The severity of aortic regurgitation is graded according to the Valve Academic Research consortium statement [9]. All three assessments should be considered to quantify the severity of aortic regurgitation. Aortic regurgitation tends to improve quickly overtime as the CoreValve expands. Therefore, waiting 5–15 min and reassessing the situation before performing any additional intervention is recommended. If the paravalvular regurgitation is moderate or severe or the patient's

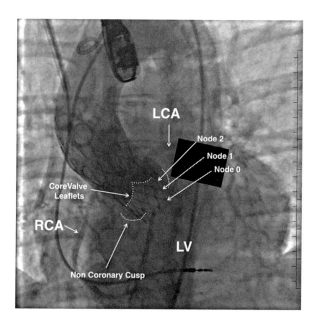

Fig. 3.9 Post-deployment aortography. An aortogram is performed with the pigtail in the outflow portion of the frame to evaluate patency of the coronary arteries (RCA, right coronary artery; LCA, left coronary artery), height of implantation, stent expansion, and competency of the valve. Note that there is trivial aortic regurgitation. The depth of implantation is at 3 mm (a little less than node 1) for both the non and left annulus. LV: left ventricle. Note the line of coaptation of the CoreValve leaflets in the constrain portion of the valve, above the level of the native aortic valves

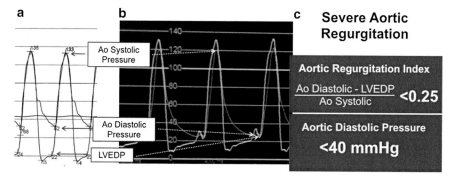

Fig. 3.10 Post CoreValve implantation hemodynamic assessment is performed by simultaneously measuring aortic and left ventricular pressure with pigtail catheters (**a**). It evaluates the complete relief of the aortic stenosis and helps to assess the degree of aortic regurgitation. The aortic (Ao) diastolic pressure, the left ventricular end-diastolic pressure (LVEDP), and the aortic regurgitation index are used to assess the severity of aortic regurgitation. An aortic diastolic pressure <40 mmHg, an aortic regurgitation index <0.25, and an elevated LVEDP suggest the presence of severe aortic regurgitation (**b, c**) [8]

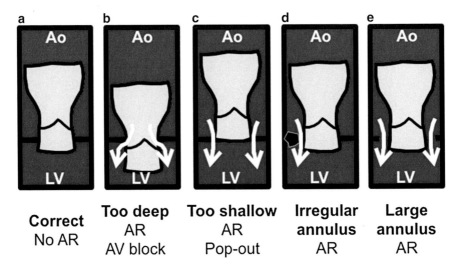

Fig. 3.11 Mechanisms of paravalvular regurgitation (AR). Paravalvular regurgitation is common after TAVR. (**a**) Achieving the optimal landing depth (2–6 mm) assures that the covered portion of the stent opposes and seals the annulus preventing paravalvular regurgitation. There are several mechanisms responsible for paravalvular regurgitation: (1) The valve is too low (**b**, too ventricular, deeper than 12 mm). The pericardial skirt is below the annulus leading to paravalvular regurgitation and also to conduction abnormalities. (2) The valve is too high (**c**, too aortic); the bottom of the inflow portion is above the annulus, and thus, it does not seal. There is also risk of the valve dislodging into the aorta (pop-out). (3) Valve underexpansion because of asymmetric calcification of the annulus (**d**). (4) Valve undersizing will also lead to paravalvular regurgitation since the stent does not contact the annulus (**e**)

hemodynamics are compromised, an intervention should be considered. The mechanism for the paravalvular leak should be assessed (Fig. 3.11). If the valve is too low, then a second valve or snaring should be considered. If the valve height is appropriate, but it is under-expanded or there is calcium that prevents the expansion and apposition of the inflow portion to the annulus, then a post-dilatation valvuloplasty or a second valve should be considered. If the valve is too high, a second valve positioned lower should be considered. The dimensions of the STJ and the sinuses of Valsalva and the potential space between the open leaflets of the first valve and the aortic wall should be considered before inserting a second valve. The size of the balloon is selected using the mean diameter of the aortic annulus as determined by MDCT. Balloon size should not exceed the diameter of the CoreValve minus one mm.

Vascular Access Repair

The delivery sheath is removed while carefully monitoring for arterial access injury. An iliofemoral angiography is performed to demonstrate the integrity of the vessels and the femoral vessels are repaired. Anticoagulation is then reversed.

Postoperative Care

Patients are extubated in the OR and monitored in the ICU for 12 h. The temporary pacemaker is maintained for 48 h. Management of congestive heart failure, renal function, pulmonary comorbidities, and delirium is essential in these patients [10]. Aspirin and clopidogrel are prescribed for 3 months. Echocardiography is performed before discharge. Most patients are discharged 3–5 days after the procedure. Patients are followed up at 1 month, 6 months, and yearly thereafter.

Outcomes

The US CoreValve Pivotal trials studied TAVR in patients with severe aortic stenosis who were at high risk or at extreme risk for surgery [1, 2]. In the extreme risk study, the rate of death and stroke at 12 months was lower than that estimated for patients treated medically (Fig. 3.12). At 30 days, 21.6 % needed permanent pacemaker, 12.7 % had bleeding, 8.2 % had vascular complications, and 4.0 % had stroke. The rate of moderate or severe paravalvular regurgitation was 10.2 % at discharge and 4.2 % at 12 months. Moderate regurgitation was not associated with

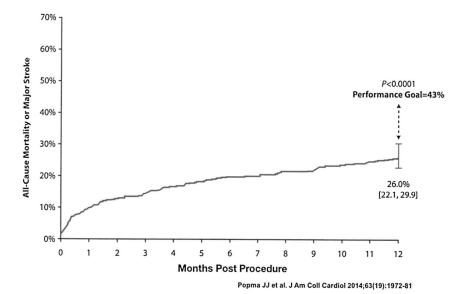

Popma JJ et al. J Am Coll Cardiol 2014;63(19):1972-81

Fig. 3.12 Extreme risk cohort of the US CoreValve Pivotal trial results: Kaplan-Meier cumulative event curve for all-cause mortality or major stroke. In inoperable patients with severe symptomatic aortic stenosis treated with transfemoral CoreValve, the all-cause mortality or major stroke at 12 months was lower than the estimated for patients treated with modern optimal medical therapy (OPG: optimal performance goal). The OPG data was derived from the medical arm of the PARTNER trial. From Popma et al. [1], with permission

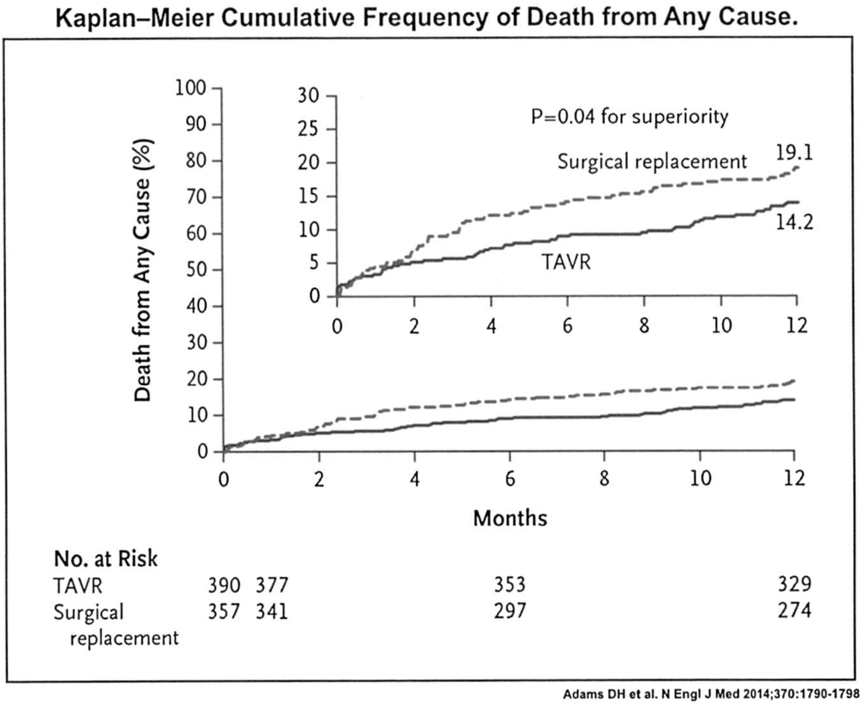

Kaplan–Meier Cumulative Frequency of Death from Any Cause.

Adams DH et al. N Engl J Med 2014;370:1790-1798

Fig. 3.13 High-risk cohort of the US CoreValve Pivotal trial results: Kaplan-Meier cumulative frequency of death from any cause. The rate of death from any cause in the TAVR group was non-inferior to that in the AVR group ($P<0.001$), and in fact it showed that TAVR was superior to surgical replacement at 1 year ($P=0.04$). From Adams et al. [2], with permission

increased mortality. At 12 months, 90 % of patients were in NYHA functional class I or II [1]. In the high risk study, patients were randomized either to TAVR or to surgical aortic valve replacement (AVR) [2]. Mortality at 1 year was lower in the TAVR group than in the AVR group (Fig. 3.13), while the improvement in NYHA class was similar. There was a trend for a lower stroke rate in the TAVR groups than in the surgical group. Permanent pacemaker at 1 year was required in 22.3 % after TAVR vs. 11.3 % after AVR ($p<0.001$). The rate of moderate or severe paravalvular regurgitation with TAVR was 9.0 % vs. 1.0 % with AVR ($p<0.001$) [2].

Conclusion

Transfemoral TAVR with the CoreValve system is indicated for patients at high risk for surgery and for those who are not candidates for surgical replacement. Meticulous preprocedure planning with assessment of the aortic root, aortic annulus, sinuses of Valsalva, access, and device size selection is essential for the success of the procedure. The short- and intermediate-term results are excellent in these cohorts. Reduction in the rate of stroke rate, access complications, need for permanent pacemaker, and paravalvular regurgitation are the main challenges ahead.

References

1. Popma JJ, Adams DH, Reardon MJ, Yakubov SJ, Kleiman NS, Heimansohn D, Hermiller Jr J, Hughes GC, Harrison JK, Coselli J, Diez J, Kafi A, Schreiber T, Gleason TG, Conte J, Buchbinder M, Deeb GM, Carabello B, Serruys PW, Chenoweth S, Oh JK, CoreValve United States Clinical Investigators. Transcatheter aortic valve replacement using a self-expanding bioprosthesis in patients with severe aortic stenosis at extreme risk for surgery. J Am Coll Cardiol. 2014;63:1972–81.

2. Adams DH, Popma JJ, Reardon MJ, Yakubov SJ, Coselli JS, Deeb GM, Gleason TG, Buchbinder M, Hermiller Jr J, Kleiman NS, Chetcuti S, Heiser J, Merhi W, Zorn G, Tadros P, Robinson N, Petrossian G, Hughes GC, Harrison JK, Conte J, Maini B, Mumtaz M, Chenoweth S, Oh JK, U.S. CoreValve Clinical Investigators. Transcatheter aortic-valve replacement with a self-expanding prosthesis. N Engl J Med. 2014;370:1790–8.

3. Jilaihawi H, Kashif M, Fontana G, Furugen A, Shiota T, Friede G, Makhija R, Doctor N, Leon MB, Makkar RR. Cross-sectional computed tomographic assessment improves accuracy of aortic annular sizing for transcatheter aortic valve replacement and reduces the incidence of paravalvular aortic regurgitation. J Am Coll Cardiol. 2012;59:1275–86.

4. Litmanovich DE, Ghersin E, Burke DA, Popma J, Shahrzad M, Bankier AA. Imaging in Transcatheter Aortic Valve Replacement (TAVR): role of the radiologist. Insights Imaging. 2014;5:123–45. PMID: 24443171.

5. Achenbach S, Delgado V, Hausleiter J, Schoenhagen P, Min JK, Leipsic JA. SCCT expert consensus document on computed tomography imaging before transcatheter aortic valve implantation (TAVI)/transcatheter aortic valve replacement (TAVR). J Cardiovasc Comput Tomogr. 2012;6:366–80.

6. Fröhlich GM, Lansky AJ, Webb J, Roffi M, Toggweiler S, Reinthaler M, Wang D, Hutchinson N, Wendler O, Hildick-Smith D, Meier P. Local versus general anesthesia for transcatheter aortic valve implantation (TAVR)--systematic review and meta-analysis. BMC Med. 2014;12:41. PMID: 24612945.

7. Grube E, Naber C, Abizaid A, Sousa E, Mendiz O, Lemos P, Kalil Filho R, Mangione J, Buellesfeld L. Feasibility of transcatheter aortic valve implantation without balloon pre-dilation: a pilot study. JACC Cardiovasc Interv. 2011;4:751–7.

8. Sinning JM, Vasa-Nicotera M, Chin D, Hammerstingl C, Ghanem A, Bence J, Kovac J, Grube E, Nickenig G, Werner N. Evaluation and management of paravalvular aortic regurgitation after transcatheter aortic valve replacement. J Am Coll Cardiol. 2013;62:11–20.

9. Kappetein AP, Head SJ, Généreux P, Piazza N, van Mieghem NM, Blackstone EH, Brott TG, Cohen DJ, Cutlip DE, van Es GA, Hahn RT, Kirtane AJ, Krucoff MW, Kodali S, Mack MJ, Mehran R, Rodés-Cabau J, Vranckx P, Webb JG, Windecker S, Serruys PW, Leon MB, Valve Academic Research Consortium-2. Updated standardized endpoint definitions for transcatheter aortic valve implantation: the Valve Academic Research Consortium-2 consensus document. J Thorac Cardiovasc Surg. 2013;145:6–23.

10. Raiten JM, Gutsche JT, Horak J, Augoustides JG. Critical care management of patients following transcatheter aortic valve replacement. F1000Res. 2013;2:62.

Chapter 4
Transfemoral: Upcoming Valves

Matthew C. Henn, Alan Zajarias, and Hersh S. Maniar

Introduction

Since the introduction of transcatheter aortic valve implantation (TAVI) over 10 years ago [1], transfemoral devices have steadily evolved. The first-generation transfemoral devices—the balloon-expandable SAPIEN valve (Edwards Lifesciences, Irvine, CA) and the self-expandable CoreValve (Medtronic Inc., Minneapolis, MN)—achieved CE (*Conformité Européenne*) mark in Europe in 2007 and have been thoroughly tested in the United States by large, multicenter trials demonstrating their safety and efficacy [2–5]. These trials have led to FDA approval of TAVI for the treatment of nonsurgical patients in November of 2011 and high-risk surgical patients in 2012 [6]. However, these same trials have highlighted the shortcomings of the first-generation devices including increased cerebrovascular accidents, vascular complications, rhythm disturbances, malposition, and a higher incidence of paravalvular regurgitation than those treated with surgery.

Under current indication guidelines, there are a projected ~190,000 TAVI candidates in 19 European countries with an additional 100,000 in North America. Those numbers are anticipated to grow with nearly 18,000 and 9,200 new TAVI candidates annually in Europe and North America, respectively. This represents an estimated $14 billion industry that will undoubtedly expand as the indications for TAVI grow

M.C. Henn, MD • H.S. Maniar, MD (✉)
Division of Cardiothoracic Surgery, Department of Surgery, Barnes-Jewish Hospital,
Washington University School of Medicine, 660 South Euclid Avenus,
Campus Box 8234, St. Louis, MO 63110, USA
e-mail: hennm@wudosis.wustl.edu; maniarh@wustl.edu

A. Zajarias, MD
Division of Cardiovascular Diseases, Department of Medicine, Barnes-Jewish Hospital,
Washington University School of Medicine, 660 South Euclid Avenue,
Campus Box 8086, St. Louis, MO 63110, USA
e-mail: azajaria@wustl.edu

© Springer Science+Business Media New York 2016
G. Ailawadi, I.L. Kron (eds.), *Catheter Based Valve and Aortic Surgery*,
DOI 10.1007/978-1-4939-3432-4_4

to include low- and moderate-risk patients [7]. This fertile economic environment combined with the success of the first-generation devices has stimulated the development of new devices at an exponential rate. The majority of these devices are aimed at overcoming the shortcomings of the first-generation devices with the ultimate goal of achieving the safest, most effective treatment of aortic valve disease. The aim of this chapter is to give an overview of upcoming transfemoral devices that are in various stages of development.

Edwards Lifesciences (Irvine, CA)

SAPIEN III

The SAPIEN III is the third version of the Edwards SAPIEN valve and is their newest balloon-expandable device. This valve improves on the previous versions of the SAPIEN and SAPIEN XT by allowing for a reduced crimped profile of 6.7 mm (compared to 8 mm), which allows delivery through a 14Fr sheath [8]. Like the previous versions, the SAPIEN III has bovine pericardial leaflets mounted on a cobalt chromium stent with an internal polyethylene terephthalate skirt. However, the SAPIEN III has an additional outer polyethylene terephthalate cuff designed to reduce paravalvular leak (Fig. 4.1i) (Table 4.1) [8].

The SAPIEN III is in the early stages of clinical investigation, but has promising early results leading to achieving CE mark in Europe in early 2014. In the first 15 patients studied, no patient had greater than mild paravalvular regurgitation with comparable hemodynamic results as earlier iterations of the Edwards valves [8]. Furthermore, in a comparison with the Edwards second-generation valve the SAPIEN XT, the SAPIEN III showed significantly reduced mild and moderate paravalvular leak (7 % vs. 42 % and 0 % vs. 8 %, respectively; $p=0.002$) [10]. Further investigation of the SAPIEN III is currently under way in the United States in the phase 3 clinical trial PARTNER II [11].

HELIO Transcatheter Aortic Dock

In an effort to broaden the use of their newer balloon-expandable valves, Edwards designed the HELIO transcatheter aortic dock to assist in the treatment of aortic regurgitation. This device consists of a self-expanding nitinol stent wrapped in polyethylene terephthalate that is implanted into the aortic sinuses, but outside of the native aortic valve cusps. Then, a balloon-expandable SAPIEN XT is placed within the native valve, which captures the native aortic valve cusps between the prosthesis and the dock. The dock can be delivered through a 16Fr sheath and has theoretical advantages of decreasing paravalvular regurgitation, decrease ongoing root dilation, and the ability to treat large annular aortic stenosis patients. There is a lack of clinical data on the device, but the first-in-man transfemoral approach demonstrates feasibility [12].

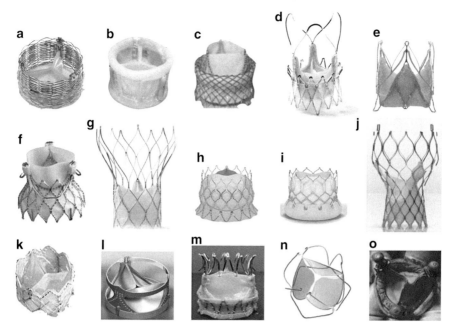

Fig. 4.1 Second-generation TAVI systems: (**a**) Lotus Valve System (Boston Scientific, Natick, MA, USA), (**b**) Direct Flow Medical (Direct Flow Medical Inc., Santa Rosa, CA, USA), (**c**) HLT valve (Heart Valve Technologies Inc., Maple Grove, MN, USA), (**d**) Symetis ACURATE™ (Symetis SA, Ecublens, Switzerland), (**e**) JenaValve (JenaValve Incorporated, Munich, Germany), (**f**) Engager (Medtronic Inc., Minneapolis, MN, USA), (**g**) Portico valve (St Jude Medical, St Paul, MN, USA), (**h**) CENTERA (Edwards Lifesciences, Irvine, CA, USA) (**i**) SAPIEN III (Edwards Lifesciences, Irvine, CA, USA), (**j**) CoreValve Evolut R (Medtronic Inc., Minneapolis, MN, USA), (**k**) Colibri valve (Colibri Heart Valve, LLC, Broomfield, CO, USA), (**l**) AorTx (Hansen Medical Inc., Mountain View, CA, USA), (**m**) Trinity TriFlexx (Transcatheter Technologies, Regensburg, Germany), (**n**) UCL (University College of London, London, UK), and (**o**) Vanguard™ II valve (ValveXchange Inc., Greenwood Village, CO, USA). Reprinted with permission from Elsevier [9]

CENTERA Transcatheter Heart Valve

In addition to the SAPIEN III, Edwards has developed their first self-expandable valve, the CENTERA transcatheter heart valve (THV) [13]. This device was designed to facilitate easy deployment with a unique motorized delivery system as well as the ability to reposition the valve via the transfemoral or subclavian routes [14]. The valve itself is composed of trileaflet bovine pericardial tissue mounted on a nitinol stent. The stent is shorter than other self-expanding valves (20 mm expanded height) in an effort to minimize impedance of the left ventricular outflow tract and decrease arrhythmias. There is also a polyethylene terephthalate skirt that is specifically designed to reduce paravalvular regurgitation (Fig. 4.1h) [13]. The valve is available in 23, 26, and 29 mm sizes—all of which are compatible with a 14Fr sheath for delivery [6, 14]. The CENTERA THV delivery system is designed

Table 4.1 Characteristics of second-generation transfemoral devices

Valve	Frame	Deployment	Sheath size	Repositionable/ retrievable	Special features	Current status
SAPIEN III	Cobalt chromium stent	Balloon expanding	14Fr	No/No	Inner and outer polyethylene cuff to reduce PVR	European CE mark 2014; current multicenter phase 3 clinical trial in the United States (PARTNER II trial)
CENTERA	Nitinol	Self-expanding	14Fr	Yes/Yes	Motorized delivery; low frame height to reduce conduction disturbances; polyethylene skirt to reduce PVR	Multicenter, prospective safety and device success trial under way in Europe
CoreValve Evolut R	Nitinol	Self-expanding	14Fr	Yes/Yes	Reduced height; more consistent radial force of nitinol stent	European CE mark 2014
Portico	Nitinol	Self-expanding	18Fr	Yes/Yes	Porcine pericardial cuff at annular level to reduce PVR; large tissue-to-frame ratio and valve is low in stent to reduce conduction disturbances and for ease of coronary access	European CE mark 2012; current multicenter phase 3 clinical trials in the United States and Europe

Lotus Valve System	Nitinol	Mechanical expanding	18Fr	Yes/Yes	Braided stent that is axially compressed to form a skirt to prevent PVR and create adaptive seal; Radiopaque marker for easier positioning; controlled mechanical release	European CE mark 2013; current multicenter trial under way in Europe; randomized control trial in the United States is in the planning phase
Symetis ACURATE TF™	Nitinol	Self-expanding	18Fr	Partial/No	Inner and outer synthetic polymer skirt to reduce PVR; stabilization arches with upper and lower crown for stable supra-annular positioning	European CE mark 2014
JenaValve	Nitinol	Self-expanding	18Fr	Partial/No	Low-profile, crown-shaped nitinol stent with three "feelers" designed to seed in the sinuses of the native valve to form clips around the native valve; also indicated for aortic insufficiency	European CE mark for transapical approach; first-in-man for transfemoral approach under way in Europe

(continued)

Table 4.1 (continued)

Valve	Frame	Deployment	Sheath size	Repositionable/retrievable	Special features	Current status
Direct Flow Medical	Polymer (metal free)	Solidifying polymer	18Fr	Yes/Yes	Polyester fabric skirt to reduce PVR; first nonmetal percutaneous valve; frame can be filled with contrast to confirm positioning prior to exchange for solidifying polymer	European CE mark 2013; current multicenter phase 3 clinical trial in the United States
Colibri Heart Valve	Stainless steel alloy	Balloon expanding	14Fr	No/No	Conical leaflets for maximal orifice area during systole; prepackaged valve ready for immediate use	First-in-man completed to 6-month follow-up; larger clinical evaluation targeting CE mark is planned in Europe

PVR, paravalvular regurgitation; CE, *Conformité Européenne*

Fig. 4.2 Edwards
CENTERA transcatheter
heart valve motorized
single-hand deployment.
Reprinted with permission
from Elsevier [13]

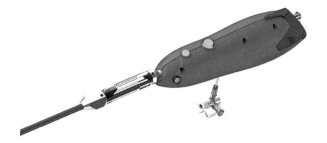

for single-operator use with two motorized buttons that retract or deploy the valve, which allows smooth, controlled repositioning of the valve (Fig. 4.2) [13]. The valve can be up to 70 % deployed with the ability to retract and redeploy [14].

The CENTERA THV has also had limited clinical evaluation. The only published report to date is the successful implantation of the CENTERA THV in 15 patients [13]. Four patients (27 %) had complete heart block after the procedure necessitating permanent pacemaker, and only one patient had moderate to severe paravalvular regurgitation at discharge. One of the 15 patients had successful redeployment after malposition [13]. After these results, the same group is currently testing a newer iteration of the valve. In unpublished data, they have implanted the valve in 14 patients with zero permanent pacemaker implantations and 100 % of the patients had less than moderate aortic regurgitation using this new configuration [6, 15]. These encouraging results have stimulated a large, nonrandomized, prospective, multicenter safety and device success study seeking to enroll 150 patients at up to 15 participating investigational centers in Europe that is currently under way [16].

Medtronic Inc. (Minneapolis, MN)

Medtronic has also evolved since the first iteration of their CoreValve. Their newest valve, the 23 mm CoreValve Evolut R, has recently achieved CE mark approval for valve-in-valve procedures and features a redesigned nitinol stent that is intended to improve conformability to the aortic annulus with consistent radial force (Fig. 4.1j) [6, 17]. This valve was specifically designed for small aortic annuli (18–20 mm) and has an overall height that is roughly 10 mm shorter than the first-generation CoreValve—allowing for easier deployment during valve-in-valve procedures in patients with failing xenografts and small internal diameters. The device can be delivered by a new 14Fr EnVeo R delivery catheter that allows the valve to be recaptured and repositioned during deployment [17].

The clinical experience with the CoreValve Evolut R is quite limited. Two groups have reported experience in a valve-in-valve setting for degenerated bioprostheses [18, 19]. The two studies had a combined total of 18 patients with successful implantation without device-related or procedure-related complications. All patients had improved hemodynamics without the need for pacemaker implantation [18, 19].

St Jude Medical (St Paul, MN)

The limitations of the first-generation devices from Edwards and Medtronic led to the development of the Portico TAVI system (St Jude Medical, St Paul, MN). Similar to the CoreValve, the Portico valve is a trileaflet pericardial valve mounted on a self-expanding nitinol stent (Fig. 4.1g) [20]. The valve is designed with a porcine pericardial cuff at the annular level to help with sealing and prevent paravalvular regurgitation. The leaflets utilize the same anti-calcification technology (Lynx) as the St Jude Medical surgical aortic valves. In an effort to reduce conduction complications and to allow easy coronary access postimplantation, the functioning valve is placed low in the nitinol stent and is designed to be placed at the annulus. The stent itself also has large tissue-to-frame ratio to encourage tissue conformation and ingrowth and minimize paravalvular regurgitation [20]. The valve is deployed through an 18Fr sheath and is fully retrievable, re-sheathable, and repositionable in situ until it has been fully deployed [6, 21, 22].

Early feasibility studies demonstrating the device safety were completed in Canada and Europe [20, 22, 23]. One group published their 30-day results following successful implantation in 10 subjects. Successful device recapture and repositioning was performed in 4 patients. One patient required second transcatheter valve secondary to leaflet dysfunction and one patient had a minor stroke. No patients required pacemaker implantation, but one patient had moderate paravalvular regurgitation. All patients had comparable hemodynamic improvements to first-generation devices [22].

The European group recently presented their acute and 1-year follow-up data on 83 patients [23]. At 6 months, the valve showed average peak gradient that decreased from 72.1 to 18.2 mmHg ($p < 0.001$) with only 3 % of patients having worse than mild paravalvular regurgitation [23]. However, 10.8 % of patients required new pacemaker implantation at 30 days [23]. This study helped the Portico valve achieve CE mark for their 23 mm iteration in 2012 and 25 mm valve in 2013. The valve is currently under further evaluation in both the Unites States and Europe in large, multicenter trials [23, 24].

Boston Scientific (Boston, MA, USA)

The Lotus Valve System was designed to overcome multiple issues with the first-generation valves. The valve features a familiar trileaflet bovine pericardial prosthesis mounted on a novel braided, self-expanding nitinol stent. The stent is specially designed to be axially compressed during delivery to create a skirt at the left ventricular outflow track, which creates an adaptive seal surrounding the ventricular portion of the device in an effort to reduce paravalvular regurgitation

(Fig. 4.1a) [25, 26]. This valve also has the ability to be safely re-sheathed, reposi-tioned, and retrieved even after full expansion [25, 27]. The valve comes pre-attached to the delivery system for simplicity and is delivered through an 18Fr sheath [6]. Lastly, there is a radiopaque marker located at the vertical center of the device to aid in positioning [26].

The Lotus Valve System received CE mark for use in Europe in October 2013 [6]. The feasibility trial entitled REPRISE I enrolled 11 patients in 3 different sites in Australia. All 11 had successful implantation and 4 out of the 11 had successful re-sheathing and repositioning of the valve during the procedure. Four patients required permanent pacemaker implantation, but all patients had less than mild paravalvular regurgitation at discharge. At 1 year, there was significant improvement in valve func-tion from a mean aortic gradient of 53.9 ± 20.9 to 15.4 ± 4.6 mmHg ($p < 0.001$), no deaths, and one major stoke [28]. REPRISE II is a multicenter prospective trial evaluat-ing the valve that was completed in April of 2013, and the interim results have recently been presented [6, 29, 30]. There was successful implantation in 120 out of 120 patients enrolled, and there were no cases of severe paravalvular regurgitation at six months. However, early results demonstrated a high rate of pacemaker implantation (17 out of 58 patients, 29.3 %) and an 8.7 % stoke rate [29]. Currently, the REPRISE III, a ran-domized control trial in the United States, is in the planning phase [25, 30].

Symetis SA (Ecublens, Switzerland)

The Symetis ACURATE™ valve was originally designed as a transapical valve and achieved CE mark approval for the transapical approach in 2011 [6]. Early successes led to a similarly designed ACURATE TF™ aortic prosthesis and delivery system that can be delivered via an 18Fr transfemoral sheath. The ACURATE TF™ valve has three leaflets derived from porcine pericardium and is mounted on a nitinol stent with an inner and outer synthetic polymer skirt. The nitinol stent has several unique modifications including stabilization arches, an upper crown, and a lower crown all designed for stable supra-annular positioning of the valve (Fig. 4.1d) [31]. Lastly, it has minimal protrusion into the LV outflow tract to minimize the effect on the conduction system of the heart.

The ACURATE TF™ was first used in January 2012 as part of the TF20 trial. Successful implantation was achieved in 19 out of 20 patients (95 %) with one patient requiring a second valve to be placed in the original because of low initial placement. All achieved significant improvement in valvular hemodynamics including an increase in valve area from 0.7 to 1.8 cm². One patient had grade 2 paravalvular regurgitation and two patients (10 %) required pacemaker implantation. There were no mortalities and one stroke at 30 days of follow-up [31]. The CE Mark study for the ACURATE *neo*™ has recently been completed, and CE mark was achieved in September 2014 [32].

JenaValve Incorporated (Munich, Germany)

The JenaValve system was also originally designed for transapical delivery and has achieved CE mark for the transapical approach, but only recently has a transfemoral delivery been successful in animals [33]. The valve itself has three porcine pericardial leaflets mounted on a low-profile, crown-shaped nitinol stent (Fig. 4.1e) [34]. The valve is unique in its delivery in that it incorporates three positional "feelers" that are designed to seed in the base of the sinuses of the native valve. When the valve is deployed, these feelers and the nitinol stent base form clips around the native valve. Theoretical advantages of this clipping system are a reduction in radial force, more accurate positional deployment, secure anchoring, and decreased paravalvular regurgitation. The clipping mechanism also allows for implantation in patients who strictly have aortic insufficiency [35]. The new transfemoral device can be delivered through an 18Fr sheath and first-in-man clinical evaluation is under way.

Direct Flow Medical Incorporated (Santa Rosa, CA)

The Direct Flow Medical percutaneous aortic valve (PAV) system is the first nonmetallic percutaneous valve to be designed with a solidifying inflation medium as its support structure. The trileaflet bovine pericardial valve is attached to this inflatable support network by a polyester fabric skirt that helps prevent paravalvular regurgitation (Fig. 4.1b) [36]. The support network consists of an aortic ring and ventricular ring that are connected by vertical inflatable tubes, which are inflated and deflated

Fig. 4.3 Direct Flow Medical valve aortogram showing contrast-filled upper (aortic) and lower (ventricular) ring. Reprinted with permission from Nature Publishing Group [6]

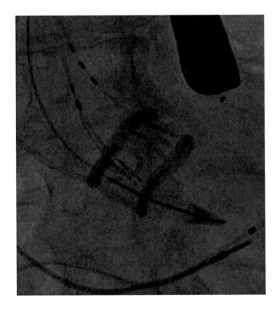

separately via three ports [37]. The aortic and ventricular inflatable rings are designed to be deployed on either side of the aortic annulus to help anchor the valve in place. To deliver the valve, the frame is filled with a mixture of contrast and saline to confirm position (Fig. 4.3), which is exchanged with a mix of water-soluble epoxy and radiopacifier that solidifies to a polymer in 90 min [37]. The device can be delivered via an 18Fr sheath and is fully retrievable prior to infusion of the epoxy medium. Of note, the epoxy medium in the liquid form is water-soluble and therefore is not at risk for embolization if a hole is created in the matrix [36].

The Direct Flow Medical valve was first evaluated in humans undergoing surgical aortic valve replacement [36]. The valve was implanted directly into the aorta in two patients and delivered by the transfemoral approach using a 22Fr sheath in six additional patients. All of these patients underwent acute echocardiographic and hemodynamic evaluation and then underwent planned standard aortic valve replacement. Of the seven patients who underwent successful implantation, the pre-procedure valve area and gradients were 0.65 cm^2 and 87.6 ± 12.4 mmHg vs. 1.65 cm^2 and 17.9 ± 12.4 mmHg post-procedure [36]. The 22Fr device was further studied in 31 patients to evaluate long-term safety and efficacy [38, 39]. The procedural success rate was 71 %, with most failures as a result of bicuspid anatomy or heavy calcification of the native valve. These patients were followed out to 3 years with a survival of 60 %. All surviving patients had none or trace aortic regurgitation [37]. Over a period of 2 years, a subset of patients underwent serial cross-sectional imaging and echocardiograms to confirm that the position and shape of the valve remained intact [40].

The newer version of Direct Flow Medical PAV can be delivered through an 18Fr sheath and is designed to have an increased radial force with stiffer inflatable frame as well as modifications to increase the ease of delivery. To evaluate the newer iteration, the multicenter, nonrandomized DISCOVER trial was recently completed, which led to achieving CE mark in 2013 [6, 41]. One hundred patients were enrolled with the first 25 patients identified as a training cohort, and the subsequent 75 patients were identified as the evaluable cohort. Survival was 99 % (99/100) at 30 days, with one patient succumbing to pneumonia on postoperative day 12. In the evaluable cohort, 70 out of 75 patients had successful device implantation. Of those that failed, two had elevated post-implant transvalvular gradient >20 mmHg or peak velocity >3 m/s while one patient had moderate aortic regurgitation. Eight patients had successful retrieval and reimplantation of misplaced valves secondary to size mismatch or migration. Three patients had major stokes and the rate of pacemaker implantation was 17 % for all 100 patients [41]. The valve is currently being studied in a large, multicenter trial in the United States.

Colibri Heart Valve, LLC (Broomfield, CO)

The Colibri valve is a newer iteration of the original Paniagua Heart Valve (EndoLumix Technology, LLC, Miami, FL) that utilizes a novel leaflet shape to produce maximal effective orifice area during systole. These leaflets are conical in shape and made out of porcine pericardium specifically manufactured as thin as possible without sacrificing tensile strength. This allows the valve to be tightly crimped onto a stainless steel balloon-expandable frame that can be delivered through a 14Fr sheath. The valve is also able to be prepackaged in a sterile fashion on the delivery balloon allowing for the catheter to be immediately ready for use (Fig. 4.1k) [42]. Early clinical results from the first-in-man implantation of the valve are promising. In the first patient, the device was successfully deployed with an immediate increase in the valve area from 0.7 to 2.3 cm^2 ($p < 0.001$). Initially the patient had mild aortic regurgitation that improved to none at 6 months with preserved excellent hemodynamics [42]. In unpublished data, the patient has 6-month follow-up demonstrating excellent valve hemodynamics with no paravalvular regurgitation, and a larger clinical evaluation targeting CE mark is planned [43].

Braile Biomédica (São Paulo, Brazil)

The Inovare valve (Braile Biomédica, São Paulo, Brazil) is a balloon-expandable device that was developed in Brazil. It was designed to increase the access and cost-effectiveness of this technology, particularly in the Brazilian population [44]. Initially tested by transapical delivery, the valve has recently been implanted via the transfemoral approach [45]. The valve is composed of bovine pericardial leaflets mounted on a stainless steel frame, which precludes repositioning at after expansion [46]. There are acceptable long-term transapical delivery results, but there are only initial feasibility results utilizing the transfemoral approach. The only series in the literature describes six patients who underwent successful implantation of the valve via a transfemoral approach with significant postoperative decrease in aortic valve gradient from 6.84 ± 15.46 mmHg to 19.74 ± 10.61 mmHg ($P = 0.002$) [47]. There were no incidences of paravalvular regurgitation; however, one patient had an iliac artery rupture likely related to the 24Fr GORE DrySeal Sheath that was utilized for delivery. Further evolution of the transfemoral delivery system and evaluation of the long-term efficacy of the valve are necessary.

Other Companies

Several other companies are in various stages of valve development, but have a lack of peer-reviewed clinical data. HLT valve (Heart Leaflet Technologies Inc., Maple Grove, MN, USA) was implanted in humans in 2009 (Fig. 4.1c) [48]. This fully repositionable and retrievable valve was implanted in 9 patients, but had significant complications that led to valve redesign [46]. The newly redesigned valve will be evaluated in the upcoming HORIZON clinical trial to determine safety and efficacy [49].

The Venus TAVI system (Hangzhou, China) is very similar to the CoreValve prosthesis except it has radiopaque markers indicating the landing zone and has increased radial force [50]. This device has been implanted in 37 patients throughout Asia with no worse than mild paravalvular regurgitation at 30 days and good hemodynamic function. However, there was a 27 % (10/37) permanent pacemaker implantation rate and 8.1 % (3/37) perioperative mortality [50].

Valve Medical TAVI system (Tel Aviv, Israel) is designed with two components: the frame module and the valve module, which allows the device to be delivered through a 12Fr delivery sheath [51]. The device is currently in animal testing and is expected to be first implanted in humans at the beginning of 2015. Another two-part valve, the Vanguard™ II valve (ValveXchange Inc., Greenwood Village, CO), is the transfemoral modification of the Vitality™ (ValveXchange Inc., Greenwood Village, CO). This valve is designed so that the leaflets are exchangeable when the valve requires replacement (Fig. 4.1o) [46].

UCL TAV (University College of London, London, UK) is a new valve currently in preclinical development, which in contrast to the other valves has polymeric leaflets. The new leaflets are mounted on a self-expanding nitinol stent that is fully retrievable (Fig. 4.1n) [52]. Optimum TAV (Thubrikar Aortic Valve Inc., Philadelphia, PA) is also currently in preclinical development [53]. This valve has a low profile and a skirt designed to prevent paravalvular regurgitation. Lastly, MyVal TAVR System (Meril Life Sciences, Gujarat, India) is a balloon-expandable valve in which the leaflets are crafted out of a single piece of bovine pericardial patch to eliminate suture lines [54]. Acute in vivo evaluation of the valve has been completed and chronic studies in animals are currently under way [54].

Conclusions

Over the past 15 years, TAVI has made tremendous progress. With established successful short- and midterm results of first-generation devices, many companies are developing new devices to challenge the first-generation devices in this rapidly expanding field. Once safety and efficacy are confirmed, indications are well established, and technology has sufficiently matured, large randomized trials will be necessary to compare each TAVI device.

References

1. Cribier A, Eltchaninoff H, Bash A, Borenstein N, Tron C, Bauer F, et al. Percutaneous transcatheter implantation of an aortic valve prosthesis for calcific aortic stenosis: first human case description. Circulation. 2002;106(24):3006–8.
2. Leon MB, Smith CR, Mack M, Miller DC, Moses JW, Svensson LG, et al. Transcatheter aortic-valve implantation for aortic stenosis in patients who cannot undergo surgery. N Engl J Med. 2010;363(17):1597–607.
3. Adams DH, Popma JJ, Reardon MJ, Yakubov SJ, Coselli JS, Deeb GM, et al. Transcatheter aortic-valve replacement with a self-expanding prosthesis. N Engl J Med. 2014;370(19):1790–8.
4. Kodali SK, Williams MR, Smith CR, Svensson LG, Webb JG, Makkar RR, et al. Two-year outcomes after transcatheter or surgical aortic-valve replacement. N Engl J Med. 2012;366(18):1686–95.
5. Smith CR, Leon MB, Mack MJ, Miller DC, Moses JW, Svensson LG, et al. Transcatheter versus surgical aortic-valve replacement in high-risk patients. N Engl J Med. 2011;364(23): 2187–98.
6. Taramasso M, Pozzoli A, Latib A, La Canna G, Colombo A, Maisano F, et al. New devices for TAVI: technologies and initial clinical experiences. Nat Rev Cardiol. 2014;11(3):157–67.
7. Osnabrugge RL, Mylotte D, Head SJ, Van Mieghem NM, Nkomo VT, LeReun CM, et al. Aortic stenosis in the elderly: disease prevalence and number of candidates for transcatheter aortic valve replacement: a meta-analysis and modeling study. J Am Coll Cardiol. 2013;62(11):1002–12.
8. Binder RK, Rodes-Cabau J, Wood DA, Mok M, Leipsic J, De Larochelliere R, et al. Transcatheter aortic valve replacement with the SAPIEN 3: a new balloon-expandable transcatheter heart valve. J Am Coll Cardiol Intv. 2013;6(3):293–300.
9. Bourantas CV, van Mieghem NM, Farooq V, Soliman OI, Windecker S, Piazza N, et al. Future perspectives in transcatheter aortic valve implantation. Int J Cardiol. 2013;168(1):11–8.
10. Amat-Santos IJ, Dahou A, Webb J, Dvir D, Dumesnil JG, Allende R, et al. Comparison of hemodynamic performance of the balloon-expandable SAPIEN 3 versus SAPIEN XT transcatheter valve. Am J Cardiol. 2014;114(7):1075–82.
11. Edwards Lifesciences. The PARTNER II trial: placement of AoRTic TraNscathetER valves. In: ClinicalTrials.gov [Internet]. Bethesda, MD: National Library of Medicine (US). 2000 [cited 2014 Sept 5]. Available from: http://clinicaltrials.gov/show/NCT01314313; NLM Identifier: NCT01314313.
12. Barbanti M, Ye J, Pasupati S, El-Gamel A, Webb JG. The Helio transcatheter aortic dock for patients with aortic regurgitation. EuroIntervention. 2013;9(Suppl):S91–4.
13. Binder RK, Schafer U, Kuck KH, Wood DA, Moss R, Leipsic J, et al. Transcatheter aortic valve replacement with a new self-expanding transcatheter heart valve and motorized delivery system. J Am Coll Cardiol Intv. 2013;6(3):301–7.
14. Ribeiro HB, Urena M, Kuck KH, Webb JG, Rodes-Cabau J. Edwards CENTERA valve. EuroIntervention. 2012;8(Suppl Q):Q79–82.
15. Schäfer U. Edwards CENTERA transcatheter heart valve. Presented at EuroPCR, May 2013.
16. Edwards Lifesciences. Safety and performance study of the Edwards CENTERA self-expanding transcatheter heart valve. ClinicalTrials.gov [Internet]. Bethesda, MD: National Library of Medicine (US). 2000 [cited 2014 Sept 4]. Available from: http://clinicaltrials.gov/ct2/show/study/NCT01808274; NLM Identifier: NCT01808274.
17. Piazza N, Martucci G, Lachapelle K, de Varennes B, Bilodeau L, Buithieu J, et al. First-in-human experience with the Medtronic CoreValve Evolut R. EuroIntervention. 2014;9(11):1260–3.
18. Diemert P, Seiffert M, Frerker C, Thielsen T, Kreidel F, Bader R, et al. Valve-in-valve implantation of a novel and small self-expandable transcatheter heart valve in degenerated small surgical bioprostheses: The Hamburg experience. Cathet Cardiovasc Interv. 2014;84(3):486–93.

19. Zavalloni D, De Benedictis M, Pagnotta P, Scrocca I, Presbitero P. New CoreValve Evolut 23 mm technology for treatment of degenerated bioprosthesis. Heart Lung Circ. 2014;23(2):183–5.
20. Manoharan G, Spence MS, Rodes-Cabau J, Webb JG. St Jude Medical Portico valve. EuroIntervention. 2012;8(Suppl Q):Q97–101.
21. Spence MS, Lyons K, McVerry F, Smith B, Manoharan GB, Maguire C, et al. New St. Jude Medical Portico transcatheter aortic valve: features and early results. Minerva Cardioangiol. 2013;61(3):263–9.
22. Willson AB, Rodes-Cabau J, Wood DA, Leipsic J, Cheung A, Toggweiler S, et al. Transcatheter aortic valve replacement with the St. Jude Medical Portico valve: first-in-human experience. J Am Coll Cardiol. 2012;60(7):581–6.
23. Manoharan G. Assessment of the St. Jude Medical Portico transcatheter aortic valve implant and the transfemoral delivery system: preliminary results: acute and 1-year outcomes. Presented at Transcatheter Cardiovascular Therapeutics, October 2013.
24. Saint Jude Medical. Portico re-sheathable transcatheter aortic valve system US IDE trial (PORTICO) (PORTICO-IDE). In: ClinicalTrials.gov [Internet]. Bethesda, MD: National Library of Medicine. 2000 [cited 2014 Sept 5]. Available from: http://clinicaltrials.gov/show/NCT02000115; NLM Identifier: NCT02000115.
25. Meredith IT, Hood KL, Haratani N, Allocco DJ, Dawkins KD. Boston Scientific Lotus valve. EuroIntervention. 2012;8(Suppl Q):Q70–4.
26. Tofield A. The Lotus valve for transcatheter aortic valve implantation. Eur Heart J. 2013;34(30):2335.
27. Gooley R, Lockwood S, Antonis P, Meredith IT. The SADRA Lotus Valve System: a fully repositionable, retrievable prosthesis. Minerva Cardioangiol. 2013;61(1):45–52.
28. Meredith IT, Worthley SG, Whitbourn RJ, Antonis P, Montarello JK, Newcomb AE, et al. Transfemoral aortic valve replacement with the repositionable Lotus Valve System in high surgical risk patients: the REPRISE I study. EuroIntervention. 2014;9(11):1264–70.
29. Meredith IT. Thirty day outcome for the first 60 patients in the REPRISE II study. Presented at EuroPCR, May 2013.
30. Meredith IT. Six-month outcomes with a fully repositionable and retrievable transcatheter aortic replacement valve in 120 high-risk surgical patients with severe aortic stenosis: results from the REPRISE II CE-Mark study. Presented at EuroPCR, May 2014.
31. Mollmann H, Diemert P, Grube E, Baldus S, Kempfert J, Abizaid A. Symetis ACURATE TF aortic bioprosthesis. EuroIntervention. 2013;9(Suppl):S107–10.
32. Symetis receives CE Mark approval for transfemoral transcatheter aortic heart valve system ACURATEneo™, and launches product with first commercial implantations [press release]. Lausanne, Switzerland; 2014 Sept 12.
33. Treede H, Mohr FW, Baldus S, Rastan A, Ensminger S, Arnold M, et al. Transapical transcatheter aortic valve implantation using the JenaValve system: acute and 30-day results of the multicentre CE-mark study. Eur J Cardiothorac Surg. 2012;41(6):e131–8.
34. Rudolph TK, Baldus S. JenaValve--transfemoral technology. EuroIntervention. 2013;9(Suppl):S101–2.
35. Seiffert M, Bader R, Kappert U, Rastan A, Krapf S, Bleiziffer S, et al. Initial german experience with transapical implantation of a second-generation transcatheter heart valve for the treatment of aortic regurgitation. J Am Coll Cardiol Intv. 2014;7(10):1168–74.
36. Low RI, Bolling SF, Yeo KK, Ebner A. Direct flow medical percutaneous aortic valve: proof of concept. EuroIntervention. 2008;4(2):256–61.
37. Bijuklic K, Tubler T, Low RI, Grube E, Schofer J. Direct flow medical valve. EuroIntervention. 2012;8(Suppl Q):Q75–8.
38. Schofer J, Schluter M, Treede H, Franzen OW, Tubler T, Pascotto A, et al. Retrograde transarterial implantation of a nonmetallic aortic valve prosthesis in high-surgical-risk patients with severe aortic stenosis: a first-in-man feasibility and safety study. Circ Cardiovasc Interv. 2008;1(2):126–33.

39. Treede H, Tubler T, Reichenspurner H, Grube E, Pascotto A, Franzen O, et al. Six-month results of a repositionable and retrievable pericardial valve for transcatheter aortic valve replacement: the Direct Flow Medical aortic valve. J Thorac Cardiovasc Surg. 2010;140(4):897–903.
40. Bijuklic K, Tuebler T, Reichenspurner H, Treede H, Wandler A, Harreld JH, et al. Midterm stability and hemodynamic performance of a transfemorally implantable nonmetallic, retrievable, and repositionable aortic valve in patients with severe aortic stenosis. Up to 2-year follow-up of the direct-flow medical valve: a pilot study. Circ Cardiovasc Interv. 2011;4(6):595–601.
41. Schofer J, Colombo A, Klugmann S, Fajadet J, DeMarco F, Tchetche D, et al. Prospective multicenter evaluation of the direct flow medical transcatheter aortic valve. J Am Coll Cardiol. 2014;63(8):763–8.
42. Fish RD, Paniagua D, Urena P, Chevalier B. The Colibri heart valve: theory and practice in the achievement of a low-profile, pre-mounted, pre-packaged TAVI valve. EuroIntervention. 2013;9(Suppl):S111–4.
43. Chevalier B. Long-term results of Colibri Heart Valve feasibility study. Presented at EuroPCR, May 2014.
44. Gaia DF, Palma JH, Ferreira CB, Souza JA, Agreli G, Guilhen JC, et al. Transapical aortic valve implantation: results of a Brazilian prosthesis. Rev Bras Cir Cardiovas. 2010;25(3):293–302.
45. Pontes JC, Duarte JJ, Silva AD, Dias AM, Benfatti RA, Gardenal N, et al. Pioneering transcatheter aortic valve Implant (Inovare(R)) via transfemoral. Rev Bras Cir Cardiovasc. 2012;27(3):469–71.
46. Bourantas CV, Farooq V, Onuma Y, Piazza N, Van Mieghem NM, Serruys PW. Transcatheter aortic valve implantation: new developments and upcoming clinical trials. EuroIntervention. 2012;8(5):617–27.
47. Pontes JC, Duarte JJ, Silva AD, Gardenal N, Dias AM, Benfatti RA, et al. Initial and pioneer experience of transcatheter aortic valve implantation (Inovare) through femoral or iliac artery. Rev Bras Cir Cardiovasc. 2013;28(2):208–16.
48. Rodes-Cabau J. Transcatheter aortic valve implantation: current and future approaches. Nat Rev Cardiol. 2012;9(1):15–29.
49. HLT Inc. HLT transfemOral Replacement of aortIc Valve Via transcatherteriZatiON (HORIZON) 2014. In: ClinicalTrials.gov [Internet]. Bethesda, MD: National Library of Medicine. 2000 [cited 2014 Sept 19]. Available from: http://clinicaltrials.gov/show/NCT02157142; NLM Identifier: NCT02157142.
50. Sievert H. The Venus TAVI system. Presented at EuroPCR, May 2014.
51. Leon MB. The Valve Medical TAVI System. Presented at EuroPCR, May 2014.
52. Rahmani B, Burriesci G, Mullen M, Seifalian A, Tzamtzis S, Yap J. TCT-109 A new generation transcatheter heart valve with a novel nanocomposite material and fully retrievable design. J Am Coll Cardiol. 2012;60(17_S):B34.
53. Thubrikar M. Optimum TAVI system. Presented at EuroPCR, May 2014.
54. Granada J. The MyVal system. Presented at EuroPCR, May 2014.

Chapter 5
Transapical Transcatheter Aortic Valve Replacement

Timothy J. George and Gorav Ailawadi

Introduction

Symptomatic aortic stenosis (AS) is associated with a precipitous functional decline and high mortality. Without valve replacement, symptomatic AS has a 5-year survival of approximately 30 %. Because of the higher perioperative mortality associated with elderly patients who suffer from multiple comorbidities, as many as 30 % of patients with severe AS do not undergo surgical treatment [1, 2]. However, patients with severe AS managed nonsurgically have a poor prognosis, with a 1-year mortality as high as 50 % [3, 4]. Given the high prevalence of AS in this high-risk cohort, transcatheter aortic valve replacement (TAVR) has been demonstrated as a superior approach over medical management in nonsurgical candidates and equivalent to traditional AVR in high-risk surgical patients [3, 5]. Additionally, TAVR is being investigated in intermediate-risk patients with promising results. As device technology has improved, the range of vascular access options for device deployment has expanded to include transapical, transaortic, trans-subclavian, transfemoral, and, recently, transcaval. As the devices have become lower profile, there has been a steady increase in the number of transfemoral TAVRs and a steady decline in the utilization of transapical access. Despite this decline in utilization, transapical TAVR remains the most common option in patients with inadequate femoral vessels for the transfemoral

T.J. George, MD (✉)
Division of Thoracic and Cardiovascular Surgery, Department of Surgery, The University of Virginia Hospital Medical Center, 735 Rainier Road, Charlottesville, VA 22903, USA
e-mail: tim.george@virginia.edu

G. Ailawadi, MD
Section of Adult Cardiac Surgery, Department of Surgery, Advanced Cardiac Valve Center, University of Virginia, 1215 Lee Street, Charlottesville, VA 22903, USA
e-mail: gorav@virginia.edu

© Springer Science+Business Media New York 2016
G. Ailawadi, I.L. Kron (eds.), *Catheter Based Valve and Aortic Surgery*,
DOI 10.1007/978-1-4939-3432-4_5

approach. Moreover, it is incumbent upon all surgeons to be familiar and facile with the transapical approach as this will likely be the initial approach in newer transcatheter interventions, including transcatheter mitral valve replacement [6].

Patient Selection

Careful patient selection is critical to a successful TAVR program. At the University of Virginia, each TAVR candidate is evaluated by the advanced valve team and discussed at a weekly conference including both surgeons and interventional cardiologists as well as other specialists. Testing is performed to deem candidacy including transthoracic echocardiography to determine severity of aortic valve pathology; a protocoled CT arteriogram of the chest, abdomen, and pelvis for access planning and valve sizing; cardiac catheterization to evaluate for concomitant coronary disease (and a right heart catheterization if indicated to evaluate for pulmonary hypertension); and pulmonary function testing. Other tests such as carotid duplex are ordered as indicated.

Currently, TAVR is FDA approved in the USA for use in patients who are high surgical risk—defined as a Society of Thoracic Surgeons Predicted Risk of Mortality Score (STS-PROM) > 10 % or surgically inoperable (e.g., porcelain aorta, prior mediastinal radiation). Two cardiac surgeons and one interventional cardiologist must agree that traditional AVR is precluded or high risk because the probability of death or serious morbidity exceeds the probability of meaningful improvement [7]. TAVR is not currently indicated for lower-risk surgical patients; however, intermediate-risk patients can undergo TAVR as part of an ongoing clinical trial (PARTNER II and SurTAVI trials).

After determining that a patient is eligible for TAVR, the heart team develops a sizing and access plan. As in most institutions, we follow a "transfemoral first" approach such that we plan for transfemoral access unless there is a contraindication. The most common contraindication for transfemoral access is inadequate size or significant calcification of the femoral and iliac arteries prohibiting insertion of the large bore valve deployment devices (Fig. 5.1). In such cases we often proceed with a transapical (TA) approach as one of our primary alternative approaches.

In order to determine an access plan, one must be familiar with the available valve sizes and the iliofemoral arterial diameters required to deploy them. In the USA, only the SAPIEN valve (Edwards Lifesciences, Irvine, California) is currently approved for transapical access. There are three generations of SAPIEN valve, the SAPIEN, the SAPIEN XT, and the recently FDA-approved S3. The valves are available in four sizes: 20, 23, 26, and 29 mm. The required sheath sizes and minimal necessary femoral artery sizes needed to accommodate these valves are shown in Table 5.1. It is important to note that heavily calcified vessels are less distensible and may need a larger diameter to accommodate a given sheath size. If the patient has inadequate femoral vessels to accommodate the required sheath for their valve size, transfemoral access is precluded and alternative access must be considered. Favorable features for TA TAVR include those without calcified left ventricular (LV) apex, those without critical lung disease in whom thoracotomy is contraindicated, and those patients who are not extremely frail.

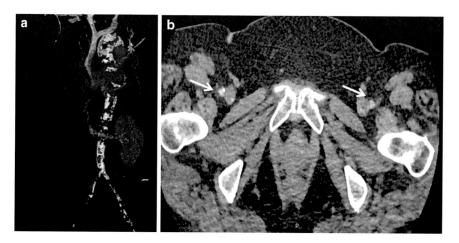

Fig. 5.1 CT arteriogram reconstruction (**a**) and axial section (**b**) demonstrating heavily calcified "porcelain aorta," with poor femoral vessels for access

Table 5.1 SAPIEN valve and required sheath sizes

Valve	Valve size (mm)	Sheath size (Fr)	Minimum necessary vessel diameter (mm)
SAPIEN S3	23	14	5.5
	26	14	5.5
	29	16	6.0
SAPIEN XT	20	14	5.5
	23	16	6.0
	26	18	6.5
	29	20	7.0

Technique

Although the majority of patients undergoing TAVR will not require cardiopulmonary bypass (CPB) support, an important part of preoperative planning is formulating a cannulation strategy should CPB become necessary. While it is difficult to predict which patients will need temporary CPB support during or after valve deployment, usually patients with ejection fraction (<25 %) with severe pulmonary hypertension, especially those requiring significant inotropes during and after anesthetic induction are at higher risk. Moreover, few patients have friable myocardium such that the ventricle can tear while securing the access site. As such, a cannulation plan for CPB must be planned. During TA TAVR, our preferred method of cannulation is through the common femoral artery and vein. Although these patients tend to have smaller or heavily calcified vessels that are inadequate to accommodate the valve deployment sheath, these vessels are often adequate for CPB cannulation as typically only 5 mm arterial vessels are needed. If we plan to use the femoral vessels for bailout CPB cannulation, we believe it is prudent to gain access to these vessels early in the case separate from the femoral arterial access for the aortogram/pigtail and from the venous access for ventricular pacing. For venous cannulation, we routinely put in a stiff wire from the femoral vein into the SVC under fluoroscopic guidance to allow for rapid cannulation.

In patients with inadequate femoral arteries to even accommodate CPB cannulae, we consider the axillary artery as a potential arterial cannulation site. Since it can be time consuming and often unnecessary to cut down on the axillary artery, we determine the risk for need for CPB to select patients in whom axillary cannulation is obtained prior to the start of TA access. A final bailout for CPB support is transapical cannulation itself putting a long arterial cannula across the aortic valve. The obvious advantage of this approach is that that area will already be readily accessible. The disadvantage is that transapical CPB cannulation involves giving up the planned site of access for TAVR device deployment.

All TAVR procedures should be performed in a hybrid operating room with CPB standby. Our patients undergo standard cardiac surgical preparation and monitoring including general anesthesia, arterial line, Swan-Ganz catheter placement, and intraoperative transesophageal echocardiography. The patient is placed on a fluoroscopically compatible operating room table such as a hybrid operating room in the supine position with both arms tucked at their side and an inflatable bump under their left chest. It is important to prep widely to include all potential CPB cannulation sites and to allow for an anterolateral thoracotomy.

All TA TAVR patients have arterial access usually in the femoral artery for a pigtail catheter for aortography and a femoral venous sheath for rapid ventricular pacing during valve deployment. As noted above, if we are planning to use the femoral vessels for CPB bailout, we place sheaths in the other femoral artery and vein and place a stiff wire through the vein into the SVC in case rapid CPB cannulation is needed.

We utilize preoperative CT imaging to identify both the rib space over the apex of the heart and the distance from the sternum to the apex laterally. These landmarks are identified on the patient and marked with a radiopaque clamp. We then use fluoroscopy to confirm the ideal location of the LV apex (Fig. 5.2). A 5 cm incision is made, usually in the 4th or 5th left intercostal space. Dissection is carried down to the pleura. Usually the LV apex is readily apparent under the ribs in patients with severe AS. We find in obese patients that placing a small soft tissue retractor is helpful in aiding in retraction. A radiolucent rib retractor is then placed. After identifying the phrenic nerve, the pericardium is incised and opened transversely. A pericardial well is developed (Fig. 5.3). In cases of a previous sternotomy, sharp dissection between the pericardium and epicardium is performed to create adequate exposure of the LV apex. We select an area on the anterior portion of the LV apex that is often free of epicardial fat and palpate the left ventricular wall under echocardiography. Ideally, we can see compression of the LV apex and the aortic valve in the same echocardiographic image in a left ventricular outflow view. After selecting our optimal site, we place two pledgeted prolenes in a competing triangle configuration (Fig. 5.4). After systemic heparinization, LV access is gained with an

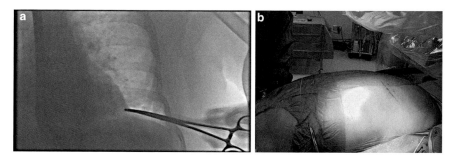

Fig. 5.2 The apex of the heart is marked fluoroscopically (**a**) with the placement of a radiopaque clamp. The small anterolateral thoracotomy is then marked on the patient in the appropriate rib space (**b**)

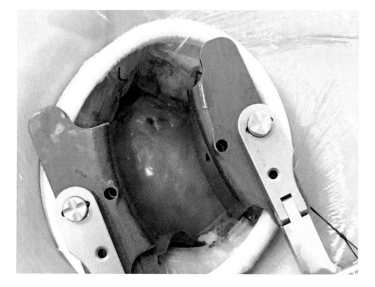

Fig. 5.3 The apex of the heart is shown after anterolateral thoracotomy, development of the peri-cardial well, and placement of retractors

introducer needle and a stiff wire. The wire should be carefully maintained perpendicular to the heart to prevent sawing of the ventricle and advanced into the descending aorta. The device sheath is advanced over the wire to a depth of about 4 cm (Fig. 5.5). If there is bleeding around the sheath at this point, the purse-string sutures can be gently snared down. If indicated, a balloon aortic valvuloplasty is performed at this time. Then the valve deployment device is guided into place under fluoroscopy and echocardiography (Fig. 5.6). It is imperative that the sheath be controlled by an assistant at all times. It can easily be dislodged due to the continuous heart motion. The valve is then deployed while rapid pacing (Fig. 5.7). The sheath is then withdrawn and the sutures are tied, again under rapid pacing to avoid tension on the purse-string sutures (Fig. 5.8).

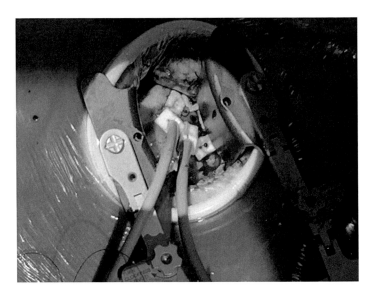

Fig. 5.4 The purse-string stitches have been placed in a "competing triangle" configuration

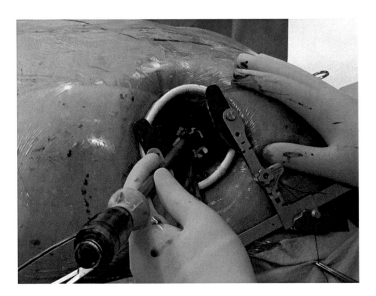

Fig. 5.5 The valve sheath has been placed through the apical purse string

Bleeding at the apical cannulation site must be assessed rapidly. Bleeding within the purse-string sutures is more easily manageable than bleeding outside the purse string. Minor venous bleeding can often be stopped with topical hemostatic agents. More significant bleeding can be managed with additional large pledgeted stitches particularly if within the purse string. It is important to induce rapid pacing as each of these stitches is placed and tied to avoid tearing the ventricle. If bleeding is outside the purse string, a bovine pericardial patch is often necessary to repair the LV without tension.

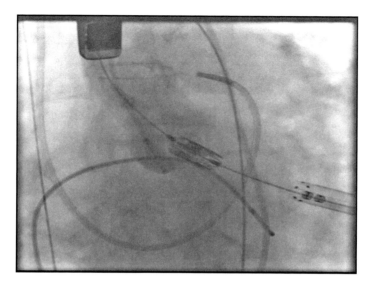

Fig. 5.6 Fluoroscopic image demonstrating pigtail in aortic annulus with aortogram in progress. Valve is being positioned under fluoroscopic guidance

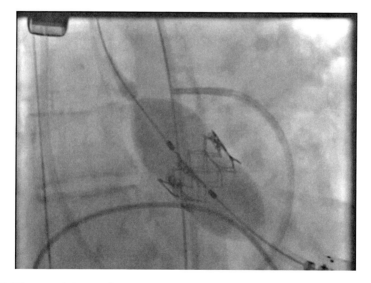

Fig. 5.7 Fluoroscopic image of valve being deployed under rapid pacing. Note that pigtail catheter has been pulled back to allow valve deployment

In cases where bleeding is not controllable or the patient is unstable hemodynamically, it may be necessary to initiate CPB while these maneuvers are being performed.

We close the pericardium with interrupted sutures to avoid having pledgeted sutures rubbing continuously against the chest wall. We leave one drain in the pericardium and one drain in the pleura. We perform an intercostal nerve block to aid in postoperative pain control. The thoracotomy is then closed in layers (Fig. 5.9).

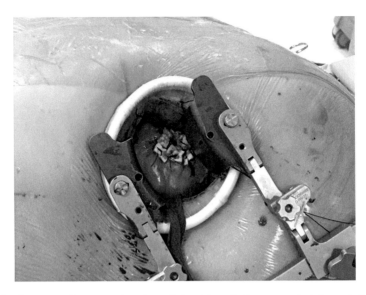

Fig. 5.8 The purse-string sutures have been tied and the apical puncture site is hemostatic

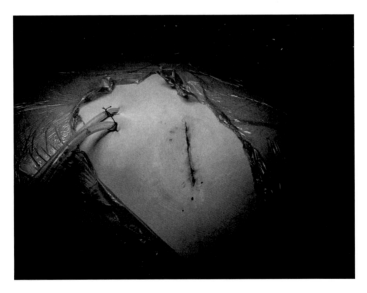

Fig. 5.9 Two drains have been placed—one in the pericardium and one in the pleural space. The thoracotomy has been closed in layers and skin glue has been applied

Outcomes

Cohorts A and B of the PARTNER trial have demonstrated the safety and efficacy of TAVR, including transapical TAVR, in both inoperable and high-risk surgical patients [3, 5]. Outcomes are highly dependent on patient comorbities and frailty. In the PARTNER trial, patients with high surgical risk who underwent a transapical TAVR had a 30-day mortality of 3.8 % and a 1-year mortality of 24.2 %. In the original as-treated analysis of the PARTNER trial, there was no difference in 1-year survival between AVR, transfemoral TAVR, or transapical TAVR. However, subsequent studies have suggested that transapical TAVR patients are at an increased risk for mortality and adverse outcomes [8]. Although transapical patients tend to be sicker and have a higher burden of atherosclerotic disease making increased morbidity and mortality, unsurprising, a recent propensity matched analysis of the PARTNER data suggests that transapical access is independently associated with higher mortality, increased adverse outcomes, more blood transfusions, and a longer length of stay [9]. In this series, neurologic events were similar regardless of access route. Despite the apparent increased risk associated with TA TAVR, there are signs that this risk has been and will continue to be mitigated over time. In a comparison of the pre-market approval cohort of the PARTNER trial to the nonrandomized continued access arm, patients undergoing transapical TAVR in the nonrandomized continued access arm had an even lower risk of stroke and a lower all-cause 1-year mortality compared with the pre-market approval group [10].

Complications

This review focuses on complications particularly relevant to the route of access chosen for TAVR including stroke, major bleeding, and vascular complications as defined by the Valve Academic Research Consortium (VARC) consensus definitions [11].

Stroke

In the only randomized trial comparing AVR to TAVR, the stroke rate at 30 days in patients undergoing TAVR was significantly higher than those undergoing traditional AVR (5.5 % vs. 2.0 %, $p=0.04$) [5]. Several studies have demonstrated that transapical TAVR has a similar stroke rate to transfemoral TAVR [12, 13]. Additionally, the rate of subclinical ischemic changes is much higher when studied with MRI [14]. Although the high stroke rate following TAVR is a major obstacle to more widespread adoption, there are several ongoing clinical trials examining the impact of cerebral protection devices on the risk of stroke after TAVR.

Vascular Complications and Major Bleeding

Vascular complications related to femoral arterial access are common after transfemoral TAVR. In cohort A of the PARTNER trial, the TAVR group had a 17.0 % risk of vascular complications [5]. Although TA TAVR obviates the need to place a large valve deployment sheath through the femoral artery, it still requires femoral access for aortography. Nonetheless, transapical TAVR is not surprisingly associated with a significantly reduced risk of vascular complications compared to transfemoral TAVR [15]. However, transapical access is associated with its own problems related to access, specifically closing the ventricle after removing the valve deployment device. It is not uncommon to have bleeding from the ventricular closure site. On multivariable analysis, the transapical approach has been shown to be associated with a threefold increase in the risk of major bleeding events as defined by the VARC definitions. There are currently several ventricular closure devices under development that may bring increased consistency to ventricular closure and thus decrease the incidence of major bleeding associated with the transapical approach.

Conclusions

Transapical TAVR can be performed safely and effectively in high-risk and inoperable patients with severe aortic stenosis. Although utilization of the transapical approach is declining as most centers have adopted a "transfemoral first" approach and approved valves are requiring smaller and smaller vessels, many TAVR-eligible patients still have inadequate anatomy to accommodate the transfemoral approach. Additionally, future transcatheter interventions will likely involve transapical access. Thus, it is incumbent on cardiac surgeons to be familiar and comfortable with transapical techniques.

References

1. Iung B, Cachier A, Baron G, et al. Decision-making in elderly patients with severe aortic stenosis: Why are so many denied surgery? Eur Heart J. 2005;26(24):2714–20. doi:10.1093/eurheartj/ehi471.
2. Bouma BJ, van Den Brink RB, van Der Meulen JH, et al. To operate or not on elderly patients with aortic stenosis: the decision and its consequences. Heart. 1999;82(2):143–8. doi:10.1136/hrt.82.2.143.
3. Leon MB, Smith CR, Mack M, et al. Transcatheter aortic-valve implantation for aortic stenosis in patients who cannot undergo surgery. N Engl J Med. 2010;363(17):1597–607. doi:10.1056/NEJMoa1008232.
4. Varadarajan P, Kapoor N, Bansal RC, Pai RG. Clinical profile and natural history of 453 non-surgically managed patients with severe aortic stenosis. Ann Thorac Surg. 2006;82(6):2111–5. doi:10.1016/j.athoracsur.2006.07.048.
5. Smith CR, Leon MB, Mack MJ, et al. Transcatheter versus surgical aortic-valve replacement in high-risk patients. N Engl J Med. 2011;364(23):2187–98. doi:10.1097/01.SA.0000410147.99581.d4.

6. Lutter G, Quaden R, Osaki S, et al. Off-pump transapical mitral valve replacement. Eur J Cardiothorac Surg. 2009;36(1):124–8. doi:10.1016/j.ejcts.2009.02.037.
7. Nishimura RA, Otto CM, Bonow RO, et al. AHA/ACC guideline for the management of patients with valvular heart disease: a report of the American college of cardiology/American heart association task force on practice guidelines. J Am Coll Cardiol. 2014;63(22):e57–185. doi:10.1016/j.jacc.2014.02.536.
8. Miller DC, Blackstone EH, MacK MJ, et al. Transcatheter (TAVR) versus surgical (AVR) aortic valve replacement: occurrence, hazard, risk factors, and consequences of neurologic events in the PARTNER trial. J Thorac Cardiovasc Surg. 2012;143(4):832–43. doi:10.1016/j.jtcvs.2012.01.055.
9. Blackstone EH, Suri RM, Rajeswaran J, Babaliaros V, Douglas PS, Fearon WF, Miller DC, Hahn RT, Kapadia S, Kirtane AJ, Kodali SK, Mack M, Szeto WY, Thourani VH, Tuzcu EM, Williams MR, Akin JJ, Leon MBSL. Propensity-matched comparison of clinical outcomes after transapical vs. transfemoral TAVR. Circulation. 2015;131(22):1989–2000.
10. Dewey TM, Bowers B, Thourani VH, et al. Transapical aortic valve replacement for severe aortic stenosis: results from the nonrandomized continued access cohort of the PARTNER Trial. Ann Thorac Surg. 2013;96(6):2083–9. doi:10.1016/j.athoracsur.2013.05.093.
11. Kappetein AP, Head SJ, Généreux P, et al. Updated standardized endpoint definitions for transcatheter aortic valve implantation. J Am Coll Cardiol. 2012;60(15):1438–54. doi:10.1016/j.jacc.2012.09.001.
12. Thomas MS. Thirty-day results of the SAPIEN aortic bioprosthesis European outcome (SOURCE) registry: a European registry of transcatheter aortic valve implantation using the Edwards SAPIEN valve. Circulation. 2010;122(1):62–9. doi:10.1161/CIRCULATIONAHA.109.907402.
13. Himbert D, Descoutures F, Al-Attar N, et al. Results of transfemoral or transapical aortic valve implantation following a uniform assessment in high-risk patients with aortic stenosis. J Am Coll Cardiol. 2009;54(4):303–11. doi:10.1016/j.jacc.2009.04.032.
14. Rodés-Cabau J, Dumont E, Boone RH, et al. Cerebral embolism following transcatheter aortic valve implantation: comparison of transfemoral and transapical approaches. J Am Coll Cardiol. 2010;57(1):18–28. doi:10.1016/j.jacc.2010.07.036.
15. Murarka S, Lazkani M, Neihaus M, Bogess M, Morris M, Gellert G, Fang HKPA. Comparison of 30-day outcomes of transfemoral versus transapical approach of transcatheter aortic valve replacement. Ann Thorac Surg. 2015;99:1539–45.

Chapter 6
Transaortic Transcatheter Aortic Valve Replacement

Michael H. Yamashita and S. Chris Malaisrie

Introduction

Aortic valve replacement (AVR) is the standard of care for patients presenting with symptomatic, severe aortic stenosis (AS). However, due to increased life expectancy and improved medical management, patients being referred for AVR are now older and generally more frail and have more medical comorbidities. As a result, new minimally invasive techniques for AVR have been developed to lower the surgical risk of these patients. Transcatheter aortic valve replacement (TAVR) is a new treatment option that has gained popularity due to demonstrated efficacy in inoperable patients and perhaps better safety in high-risk patients.

Recently, large randomized controlled trials have demonstrated that TAVR has good short-term results in selected patient populations. The PARTNER 1B trial using the Edwards SAPIEN valve demonstrated that TAVR via the transfemoral route (TF-TAVR) is superior to standard medical therapy at 1-year [1] and 2-year [2] follow-up in patients who were not suitable candidates for surgery. The PARTNER 1A trial has shown that both TF-TAVR and TAVR via the transapical route (TA-TAVR) are non-inferior to conventional AVR in high-risk surgical patients at 1-year [3] and 2-year [4] follow-up. The CoreValve High-Risk US Pivotal Trial using the Medtronic CoreValve demonstrated that, in patients with increased

M.H. Yamashita, MDCM, MPH (✉) • S.C. Malaisrie, MD
Division of Cardiac Surgery, Bluhm Cardiovascular Institute,
Northwestern University/Northwestern Memorial Hospital,
201 East Huron Street, Galter 11-140, Chicago, IL 60611, USA
e-mail: michael.yamashita@mail.mcgill.ca; cmalaisr@nm.org

© Springer Science+Business Media New York 2016
G. Ailawadi, I.L. Kron (eds.), *Catheter Based Valve and Aortic Surgery*,
DOI 10.1007/978-1-4939-3432-4_6

surgical risk, there is a better 1-year survival for patients receiving a transcatheter CoreValve (85.8 %) compared to patients receiving an open AVR (80.9 %) [5]. In most centers, TF-TAVR has become the first choice of treatment for patients determined to be at high risk for standard AVR, with TA-TAVR being an alternative choice for patients with small iliofemoral vessels, severe peripheral vascular disease, and extremely tortuous aortas. Other alternative routes include transaortic (TAo-TAVR) and transaxillary TAVR.

TAo-TAVR does have some advantages over TA-TAVR. Its main advantage is the avoidance of a large transapical puncture which can be technically challenging to close, can be a source of postoperative pseudoaneurysm, and may impair left ventricular function. It also avoids a left thoracotomy which can further impair patients with poor pulmonary function. TAo-TAVR can also be performed via a J ministernotomy or right thoracotomy, approaches much more familiar to cardiac surgeons specializing in minimally invasive valve surgery than the transapical approach. TAo-TAVR also has advantages over the transaxillary approach. The transaxillary approach can be limited by small axillary arteries. As well, for patients with patent internal mammary grafts, the transaxillary approach can cause cardiac ischemia. Lastly, particularly for patients with carotid disease who depend on the vertebral arteries for cerebral perfusion, the transaxillary approach does carry a higher risk of stroke due to interruption of blood flow to the vertebral arteries. For these reasons, TAo-TAVR is the preferred alternative to TF-TAVR in some centers.

Valves

Two companies currently have valves approved by the US Food and Drug Administration for TAVR. Edwards Lifesciences Corp. (Irvine, CA, USA) and Medtronic Inc. (Minneapolis, MN, USA) both produce transcatheter aortic valves which can be used in TAo-TAVR. Several other companies are developing valves but these are still investigational.

Edwards Lifesciences Corp. produces the SAPIEN, SAPIEN XT, and SAPIEN 3 valves (Fig. 6.1). The SAPIEN XT valve is approved in the USA for transfemoral, transapical, and transaortic TAVR. It is a balloon expandable valve composed of bovine pericardial leaflets mounted on a cobalt chromium frame. The XT valve is available in three sizes: 23, 26, and 29 mm. For TAo-TAVR, this valve is implanted using the Ascendra + Delivery System which is a 24F size sheath for the 23 mm and 26 mm valves and a 26F size sheath for the 29 mm valve. Similar to the SAPIEN XT valve, the SAPIEN 3 valve is composed of bovine pericardial leaflets mounted on a cobalt chromium frame. The SAPIEN 3 valve also has an outer skirt designed to minimize the occurrence of paravalvular leak. The valve comes in sizes 20, 23, 26, and 29 mm and is delivered transaortically using an 18F sheath. The SAPIEN 3 valve has received CE Mark and is available in Europe but as of May 2015 remains an investigational device in the USA only available in the PARTNER II trial.

Fig. 6.1 Edwards
SAPIEN, SAPIEN XT, and
SAPIEN 3 valves

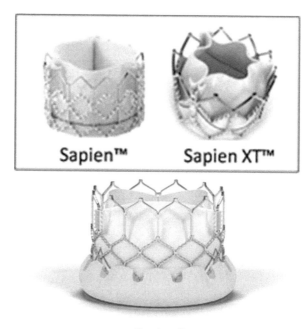

Sapien 3

Fig. 6.2 Medtronic
CoreValve

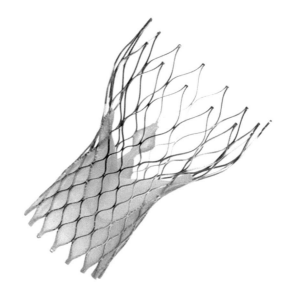

The Medtronic Inc. TAVR valve is called the CoreValve (Fig. 6.2). It has been approved in the USA for transfemoral, transaxillary, and transaortic TAVR. It is a self-expanding valve with porcine pericardial leaflets mounted on a nitinol frame. The CoreValve is available in sizes 23, 26, 29, and 31 mm.

The technique for implantation of these two valves is very similar except for during the actual valve deployment phase. These differences will be highlighted in the text below.

Technique

Ideally, TAo-TAVR is performed in a hybrid operating room where fluoroscopy and transesophageal echocardiography (TEE) are available for valve positioning. Cardiopulmonary bypass should be readily available in case there is an intraoperative complication or the patient becomes hemodynamically unstable. A general anesthetic is used and an arterial line and central venous access should be obtained. The medical team should consist of a cardiac surgeon, an interventional cardiologist, a cardiac-trained anesthesiologist, a transesophageal echocardiographer, a perfusionist, an x-ray technician and cardiac-trained nursing staff (Fig. 6.3).

TAo-TAVR can be performed via two approaches. The first is via mini-sternotomy and the second is via a right mini-thoracotomy (Fig. 6.4). The approaches are similar except for the initial incision. In the mini-sternotomy approach, a 5 cm upper sternotomy skin incision is made over the angle of Louis. A J mini-sternotomy is then performed with a sternal saw into the right 2nd intercostal space, sparing the right

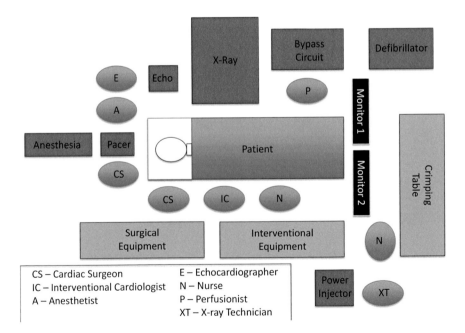

Fig. 6.3 TAo-TAVR or room setup

Fig. 6.4 Two approaches
to TAo-TAVR

Mini-Sternotomy

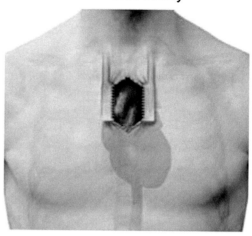

Right Mini-Thoracotomy

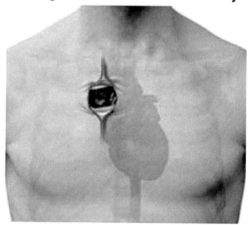

internal mammary artery. In the right mini-thoracotomy approach, a 5 cm horizontal incision is made in the right 2nd intercostal space. The incision is then carried down and the chest wall is entered, sparing the right internal mammary artery. From here, the two approaches follow the same steps. Hemostasis is obtained, the thymic fat pad is divided, and the pericardium is opened. Pericardial stay sutures are placed for retraction. The aorta is then inspected to find a suitable place for catheter insertion. This is usually on the anterolateral surface of the aorta, thereby facilitating perpendicular access to the aortic valve. It should be free from calcification and at least 6 (CoreValve) or 7–8 (SAPIEN XT) centimeters from the aortic valve (Fig. 6.5) to allow for valve deployment. When an appropriate spot is chosen, aortic purse-string

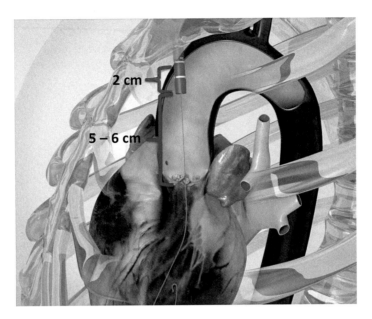

Fig. 6.5 Minimum aortic puncture to annulus distance when using the SAPIEN XT valve

sutures are placed in the standard fashion for aortic cannulation. Intravenous heparin is then administered, usually 100 units/kg, to maintain an ACT > 250 s.

Simultaneous to mini-sternotomy, femoral arterial access is obtained, and a pigtail catheter is advanced toward the aortic valve and placed in the noncoronary cusp for a CoreValve or the right coronary cusp for the SAPIEN XT valve. Femoral or internal jugular venous access is then obtained and a transvenous pacemaker wire is advanced into the tip of the right ventricle. The pacemaker is tested to ensure capture. An aortic root aortogram is then performed to find the implant angle where the right coronary cusp is directly between the other cusps and the base of all three cusps are planar (Fig. 6.6). The preoperative CT scan is often helpful in predicting the optimal implant angle.

The aorta is then punctured with a needle inside the purse string and a J-tipped wire is inserted. If using the hemi-sternotomy incision, then this is done through the sternotomy. If using the right mini-thoracotomy incision, then a separate 1.5 cm incision is made in the 1st intercostal space, directly superior to the thoracotomy incision, and the aortic needle puncture is performed through this separate incision to facilitate a perpendicular approach to the aortic valve. An 8 French sheath is then inserted over the wire. A JR4, AL, or multipurpose catheter and a straight wire are inserted into the sheath and used to direct a straight wire across the aortic valve. Once the catheter is in the left ventricle, the wire is exchanged for a stiff wire [Amplatz extra-stiff wire (Boston Scientific, Marlborough, MA, USA), Amplatz super-stiff wire (Boston Scientific, Marlborough, MA, USA), or Lunderquist stiff wire (Cook Medical, Bloomington, IN, USA)] that has been curled at the end to

Fig. 6.6 Optimal implant angle

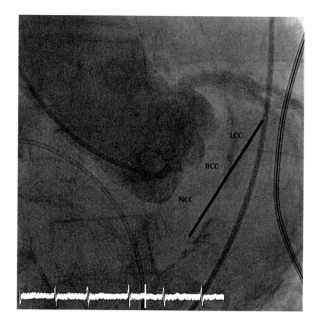

prevent cardiac perforation (Fig. 6.7). At this point, the catheter and sheath are removed, and the valve implanting sheath is inserted into the aorta and deaired. A 20 mm balloon is then inserted through the sheath and positioned 50 % in the left ventricle and 50 % in the aorta. Rapid ventricular pacing is initiated and the balloon is inflated to perform an aortic valvuloplasty. Pacing is stopped and the balloon is removed from the sheath. Correct orientation of the valve prosthesis for retrograde implantation is confirmed and the implant catheter is inserted into the sheath.

At this point, the discussion will first describe implantation using the SAPIEN XT valve and then describe implantation using the CoreValve. For the SAPIEN XT valve, the prosthesis is then positioned across the aortic valve using fluoroscopy and TEE. The recommended position of implantation for the SAPIEN valve is 50 % ventricular and 50 % aortic (Fig. 6.8); however, this may be modified based on anatomical issues. For instance, in patients with low coronary ostia, a more ventricular prosthesis position may be more appropriate keeping in mind that the prosthesis should not be placed below the hinge point of the anterior leaflet of the mitral valve. Once optimal positioning of the valve is confirmed, rapid ventricular pacing of 160–200 beats per minute is initiated to minimize cardiac output. The SAPIEN valve is then deployed by inflating the balloon for a full 3 seconds and then deflating the balloon. Rapid pacing is stopped and the valve is evaluated.

For CoreValve implantation, the prosthesis should be positioned so that the valve stent is placed 4 mm below the aortic annulus. When the valve is positioned correctly, the first phase of deployment is started by slowly turning the micro knob on the sheath and visualizing the stent flare out on fluoroscopy. Aortograms can be used to assess positioning and progress of stent deployment. Once appropriate positioning

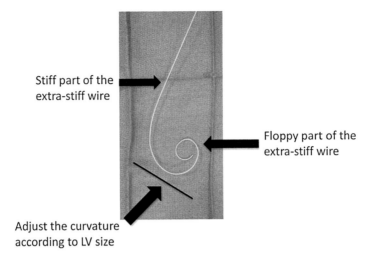

Stiff part of the
extra-stiff wire

Floppy part of the
extra-stiff wire

Adjust the curvature
according to LV size

Fig. 6.7 Curled stiff wire used for implant

Fig. 6.8 Optimal
Edwards valve implantation
position

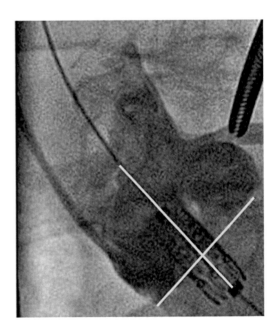

is confirmed, rapid ventricular pacing of 120 beats per minute is commenced, and the second phase of deployment is started where the stent comes in contact with the aortic annulus and aortic outflow is obstructed. At this point, deployment must be carried out quickly until 2/3 of the stent is deployed, pacing can be stopped, and cardiac output is restored. The third phase of deployment can then be carried out by releasing the remainder of the valve to complete implantation.

TEE is used to evaluate prosthesis position and the presence of any paravalvular leaks. An aortogram may also be used to evaluate paravalvular and intravalvular regurgitation, as well as patency of the coronary ostia. Subsequent balloon valvuloplasty can be employed to decrease any paravalvular leaks. When valve implantation is deemed satisfactory, the valve sheath is removed and the aortic purse-string sutures are secured and tied. Protamine is administered and hemostasis is obtained. A single mediastinal chest tube is placed. If there are rhythm abnormalities or bundle branch blocks post implant, the temporary transvenous pacemaker wire can be left in situ during the perioperative period. The chest is then closed with sternal wires in the standard fashion. The femoral arterial and venous sheaths are removed and manual pressure is applied for hemostasis. The patient is then transferred to an intensive care setting for postoperative recovery.

Discussion

Since first reported by Cribier and colleagues in 2002 [6], TAVR has revolutionized the treatment of AS in nonoperative and high-risk surgical patients. The transfemoral and transapical routes are the two most established techniques; however, the transaortic and transaxillary routes are becoming more popular. TAo-TAVR has several advantages compared to other TAVR options. First, both the SAPIEN XT and CoreValve are approved for TAo-TAVR, and therefore, there is a choice of prosthesis. As well, TAo-TAVR does not require access of the iliofemoral vessels with large catheters and sheaths, thereby remaining an option for patients with small or diseased vessels. It also decreases the possibility of vascular complications, a significant source of morbidity in TF-TAVR patients. Implantation of the prosthesis is more precise with TAo-TAVR, compared to TF-TAVR, because the short distance between the aortic puncture site and the annulus allows for accuracy in movement of the valve and the valve sheath provides a stable platform. TAo-TAVR is also performed through a mini-sternotomy incision with access to the ascending aorta, a method of exposure that is very familiar to cardiac surgeons. As well, the aortic access site can be easily controlled and repaired with conventional techniques. This is in contrast to TA-TAVR which requires a left thoracotomy and exposure of the apex which can be very challenging, particularly in obese patients. Closing the apex is difficult in patients with friable myocardium and losing control of the apex can be fatal. In patients with poor left ventricular function, the TAo-TAVR approach avoids puncture and purse-string sutures on the apex of the heart which can further impair left ventricular function. Furthermore, TAo-TAVR does not require opening of the pleural space, thereby avoiding pleural effusions. Lastly, if a serious complication were to occur in TAo-TAVR, such as annular rupture, coronary ostial obstruction, or valve embolization, the mini-sternotomy can easily be converted to a full sternotomy to facilitate cardiopulmonary bypass and open repair. The main disadvantage of TAo-TAVR is that it is an invasive approach that requires a partial sternotomy and general anesthesia. As well, this approach is difficult in a patient with previous cardiac surgery and adhesions or patent bypass grafts. It is also not a good approach for patients with COPD. Absolute contraindications to TAo-TAVR include a truly porcelain ascending aorta where there is no safe place to puncture the aorta with a valve sheath, a very short aorta less than 6 cm in length, patients who have a prohibitive anesthesia risk and those who have a low surgical risk.

The reported results of TAo-TAVR (Table 6.1), while limited, are certainly promising and seem to indicate comparable outcomes to TF-TAVR and TA-TAVR. The CoreValve Extreme Risk US Pivotal Trial alternative access arm [7] published outcomes on 80 patients who had TAo-TAVR during study enrollment and 260 patients who had TAo-TAVR through continued access following study enrollment completion. The all-cause mortality rate at 30 days was 13.7 % for the Pivotal study patients and 10.8 % in the continued access patients, $p=0.5$. The major stroke rates at 30 days were 6.5 % and 2.7 % ($p=0.14$), respectively. As well, the major adverse cardiovascular and cerebrovascular event (MACCE) rates at 30 days were 20.0 % and 16.2 % ($p=0.45$), respectively. The study also reported results for transaxillary TAVR; however, they are not comparable to the TAo-TAVR results because TAo-TAVR was only used if transaxillary TAVR was not feasible. Nonetheless, for transaxillary TAVR, the 30-day all-cause mortality rates were 8.6 % and 4.2 % ($p=0.25$), the 30-day major stroke rates were 8.6 % and 3.9 %, and the MACCE rates at 30 days were 14.3 % and 12.1 % ($p=0.67$) for the Pivotal study and continued access patients, respectively. Lardizabal et al. [8] reported on 44 consecutive patients undergoing TAo-TAVR with the Edwards SAPIEN valve and compared them to 76 consecutive patients undergoing TA-TAVR. They found that the rate of device success was similar at 89 % for the TAo-TAVR group and 84 % for the TA-TAVR group ($p=0.59$) with no difference in significant paravalvular regurgitation. Procedural mortality (TAo-TAVR=2 %, TA-TAVR=3 %, $p=0.99$) and 30-day all-cause mortality (TAo-TAVR=14 %, TA-TAVR=14 %, $p=0.99$) were also similar between the two groups. However, this group did find that the rate of major bleeding (TAo-TAVR=11 %, TA-TAVR=28 %, $p=0.04$) and incidence of total bleeding and vascular complications (TAo-TAVR=27 %, TA-TAVR=46 %, $p=0.05$) were higher in the TA-TAVR group indicating a better safety profile with TAo-TAVR. There was also a shorter median length of intensive care unit stay for the TAo-TAVR patients (3 days vs. 6 days; $p=0.01$). Interestingly, this paper also demonstrated a lower procedural adverse event rate after the first 20 cases in the TAo-TAVR group which was not seen in the TA-TAVR group. This may indicate a more favorable technical learning curve for the TAo-TAVR procedure. Bapat and Attia [9] published on 50 patients who had TAo-TAVR with the Edwards SAPIEN XT valve. The mean transaortic valve gradient decreased from 48 ± 14 mmHg to 10 ± 5 mmHg, and paravalvular regurgitation was less than or equal to grade 2 in all the patients. There were no periprocedural complications and the 30-day survival was reported to be 92 %. Spargias and colleagues [10] reported on a series of 25 patients undergoing TAo-TAVR using the Edwards SAPIEN

Table 6.1 Reported results of transaortic transcatheter aortic valve replacement

Author	No. of patients (N)	Valve	Device success (%)	Procedural mortality (%)	30-day mortality (%)
Reardon et al. [7]	80[a]	CoreValve	Not reported	Not reported	13.7
	260[b]	CoreValve	Not reported	Not reported	10.8
Lardizabal et al. [8]	44	SAPIEN	89	2	14
Bapat and Attia [9]	50	SAPIEN XT	100	0	8
Spargias et al. [10]	25	SAPIEN XT/ CoreValve	100	0	4
Amrane et al. [11]	27	SAPIEN XT/ CoreValve	92.6	4	11
Etienne et al. [12]	3	SAPIEN	100	0	Not reported
Latsios et al. [13]	2	CoreValve	100	0	Not reported
Pascual et al. [14]	2	CoreValve	100	0	0

[a]Pivotal study
[b]Continued access

XT and Medtronic CoreValve. They had a procedural and device success rate of 100 % with no procedural mortalities. The in-hospital mortality was 4 % while at 30 days there were no strokes. As well, the mean New York Heart Association (NYHA) functional class improved from 3.2±0.4 to 1.5±0.9 at 30 days postoperatively. However, 48 % of patients had a major bleeding complication, according to the Valve Academic Research Consortium (VARC) definitions. Amrane et al. [11] published on a single center experience of 27 patients having TAo-TAVR using the Medtronic CoreValve and Edwards SAPIEN XT. They had a device success rate of 92.6 %, with a 4 % intraoperative mortality rate, 11 % 30-day mortality rate, and 4 % major stroke rate at 30 days. Of particular note in this series is the low need for postoperative pacemaker implantation, only 7 %, which may suggest that TAo-TAVR facilitates more accurate valve positioning compared to TF-TAVR. Etienne et al. [12], Latsios et al. [13], and Pascual et al. [14] have also published very small case series of successful TAo-TAVR.

TAo-TAVR is a safe and feasible method of TAVR with very few contraindications. It also has several advantages compared to TA-TAVR and is therefore becoming the preferred alternative to TF-TAVR in some centers. Most notably, it is an approach that is most familiar to the cardiac surgeon and therefore can be easily adopted by those with TAVR experience. As the experience with TAVR grows and the indications expand, TAo-TAVR may become a standard method for AVR. However, this will depend on the long-term durability of transcatheter valves, which is currently unknown, and the results of randomized trials in lower-risk patients, such as PARTNER II, comparing TAVR to open surgical AVR.

References

1. Leon MB, Smith CR, Mack M, et al. Transcatheter aortic-valve implantation for aortic stenosis in patients who cannot undergo surgery. N Engl J Med. 2010;363:1597–607.
2. Makkar RR, Fontana GP, Jilaihawi H, et al. Transcatheter aortic-valve replacement for inoperable severe aortic stenosis. N Engl J Med. 2012;366:1696–704.
3. Smith CR, Leon MB, Mack MJ, et al. Transcatheter versus surgical aortic-valve replacement in high-risk patients. N Engl J Med. 2011;364:2187–98.
4. Kodali SK, Williams MR, Smith CR, et al. Two-year outcomes after transcatheter or surgical aortic-valve replacement. N Engl J Med. 2012;366:1686–95.
5. Adams DH, Popma JJ, Reardon MJ, et al. Transcathether aortic-valve replacement with a self-expanding prosthesis. N Engl J Med. 2014;370:1790–8.
6. Cribier A, Eltchaninoff H, Bash A, et al. Percutaneous transcatheter implantation of an aortic valve prosthesis for calcific aortic stenosis: first human case description. Circulation. 2002;106(24):3006–8.
7. Reardon MJ, Adams DH, Coselli JS, et al. Self-expanding transcatheter aortic valve replacement using alternative access sites in symptomatic patients with severe aortic stenosis deemed extreme risk of surgery. J Thorac Cardiovasc Surg. 2014;148:2869–76.
8. Lardizabal JA, O'Neill BP, Desai HV, et al. The transaortic approach for transcatheter aortic valve replacement: initial clinical experience in the United States. J Am Coll Cardiol. 2013;61(23):2341–5.
9. Bapat VV, Attia R. Transaortic transcatheter aortic valve implantation using the Edwards Sapien valve. Multimed Man Cardiothorac Surg. 2012;2012:mms017. doi:10.1093/mmcts/mms017.
10. Spargias K, Bouboulis N, Halapas A, et al. Transaortic aortic valve replacement using the Edwards Sapien-XT valve and the medtronic corevalve: initial experience. Hellenic J Cardiol. 2014;55:288–93.
11. Amrane H, Porta F, Head S, et al. Minimally invasive transaortic transcatheter aortic valve implantation of the CoreValve prosthesis: the direct aortic approach through a mini-sternotomy. Multimed Man Cardiothorac Surg. 2013;2013:mmt018. doi:10.1093/mmcts/mmt018.
12. Etienne P-Y, Papadatos S, El Khoury E, et al. Transaortic transcatheter aortic valve implantation with the Edwards Sapien valve: feasibility, technical considerations, and clinical advantages. Ann Thorac Surg. 2011;92:746–8.
13. Latsios G, Gerckens U, Grube E. Transaortic transcatheter aortic valve implantation: a novel approach for the truly "no-access option" patients. Catheter Cardiovasc Interv. 2010;75(7):1129–36.
14. Pascual I, Alonso-Briales JH, Llosa JC, et al. Direct transaortic access for transcatheter valve implantations with the self-expanding CoreValve prosthesis: A series of 2 cases. Rev Esp Cardiol. 2012;65:1141–2.

Chapter 7
Alternate Vessel Approaches to Transcatheter Aortic Valve Replacement (TAVR)

Hanna A. Jensen, Amjadullah Syed, Arul Furtado, Jared E. Murdock, and Vinod H. Thourani

Key Points

- Multi-access approach to transcatheter aortic valve replacement (TAVR) can be performed safely with low morbidity and mortality in high-risk and inoperable patients who are not candidates for the transfemoral approach.
- Careful selection of alternative access options (transapical, transaortic, trans-subclavian, and transcarotid) by a dedicated heart valve team can lead to excellent postoperative outcomes.
- Larger and longer-term studies are needed in order to differentiate outcomes between different access routes and to define the optimal target population for each TAVR approach.

Introduction

Aortic stenosis (AS) is the most common acquired valve disease in elderly patients with a prevalence of approximately 2.8 % in ages 75 or older [1]. Surgical aortic valve replacement (SAVR) utilizing cardiopulmonary bypass is the gold standard treatment for severe symptomatic AS, as it leads to excellent results with low morbidity and long-term survival [2–6]. However, as the elderly population expands, more patients

H.A. Jensen, MD, PhD • A. Syed, MD • A. Furtado, MD • J.E. Murdock, MD
V.H. Thourani, MD (✉)
Joseph B. Whitehead Department of Surgery, Emory University School of Medicine,
Atlanta, GA, USA

Department of Cardiothoracic Surgery, Structural Heart and Valve Center,
Emory University Hospital Midtown, 550 Peachtree Street NE, 6th Floor,
Medical Office Tower, Atlanta, GA 30308, USA
e-mail: hjensen@emory.edu; amjadsyed@emory.edu; adfurtado@emory.edu;
jaredmurdock@emory.edu; vthoura@emory.edu

© Springer Science+Business Media New York 2016
G. Ailawadi, I.L. Kron (eds.), *Catheter Based Valve and Aortic Surgery*,
DOI 10.1007/978-1-4939-3432-4_7

are presenting with multiple comorbidities. Many patients referred for SAVR are deemed "inoperable" due to high perioperative risk, age, multiple comorbidities, and/ or patient or family refusal despite good clinical data demonstrating satisfactory clinical outcomes [2, 4, 5, 7]. Patients with severe AS have an exponential increase in mortality that, if left untreated, can reach 50 % in 2 years [8]. Transcatheter aortic valve replacement (TAVR) was thus developed as an alternative to SAVR with particular benefit in the cohort of patients whose operative risk is prohibitive [8–11].

The Placement of Aortic Transcatheter Valve (PARTNER) trial was the first multicenter randomized trial comparing TAVR versus medical therapy or TAVR versus SAVR in inoperable or high-risk surgical patients, respectively [8, 11]. This study demonstrated superiority of TAVR over medical therapy in inoperable patients and noninferiority of TAVR to SAVR in high-risk surgical candidates [8, 10–12]. These results have since been validated in several studies exploring 30-day and 1-year mortality and 30-day stroke in TAVR vs. SAVR in high-risk patients [13, 14]. As a result there has been an exponential increase of TAVR with more than 60,000 procedures performed via transfemoral (TF), transapical (TA), transaortic (TAo), trans-subclavian (TS), trans-carotid (TC), and most recently transcaval (TCvl) approaches over the last decade.

The first TAVR was performed via a transvenous, transseptal technique in 2002 by Cribier [15], with other variations subsequently developed. The retrograde transfemoral approach remains the least invasive and has become the preferred initial choice of most operators. Its advantages include its ability to be performed under local anesthesia in most instances and the patient's ease of recovery and brief hospital stay [16]. Some patients, however, are not good candidates for this approach due to small-caliber vessels, significant tortuosity, calcification, or peripheral artery disease. Studies estimate that up to 30 % of patients screened for TAVR are not suitable for a TF approach [17, 18] and instead should be considered for alternative access. Appropriate patient selection for each access route is the key to success in any subgroup, and thus the role of a dedicated, multispecialty structural heart team consisting of interventional cardiologists, cardiac surgeons, echocardiographers, cardiac anesthesiologists, and imaging specialists cannot be overemphasized. We aim to examine these techniques in detail and provide tools for clinical decision-making as well as practical guidelines for their execution.

The SAPIEN valve (Edwards Lifesciences Corporation, Irvine, CA, USA) and the CoreValve (Medtronic, Minneapolis, MN, USA) are the only transcatheter aortic valves currently approved by the Food and Drug Administration (FDA) in the USA; however, several new transcatheter valves are in development. The eligibility and suitability for alternative access TAVR can be dependent on the type of valve and delivery system used, thus the future will undoubtedly bring intriguing new research and data about each valve type and the preferred access routes.

Preoperative Assessment and Planning

TAVR is currently indicated for those patients with severe AS and a life expectancy greater than 1 year, who are also considered either high risk or inoperative by a multidisciplinary heart team. Under current guidelines these are patients who have a Society of Thoracic Surgeons (STS) predicted risk score of mortality (PROM) ≥8 % or coexisting conditions that would be associated with a predicted 30-day surgical mortality of ≥15 %.

Potential TAVR candidates must undergo a multi-image evaluation using transthoracic echocardiography (TTE), transesophageal echocardiography (TEE), cardiac multi-detector computed tomography (MDCT), noncontrast CT of the abdomen and pelvis, and angiography of the coronary and iliofemoral arteries. Initial TAVR evaluation should include an assessment of the following patient variables: (1) severity of aortic stenosis; (2) ileofemoral vessel size, calcification, and tortuosity; (3) anatomic details of the aortic valve leaflets; (4) annular, sinotubular, and sinus of Valsalva dimensions; (5) ventricular function; and (6) extent of coronary artery disease. At our institution we utilize 3D computed tomography (CT) of the chest, abdomen, and pelvis and echocardiography as our primary imaging modalities due to their accuracy and reproducibility.

Echocardiography, usually done prior to initial patient evaluation, is primarily used to delineate the severity of aortic stenosis, aortic regurgitation, and ventricular dysfunction. Measurements of the annulus as well as the sinuses of Valsalva, the sinotubular junction, and the coronary heights are also obtained. The aortic annulus is sized at mid-systole, and the valve size is selected based upon 10 % over-sizing of the annular diameter [19]. Accurate measurement is essential, as failure to properly size the annulus may result in improper valve selection, with subsequent paravalvular leak or embolization. In addition, there is risk for coronary obstruction if the sinus of Valsalva is narrow or there is a short distance between the annulus and the coronary ostia (<10 mm) or bulky leaflet calcification exists. A sinus of Valsalva greater than 27 mm should accommodate smaller valves, while a sinus > 29 mm is adequate for all devices. If calcification, body habitus, or other factors preclude the accurate measurement of the annulus, a TEE ought to be performed. The use of supravalvular aortography during balloon aortic valvuloplasty (BAV) may provide additional information when the aortic annulus size remains questionable [20].

All patients should have a CT scan from the aortic valve to the femoral arterial bifurcation with 3D reconstruction of the aortic root. This includes annular, sinotubular, and sinus of Valsalva dimensions, as well as annulus to coronary distances. At our institution, CT measurements of the annular area and perimeter have supplanted two-dimensional echocardiography in guiding appropriate valve selection. In those with chronic kidney disease, a 3D TEE can be employed to calculate the aortic annulus area and perimeter. CT also provides accurate measurements of peripheral arterial vessel diameter, tortuosity, and calcification and is the preferred imaging method for delineating aorto-bifemoral anatomy.

Assessment of the lower extremity vasculature begins with a CT scan or lower extremity angiogram at the time of cardiac catheterization. The first consideration in the transfemoral approach is vessel size. The latest generation of FDA-approved valves requires sheaths ranging from 16 to 20 French, which in turn mandate minimum vessel sizes ranging from 6 to 7 mm. Calcification of the large iliac arteries is common but generally is not a contraindication to the transfemoral approach unless the calcification is circumferential and significantly reduces the arterial lumen diameter. However, calcification in the smaller common femoral arteries is more problematic and may preclude the safe insertion and removal of the TF sheath as well as arterial closure. Tortuosity, particularly in the external iliac artery, may complicate the advancement of the sheath. Consequently, moderate calcification in tortuous external iliac arteries (which tend to dive deep into the pelvis) may increase the likelihood of major vascular complications. Compliant arteries can usually accommodate sheaths that are 1 to 2 mm larger than their internal diameters, though not in the case of severe atheromatous disease, calcification, or tortuosity [21]. If there are significant concerns with any of these (size, calcification, tortuosity), then alternative access is used. This is always a consensus decision among the dedicated heart valve team.

Patients with severe coronary artery disease and significant lesions that are amenable to percutaneous coronary intervention can undergo implantation of a bare metal or drug-eluting stent prior to TAVR. If coronary stenting is performed with a bare-metal stent, the patient is treated with clopidogrel for 30 days, followed by TAVR. In those with a drug-eluting coronary stent, the TAVR procedure is performed on two antiplatelet anticoagulation regimen. Lastly, severe hemodynamically significant carotid disease should be treated prior to TAVR. Preoperative workup also includes the performance of pulmonary function testing (PFT). Patients with a predicted FEV1 % of less than 30 and DLCO less than 30 % may be less tolerant to a left anterior thoracotomy. A transaortic (TAo) approach might be an optimal alternative access choice in this group.

Alternative approaches are considered when preoperative imaging workup shows a TF approach to be contraindicated or less desirable. A TA approach, via an anterior left mini-thoracotomy, has traditionally been employed as the alternative in these patients. However, this approach comes with additional challenges and may not be appropriate for all patients, particularly those with significant parenchymal lung disease or a low ejection fraction. TAo approach is an additional feasible approach for TAVR in patients who have not had a previous sternotomy [22–24]. It is important to evaluate the degree of ascending and aortic arch calcification and the distance of the cannulation (>7 cm) site to the aortic annulus to ensure adequate space for balloon inflation and valve deployment. The transcarotid [25, 26] and trans-subclavian [27–29] approaches have been utilized successfully in those who are not candidates for TF, TA, or TAo.

The Transapical Approach

The TA approach offers several advantages over its TF counterpart: (1) it is not limited by peripheral vascular anatomy and size, (2) the valve is easily crossed in the antegrade direction (vs. retrograde), and (3) the device does not cross aortic arch and (4) allows for improved fine adjustment prior to valve deployment. The TA approach further allows for a more coaxial alignment of the stent valve in the AV annulus and has been shown to have less paravalvular leaks than in those undergoing TF-TAVR [30, 31]. Other potential advantages of the TA approach generally include shorter time for insertion and lesser contrast use. However, the effect of a thoracotomy on patient recovery and the possibility of bleeding after direct cardiac cannulation make this a potentially higher-risk procedure than TF, which may not be suitable for those with significant parenchymal lung disease (forced expiratory volume in 1 s < 35 %) or low ejection fraction (<15–20 %) [32]. However, new sutureless apical closure devices have been utilized to minimize incision and blood loss following TA-TAVR [33].

TA-TAVR requires general anesthesia, and the procedure should be performed in a hybrid room with both fixed fluoroscopic imaging and TEE. Cardiopulmonary bypass should be readily available in case emergent conversion to open AVR is required.

The patient is placed supine on the operating room table, and femoral artery and vein access is achieved. A femoral transvenous pacer is placed in the right ventricle through a Mullins sheath, and a pigtail catheter is placed in the aortic root via the femoral artery. Using fluoroscopic guidance, an anterolateral thoracotomy is made in the fifth or sixth intercostal space, a soft tissue retractor and then a rib spreading retractor are inserted, and the pericardium is incised and retracted with stay sutures to expose the left ventricular apex (Fig. 7.1). Two apical concentric pledgeted 3-0 PROLENE purse-string sutures are placed just cephalad to the apex and lateral to the LAD (Fig. 7.2). The purse-string sutures must be deep into the myocardium as they are prone to tearing through the ventricular tissue.

The patient is heparinized to maintain an ACT to 250 s. Fluoroscopy is used to position the aortic root and annulus perpendicular to each other and to align all three aortic cusps in the same plane in a similar fashion to the TF approach. At Emory, we generally have performed this with the angled pigtail in the non-coronary cusp. The

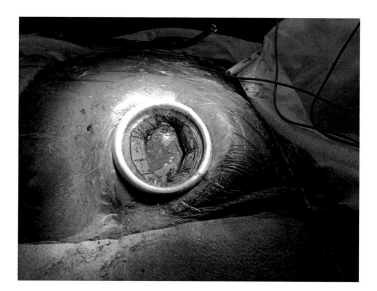

Fig. 7.1 Exposure for transapical approach

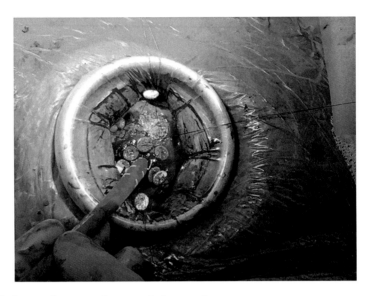

Fig. 7.2 Purse-string sutures for transapical approach

importance of achieving proper alignment cannot be overstated as this is crucial for accurate valve implantation. The LV cavity is punctured with a needle and a 0.035″ J wire is passed into the left ventricle, across the aortic valve, and into the ascending aorta. The wire is maintained in the ascending aorta without entry into the carotid arteries as the needle is exchanged for a 7-French sheath. A right Judkins catheter is used through the sheath to position the 0.035″ J wire into the descending aorta. The 0.035″ guide wire is then exchanged for an Amplatz super-stiff wire (Boston Scientific, Natick, MA) over which the valve will be delivered. The 7-French sheath is exchanged for the appropriate transapical delivery sheath which is positioned at 4 cm at the LV apex. If a BAV is indicated, a valvuloplasty balloon is threaded over the wire and inflated under rapid ventricular pacing of 180–200 beats per second. Most recently, we have not routinely performed a BAV in our TA cases, except in those circumstances where a balloon sizing is required. Following BAV, the balloon is removed and the valve is delivered through the sheath, de-airing done and positioned across the valve.

Positioning of the valve is a critically important aspect of any TAVR procedure. Using both echocardiographic and fluoroscopic imaging, the valve is aligned parallel to the long axis of the aorta and perpendicular to the aortic annulus [19]. Both TEE and aortic root injection can be used to confirm the position of the valve and its spatial orientation. The SAPIEN valve, a balloon-expandable valve, is ideally positioned so that its upper margin covers the aortic leaflet tips, while the ventricular end covers the aortic annulus. Once the optimal position is confirmed, the valve is deployed during rapid ventricular pacing. The valve delivery apparatus is then removed leaving the stiff wire across the bioprosthesis. Echocardiography with color Doppler and angiography is employed to evaluate valve position and assess the amount of paravalvular leak. Repeat balloon dilation may be performed for ≥2+ paravalvular leak; however, most pericardial valves will have a small central aortic regurgitant jet.

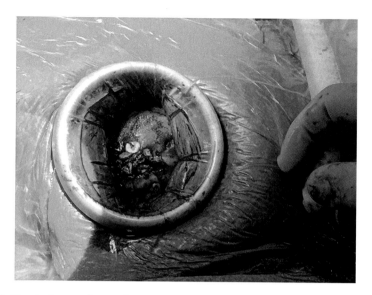

Fig. 7.3 Ventriculotomy closure after transapical approach

Once satisfactory valve function and position is confirmed, all catheters and wires are removed from the apex, and purse-string sutures are tightened during rapid ventricular pacing. Protamine is administered, and additional pledgeted sutures may be placed in the LV apex to achieve hemostasis (Fig. 7.3). The pericardium can be loosely closed over the LV apex, and a flexible Blake drain is placed in the left pleural space with part of it draining the pericardium as well. After complete hemostasis has been achieved, local anesthetic is injected into the intercostal bundle and the chest is closed in multiple layers.

The Transaortic Approach

The TAo approach is the third most common TAVR technique and has several practical advantages when compared to TA. It avoids a thoracotomy which potentially impedes pulmonary function in COPD patients, and it avoids cannulation of the ventricular apex in patients with a low left ventricular ejection fraction. Cannulation of the aorta, instead of suturing the ventricular apex, provides a more hemostatic closure especially in those with fragile myocardium, and it is compatible with both the SAPIEN valve and CoreValve. If needed, direct visualization of the aorta permits rapid cannulation and initiation of cardiopulmonary bypass for support. In TAo techniques, there are technical challenges when considering patients with a previous sternotomy and internal mammary artery or saphenous vein grafts that overlie the aorta and those with a severe porcelain aorta [34].

The patient is placed in supine position on the operating room table with the lower neck remaining exposed to allow for a counterincision for the delivery sheath.

Arterial access is obtained, an angled pigtail catheter is placed in the aortic root and a femoral transvenous pacer is placed in the right ventricle. Preoperative CT shows the relationship of the distal ascending aorta to the sternum, the extent of calcification, and the distance from the distal aortic cannulation site to the aortic root. This distance should be ideally >7 cm allowing enough space between balloon and delivery system for free inflation during the valve implantation.

A 5–6-cm sternotomy incision overlying the manubrium is made, and a mini-sternotomy is performed dividing the sternum down to the second intercostal space, where the "J" is completed with a transverse sternotomy. The distal ascending aorta is exposed and two aortic purse strings are placed at the base of the innominate artery.

The patient is heparinized to maintain an ACT >250 s. An 18-gauge needle with a 0.035″ soft J guide wire is passed through the counterincision in the lower neck and used to puncture the aorta through the purse strings. The needle is exchanged for a 7-F sheath (Fig. 7.4), and a multipurpose (MP) catheter with a straight soft wire is used to cross the valve. This is exchanged for a 260-cm-long, 0.035″ Amplatz extra-stiff J guide wire which has an exaggerated pigtail bend at the proximal end. The appropriate valve sheath is placed 2–4 cm into the aorta.

A BAV is performed under rapid ventricular pacing. The balloon is removed and the valve is placed through the delivery sheath and positioned across the valve. Positioning, deployment, and assessment of the deployed valve are as described in the TA section. Some views from fluoroscopy and echocardiography images for valve alignment are shown in Figs. 7.5 and 7.6.

After adequate evaluation, all catheters and wires are removed and the aortic sutures are tightened under rapid ventricular pacing. Protamine is administered and

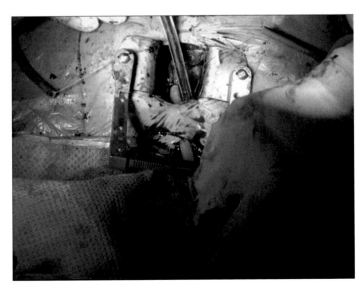

Fig. 7.4 Exposure for transaortic approach

Fig. 7.5 Valve alignment
in conjunction with
transaortic approach.
Echocardiography image

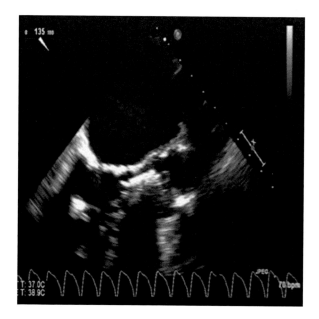

Fig. 7.6 Valve deployment
in conjunction with
transaortic approach.
Fluoroscopy image

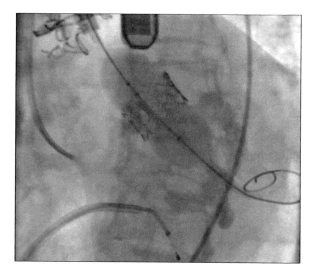

generally the pericardium is left open. A small flexible chest tube is placed in the
mediastinum and the sternum is re-approximated with stainless steel wires.

A right mini-thoracotomy (through second intercostal space) is an additional
option if a surgeon wants to avoid sternotomy or improve visualization in the case
of a horizontal or a right-sided aorta. Approaching from a mini-thoracotomy can
provide a better coaxial prosthesis deployment, but access to major cardiac structures such as ascending aorta, right atrium, and SVC is limited.

The Trans-subclavian (Axillary) Approach (TS)

The trans-subclavian approach was first used as an alternative to transfemoral deployment of the Medtronic CoreValve in patients with unfavorable femoral anatomy. It is less invasive when compared to a TA or TAo approach as it does not require thoracotomy or sternotomy. This makes it appealing for the older, debilitated patient in whom the TF approach is limited by anatomy or the aorta is severely calcified. However, the subclavian artery is often less compliant and more friable, especially in the elderly [29, 35]. It is also subject to the same concerns regarding caliber and calcification as the ileofemoral vessels in the TF approach. A review of TAVR using the TS approach suggested that subclavian access is not advisable in patients with subclavian artery diameter <7 mm, significant tortuosity, or prior CABG and patent in situ internal mammary artery grafts [36].

Standard femoral artery and vein access is obtained and an angled pigtail catheter is placed in the aortic root and a femoral transvenous pacer is placed in the right ventricle. Surgical cutdown for the left axillary artery is familiar to most cardiac surgeons as it is routinely employed as an arterial inflow cannulation site in the setting of aortic surgery. An oblique incision is made in the deltopectoral groove. The first portion of the axillary artery can be exposed with lateral retraction of the pectoralis minor. Division of the head of pectoralis minor can be performed with minimal morbidity if necessary to obtain optimum exposure. Great care is taken to avoid injury to the medial and lateral cords of the brachial plexus, as they often travel in close association with the artery, particularly in its second portion. The patient is heparinized to maintain an ACT > 250 s. The use of an 8-mm synthetic graft anastomosed in an end-to-side fashion and then cannulated with the delivery sheath is favored by some, while others use direct access via a purse-string suture. Using the Seldinger technique, the access site is dilated to accommodate the appropriate caliber delivery sheath for the chosen device. This is advanced over a stiff wire, using fluoroscopic guidance with the tip of the sheath left at the origin of the innominate artery when approached from the left. When approaching from the right, the concern for potential occlusion of the right common carotid artery has led some high-volume centers to position the sheath tip at the origin of the right subclavian artery. Once the sheath is appropriately placed, TAVR deployment proceeds using the same protocol as the transaortic TAVR. At the conclusion of the procedure, following removal of the delivery sheath, vascular control of the access site is obtained and selective angiography can be used to confirm vessel integrity.

The Transcarotid Approach (TC)

Currently the TC approach is used only for patients who have contraindications to all other access routes. Any patient considered for this technique must have a common carotid artery diameter > 8 mm without evidence of calcification, stenosis, or

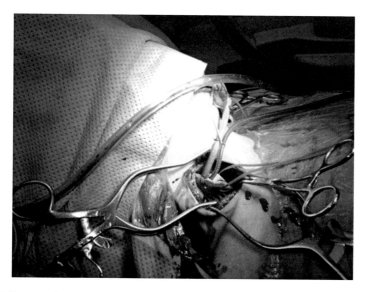

Fig. 7.7 Exposure for transcarotid approach

severe tortuosity. All patients have a comprehensive neurovascular imaging workup to rule out significant atherosclerotic disease and to assess patency of the circle of Willis and cerebral circulation. Modine reported a successful series of 12 patients who underwent CoreValve TAVR with no access site complications, no stroke, and only 1 TIA contralateral to the accessed side [37].

A 6-F sheath is placed in the femoral artery and an angled pigtail catheter is utilized for ascending aortography. In the contralateral femoral artery, a 16-F Fem-Flex II cannula (Edwards Lifesciences, Irvine, CA) is placed percutaneously. This cannula is connected to perfusion tubing and a 14/15 Sundt carotid bypass shunt (Covidien, Mansfield, MA). A pacing catheter is placed via the femoral vein. The right common carotid artery is exposed using a 5-cm vertical lower neck incision. After proximal cross-clamping of the common carotid artery, it is opened longitudinally for 2.5 cm (Fig. 7.7). The de-aired bypass shunt is placed through the arteriotomy into the distal carotid to maintain cerebral perfusion. Cerebral oximetry from the left and right hemispheres is monitored throughout the procedure. Through the proximal portion of the arteriotomy, a 0.035-inch J-tipped wire and 7-F introducer are placed in the ascending aorta. A multipurpose catheter is then inserted and a straight wire is used to cross the native aortic valve. The straight wire is exchanged for an Amplatz extra-stiff wire and a retroflex sheath is introduced into the ascending aorta. Similar to the transfemoral TAVR, a BAV is followed by the implantation of the valve. Finally, the wires, catheters, and sheath are removed, and the carotid artery is repaired with a bovine pericardial patch.

The Transcaval Approach (TCvl)

In the transcaval approach, the delivery system is inserted through the femoral vein and crossed to the arterial system by creating an aorto-caval fistula, which is closed with an Amplatzer device (St. Jude Medical) after the valve is deployed. A schematic diagram of the transcaval access route is illustrated in Fig. 7.8. The location of the fistula is determined by a careful evaluation of the CT abdomen and pelvis prior to the procedure. A case series demonstrated the feasibility of the transcaval TAVR, revealing a successful valve deployment in 17 of 19 patients despite a 79 % rate of transfusion and a 33 % rate of vascular complications [38]. This access is currently being investigated in a multicenter clinical trial and more results should become available in the near future.

Figure 7.9 summarizes the most common access routes for TAVR.

Outcomes

Mortality

The PARTNER trial reported a 30-day mortality rate of 5.0 % in nonoperative TAVR patients [8] and 3.4 % in high-risk TAVR patients [11]. Since then, all-cause 30-day mortality rates for TF-TAVR have been reported to be 1.7–14.5 % [39]. Published data since the first TA-TAVR in 2006 show these alternative routes of access can have results similar to those in TF- TAVR cohorts.

Several studies focusing on the TA approach have outcomes after TA-TAVR comparable to TF-TAVR, particularly in centers where significant experience with both approaches exists [40–43]. The proportion of patients having TF versus TA varies widely ranging from 30 to 80 % TF, and most clinicians agree that patients undergoing TA are a different higher-risk population. An early report by Bleiziffer and colleagues [44] compared a large series of 153 TF with 50 TA patients who were selected based only on access and reported no difference in 30-day mortality (11.2 % TF vs. 8.3 % TA, $P=0.918$). Results of the multicenter PREVAIL TA European study using the SAPIEN XT valve and Ascendra 2 TA delivery system demonstrated a 30-day mortality rate of 8.7 % in 150 patients [45], similar to an 8.0 % postoperative rate of death from any cause reported by from the national Transcatheter Valve Therapy (TVT) registry [46]. By comparison, the all-cause 30-day mortality rates for TF-TAVR have been reported to be 1.7–14.5 % by Genereux [39], and other studies have reported 30-day mortality for TA-TAVR ranging from 5.7 to 17.5 % [47–49].

Rapid improvement in outcomes continues as surgical experience increases, patient selection is refined, and TA-TAVR delivery systems improve. However, it is consistent among all series that there is a learning curve period required to achieve good outcomes in TA-TAVR. In a recent report from a high-volume TAVR center, the 1-year mortality of TA-TAVR patients was significantly improved when patients from 2007 to 2010 were compared with those from 2011 to 2013 (16.9 % vs. 4.7 %, respectively, $p=0.002$) [50].

Our institution has retrospectively reviewed all patients who underwent TA, TAo, and TC-TAVR from September 2007 to May 2013 [51]. 139 patients underwent TA, 35 TAo, and 11 TC-TAVR. While there were no preoperative differences in ejection fraction, NYHA class, significant COPD, and STS predicted risk of mortality between the different access groups, TC patients were younger than TA and

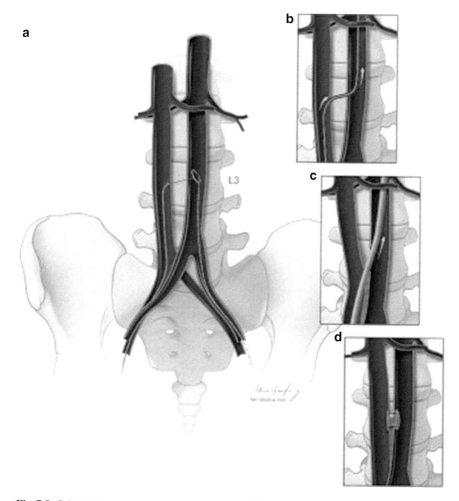

Fig. 7.8 Schematic depiction of caval-aortic access [38]. (**a**) A catheter directs a transfemoral vein guide wire from the inferior vena cava toward a snare target positioned in the adjoining abdominal aorta. (**b**) A catheter is advanced over the guide wire into the aorta and used to introduce a more rigid guide wire. (**c**) The valve introducer sheath is advanced from the vena cava into the aorta. (**d**) After completion of transcatheter aortic valve replacement, the aorto-caval access tract is closed with a nitinol occluder [38]

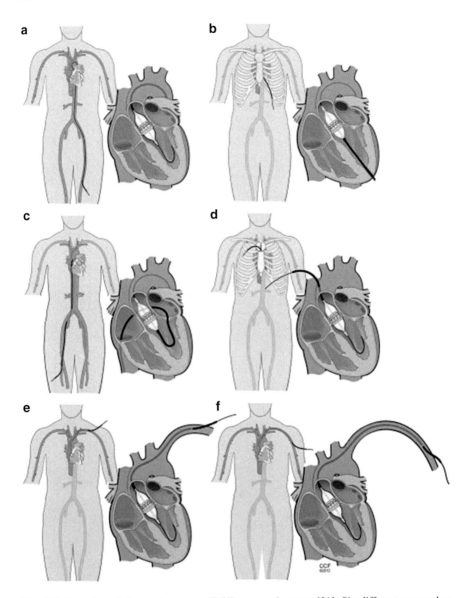

Fig. 7.9 Overview of the most common TAVR approach routes [21]. Six different approaches used for transcatheter aortic valve replacement (TAVR) with a stent valve. (**a**) Retrograde transfemoral arterial approach from femoro-iliac vessels. (**b**) Antegrade left ventricular transapical approach via anterolateral mini-thoracotomy. (**c**) Antegrade transfemoral venous approach, used during initial experience. (**d**) Retrograde transaortic approach via mini-anterior thoracotomy. (**e**) Retrograde trans-subclavian artery approach via surgical cutdown. (**f**) Retrograde trans-axillary artery approach via percutaneous Seldinger method [21]

Table 7.1 Results from the national TVT registry—transapical and transaortic TAVR [53]

All patients	Overall (N=4953)	Transapical (N=4085)	Transaortic (N=868)	p value
STS PROM score (median, IQR)	7.6 (5.1, 11.5)	7.4 (5.0, 11.1)	8.8 (5.8, 13.0)	<0.001
Operative mortality, n (%)	347 (7.0)	277 (6.8)	70 (8.1)	0.178
O/E mortality	0.759	0.756	0.771	0.177
Post-op stroke, n (%)	108 (2.2)	86 (2.1)	22 (2.5)	0.433
Major vascular complication n (%)	17 (0.3)	14 (0.3)	3 (0.3)	0.990
New post-op dialysis, n (%)	124 (2.5)	100 (2.5)	24 (2.8)	0.588
Post-op LOS (days), mean±SD	8.5±6.6	8.5±6.6	8.9±6.4	<0.001

TAVR transcatheter aortic valve replacement, *STS PROM* Society of Thoracic Surgeons predicted risk of mortality, *O/E* observed/expected, *LOS* length of stay

TAo patients. There were 13 (9.4 %) and 4 (11.4 %) operative deaths in the TA and TAo groups, respectively, while no deaths were observed in the TC group.

The reported 30-day mortality for TAo patients currently ranges from 7.4 to 14 % [22–24]. The initial results of the national TVT registry show that in inoperative patients, mortality associated with the TAo technique (10.4 %) seemed to be higher than the TA technique (5.6 %, $p=0.055$); however, this patient cohort had higher STS PROM scores, and no differences were found in terms of mortality at 1 year in propensity-adjusted analysis [52]. In a more recent TVT registry report focusing on these two alternative access routes, operative mortality was reported as 6.8 % for the TA and 8.1 % for TAo ($p=0.178$, Table 7.1), and again no differences were found in 1-year mortality in adjusted analysis [53]. Correspondingly, contemporary outcomes between patients operated with the TA or TAo have been comparable in our results and other series [22, 24].

Published literature about the transcarotid and trans-subclavian/trans-axillary approaches is scarce and includes only small series. Since the initial report of the transcarotid procedure from our institution [25], a report of 12 patients who underwent TC-TAVR was published with no deaths in the perioperative or 30-day follow-up period [37]. In another study, 19 TC-TAVR patients were operated under local anesthesia [26]. Although feasible with the SAPIEN valve, most of the trans-subclavian/trans-axillary reports come from Europe in patients implanted with the CoreValve [27, 28]. A single-center experience from Milan, Italy, reported six SC-TAVR patients with procedural success obtained in all patients and no 30-day mortality [29].

Morbidity

Although TA-TAVR largely avoids the risk of peripheral vascular complications, concern for LV apex complications, such as bleeding, rupture, and pseudoaneurysm formation, makes this a potentially higher-risk procedure [42]. However, in the

European PREVAIL TA study with the SAPIEN XT valve, apical injury occurred in only one of 150 patients (0.7 %) [45], and results from the US TVT registry have not demonstrated significant differences in major vascular complications between the access routes (Table 7.1) [52, 53]. Some studies have demonstrated significant LV function impairment after TA-TAVR compared with TF-TAVR [54–56]. Overall longer recovery time coupled with these findings may explain why health-related quality of life in high-risk AS patients seems to improve faster in patients treated with the transfemoral approach compared with patients treated with TA-TAVR [56]. In small series, pacemaker implantation has been reported as the most common morbidity in the immediate postoperative period after TC-TAVR [26] and SC-TAVR [29].

The hemodynamic results measured by post-procedural echocardiography in our in-hospital cohort of TA, TAo, and TC-TAVR [51] were excellent with increases in the aortic valve area and decreases in mean AV gradient consistent with the PARTNER trial results. These results suggest that alternative TAVR approaches can reproduce comparable hemodynamic results and benefits.

Paravalvular Leak

Paravalvular leak (PVL) may be an independent predictor of mortality, with increased morbidity and mortality in patients with greater than mild PVL [10, 57, 58]. In our institutional study, 2.2 % of patients had moderate or severe PVL (2.2 % of TA patients, 2.9 % of TAo, and no TC patients) postoperatively [51]. This is comparable to the PARTNER trial, where moderate or severe paravalvular aortic regurgitation was found in 11.8 % of inoperable patients and 12.2 % of high-risk patients [8, 11] and to the TVT registry results reporting moderate or severe PVL in approximately 6 % of patients operated via TA or TAo access [53]. These results are also consistent with a review by Sinning and colleagues where PVL rate was reported at 3–21 % [58]. While two big European registries, the France 2 registry [30] and the UK TAVI registry [31], suggest that the antegrade transapical approach had a significantly lower incidence of PVL when compared with all retrograde routes, this finding has not been supported by all investigators [59].

Neurological Complications

The differing risks for adverse neurological events between TAVR techniques remains poorly described [13, 60]. Many hypothesize, and some initial findings suggest TA-TAVR could have a lower neurologic risk profile due to its avoidance of the often heavily calcified aortic arch [55, 61, 62]. In the first report from the national TVT registry, high-risk patients operated with the TAo approach demonstrated a stroke rate twice as high as the TA group (3.0 % vs. 1.6 %, $p=0.004$), but at 1 year after the procedure, no differences between the groups were detected in adjusted analysis [52]. This operative stroke rate difference was, however, not present in a more recent TVT registry report focusing on alternative access, where operative strokes occurred in 2.1 % of TA patients and 2.5 % of TAo patients ($p=0.433$, Table 7.1) [53]. Other series have not reported major differences in stroke rates between approach routes [41, 63, 64]. The prospective Australian SANITY study should provide comprehensive information about neurological and neurocognitive outcomes from the different contemporary TAVR approaches [65].

Conclusions

In conclusion, a multi-access approach to TAVR can be performed safely with low morbidity and mortality in high-risk and inoperable patients who are not candidates for TF-TAVR. Careful patient and procedure selection leads to excellent and comparable immediate postoperative outcomes. Essential to this success is having a consistent, dedicated heart valve team familiar with the risks and benefits of each approach. Undoubtedly as experience and data accumulate, the optimal approach for these high-risk patients will be clarified, and standardized algorithms for optimal patient care will be created.

Disclosures Dr. Jensen has no disclosures.
Dr. Murdock has no disclosures.
Dr. Syed has no disclosures.
Dr. Furtado has no disclosures.
Dr. Thourani: Advisory Board, St. Jude Medical, Edwards Lifesciences, Boston Scientific. Research: Medtronic, Edwards Lifesciences, St. Jude, and Sorin Medical.

References

1. Go AS, Mozaffarian D, Roger VL, et al. Heart disease and stroke statistics – 2013 update: a report from the American Heart Association. Circulation. 2013;127:e6–245.
2. Thourani VH, Myung R, Kilgo P, et al. Long-term outcomes after isolated aortic valve replacement in octogenarians: a modern perspective. Ann Thorac Surg. 2008;86:1458–64.
3. Thourani VH, Suri R, Gunter RL, et al. Contemporary real-world outcomes of surgical aortic valve replacement in 141,905 low-, intermediate, and high-risk patients. Ann Thorac Surg. 2015;99(1):55–61.
4. Grossi EA, Schwartz CF, Yu PJ, et al. High-risk aortic valve replacement: are the outcomes as bad as predicted? Ann Thorac Surg. 2008;85:102–7.
5. Brennan JM, Edwards FH, Zhao Y, et al. Developing evidence to inform decisions about effectiveness–aortic valve replacement (DEcIDE AVR) research team. Long-term survival after aortic valve replacement among high-risk elderly patients in the United States: insights from the Society of Thoracic Surgeons Adult Cardiac Surgery Database, 1991 to 2007. Circulation. 2012;126:1621–9.
6. Brown JM, O'Brien SM, Wu CW, et al. Isolated aortic valve replacement in North America comprising 108,687 patients in 10 years: changes in risks, valve types, and outcomes in the Society of Thoracic Surgeons National Database. J Thorac Cardiovasc Surg. 2009;137:82–90.

7. Iung B, Cachier A, Baron G, et al. Decision-making in elderly patients with severe aortic stenosis: why are so many denied surgery? Eur Heart J. 2005;26:2714–20.
8. Leon MB, Smith CR, Mack M, et al. Transcatheter aortic valve implantation for aortic stenosis in patients who cannot undergo surgery. N Engl J Med. 2010;363:1597–607.
9. Reynolds MR, Magnuson EA, Lei Y, et al. Health-related quality of life after transcatheter aortic valve replacement in inoperable patients with severe aortic stenosis. Circulation. 2011;124:1964–7.
10. Kodali SK, Williams MR, Smith CR, et al. Two-year outcomes after transcatheter or surgical aortic valve replacement. N Engl J Med. 2012;366:1686–95.
11. Smith CR, Leon MB, Mack M, et al. Transcatheter versus surgical aortic valve replacement in high-risk patients. N Engl J Med. 2011;364:2187–98.
12. Makkar RR, Fontana GP, Jilaihawi H, et al. Transcatheter aortic-valve replacement for inoperable severe aortic stenosis. N Engl J Med. 2012;366:1696–704.
13. Eggebrecht H, Schmermund A, Voigtlander T, Kahlert P, Erbel R, Mehta RH. Risk of stroke after transcatheter aortic valve implantation (TAVI): a meta-analysis of 10,037 published patients. EuroIntervention. 2012;8:129–38.
14. Iung B, Laouénan C, Himbert D, et al. Predictive factors of early mortality after transcatheter aortic valve implantation: individual risk assessment using a simple score. Heart. 2014;100:1016–23.
15. Cribier A, Eltchaninoff H, Bash A, et al. Percutaneous transcatheter implantation of an aortic valve prosthesis for calcific aortic stenosis: first human case description. Circulation. 2002;106:3006–8.
16. Babaliaros V, Devireddy C, Lerakis S, et al. Comparison of transfemoral transcatheter aortic valve replacement performed in the catheterization laboratory (minimalist approach) versus hybrid operating room (standard approach): outcomes and cost analysis. JACC Cardiovasc Interv. 2014;7:898–904.
17. Descoutures F, Himbert D, Lepage L, et al. Contemporary surgical or percutaneous management of severe aortic stenosis in the elderly. Eur Heart J. 2008;29:1410–7.
18. Rodés-Cabau J, Webb JG, Cheung A, et al. Transcatheter aortic valve implantation for the treatment of severe symptomatic aortic stenosis in patients at very high or prohibitive surgical risk. J Am Coll Cardiol. 2010;55:1080–90.
19. Walther T, Dewey T, Borger MA, et al. Transapical aortic valve implantation: step by step. Ann Thorac Surg. 2009;87:276–83.
20. Babaliaros VC, Junagadhwalla Z, Lerakis S, et al. Use of balloon aortic valvuloplasty to size the aortic annulus before implantation of a balloon-expandable transcatheter heart valve. JACC Cardiovasc Interv. 2010;3(1):114–8. doi:10.1016/j.jcin.2009.09.017.
21. Alfirevic A, Mehta AR, Svensson LG. Transcatheter aortic valve replacement. Anesthesiol Clin. 2013;31:355–81.
22. Bapat V, Khawaja MZ, Attia R, et al. Transaortic transcatheter aortic valve implantation using Edwards Sapien valve: a novel approach. Catheter Cardiovasc Interv. 2012;79:733–40.
23. Hayashida K, Romano M, Lefèvre T, et al. The transaortic approach for transcatheter aortic valve implantation: a valid alternative to the transapical access in patients with no peripheral vascular option. A single center experience. Eur J Cardiothorac Surg. 2013;44:692–700.
24. Lardizabal JA, O'Neill BP, Desai HV, et al. The transaortic approach for transcatheter aortic valve replacement: initial clinical experience in the United States. J Am Coll Cardiol. 2013;61:2341–5.
25. Guyton RA, Block PC, Thourani VH, Lerakis S, Babaliaros V. Carotid access for transcatheter aortic valve replacement. Catheter Cardiovasc Interv. 2013;82:E583–6.
26. Azmoun A, Amabile N, Ramadan R, et al. Transcatheter aortic valve implantation through carotid artery access under local anaesthesia. Eur J Cardiothorac Surg. 2014;46(4):693–8.
27. Ruge H, Lange R, Bleiziffer S, et al. First successful aortic valve implantation with the CoreValve ReValving System via right subclavian artery access: a case report. Heart Surg Forum. 2008;11:E323–4.
28. Fraccaro C, Napodano M, Tarantini G, et al. Expanding the eligibility for transcatheter aortic valve implantation: the trans-subclavian retrograde approach using the III generation Corevalve revalving system. J Am Coll Cardiol Interv. 2009;2:828–33.

29. Bruschi G, Fratto P, de Marco F, et al. The trans-subclavian retrograde approach for transcatheter aortic valve replacement: single-center experience. J Thorac Cardiovasc Surg. 2010;140:911–5.
30. Gilard M, Eltchaninoff H, Iung B, et al. Registry of transcatheter aortic-valve implantation in high-risk patients. N Engl J Med. 2012;366:1705–15.
31. Moat NE, Ludman P, de Belder MA, et al. Long-term outcomes after transcatheter aortic valve implantation in high-risk patients with severe aortic stenosis: the UK TAVI (United Kingdom Transcatheter Aortic Valve Implantation) Registry. J Am Coll Cardiol. 2011;58:2130–8.
32. Thourani VH, Gunter RL, Neravetla S, et al. Use of transaortic, transapical, and transcarotid transcatheter aortic valve replacement in inoperable patients. Ann Thorac Surg. 2013;96:1349–57.
33. Blumenstein J, Kempfert J, Van Linden A, et al. First-in-man evaluation of the transapical APICA ASC™ access and closure device: the initial 10 patients. Eur J Cardiothorac Surg. 2013;44:1057–62.
34. Russo M, Tartara P. Trans-aortic transcatheter aortic valve replacement with edwards Sapien-Ascendra 3. 10 Apr 2014, The Cardiothoracic Surgery Network. http://www.ctsnet.org/print/article/trans-aortic-transcatheter-aortic-valve-replacement-edwards-sapien-ascendra-3. Accessed 07-14-2014.
35. Asgar AW, Mullen MJ, Delahunty N, et al. Transcatheter aortic valve intervention through the axillary artery for the treatment of severe aortic stenosis. J Thorac Cardiovasc Surg. 2009;137:773–5.
36. Caceres M, Braud R, Roselli EE. The axillary/subclavian artery access route for transcatheter aortic valve replacement: a systematic review of the literature. Ann Thorac Surg. 2012;93:1013–8.
37. Modine T, Sudre A, Delhaye C, et al. Transcutaneous aortic valve implantation using the left carotid access: feasibility and early clinical outcomes. Ann Thorac Surg. 2012;93:1489–94.
38. Greenbaum AB, et al. Caval-aortic access to allow transcatheter aortic valve replacement in otherwise ineligible patients: initial human experience. J Am Coll Cardiol. 2014;63(25 Pt A):2795–804.
39. Généreux P, Head SJ, Van Mieghem NM, et al. Clinical outcomes after transcatheter aortic valve replacement using valve academic research consortium definitions: a weighted meta-analysis of 3,519 patients from 16 studies. J Am Coll Cardiol. 2012;59:2317–26.
40. D'Onofrio A, Salizzoni S, Agrifoglio M, et al. Medium term outcomes of transapical aortic valve implantation: results from the Italian registry of trans-apical aortic valve implantation. Ann Thorac Surg. 2013;96:830–6.
41. Johansson M, Nozohoor S, Kimblad PO, Harnek J, Olivecrona GK, Sjögren J. Transapical versus transfemoral aortic valve implantation: a comparison of survival and safety. Ann Thorac Surg. 2011;91:57–63.
42. Ewe SH, Delgado V, Ng AC, et al. Outcomes after transcatheter aortic valve implantation: transfemoral versus transapical approach. Ann Thorac Surg. 2011;92:1244–51.
43. Greason KL, Suri RM, Nkomo VT, Rihal CS, Holmes DR, Mathew V. Beyond the learning curve: transapical versus transfemoral transcatheter aortic valve replacement in the treatment of severe aortic valve stenosis. J Card Surg. 2014;29:303–7.
44. Bleiziffer S, Ruge H, Mazzitelli D, et al. Results of percutaneous and transapical transcatheter aortic valve implantation performed by a surgical team. Eur J Cardiothorac Surg. 2009;35:615–20.
45. Walther T, Thielmann M, Kempfert J, et al. One-year multicentre outcomes of transapical aortic valve implantation using the SAPIEN XT™ valve: the PREVAIL transapical study. Eur J Cardiothorac Surg. 2013;43:986–92.
46. Mack MJ, Brennan J, Brindis R, et al. Outcomes following transcatheter aortic valve replacement in the United States. JAMA. 2013;310:2069–77.
47. Beller CS, Schmack B, Seppelt P, et al. The groin first approach for transcatheter aortic valve implantation: are we pushing the limits for transapical implantation? Clin Res Cardiol. 2013;102:111–7.
48. Svensson L, Dewey T, Kapadia S, et al. United States feasibility study of transcatheter insertion of a stented aortic valve by the left ventricular apex. Ann Thorac Surg. 2008;86:46–54.
49. Pasic M, Buz S, Dreysse S, et al. Transapical aortic valve implantation in 194 patients: problems, complications and solutions. Ann Thorac Surg. 2010;90:1463–70.

50. Aguirre J, Waskowski R, Poddar K, et al. Transcatheter aortic valve replacement: experience with the transapical approach, alternate access sites, and concomitant cardiac repairs. J Thorac Cardiovasc Surg. 2014;148(4):1417–22.

51. Thourani VH, Li C, Devireddy C, Kilgo P, et al. High-risk and inoperative aortic stenosis patients: use of transapical, transaortic, and transcarotid techniques. Ann Thorac Surg. 2015;99(3):817–23.

52. Thourani VH, Babaliaros VC, Suri R et al. Comparison of alternative access TAVR techniques in the US for patients considered high-risk or inoperative for aortic valve replacement and with severe aortic stenosis: an analysis from the STS/ACC TVT database. Presentation. The society of thoracic surgeons annual meeting, Jan 2015, San Diego, CA.

53. Thourani VH, Jensen HA, Babaliaros VC et al. Transapical and transaortic transcatheter aortic valve replacement in the United States. Presentation at the 51st annual meeting of the Society of Thoracic Surgeons, San Diego, CA, Jan 2015. Abstract available at: http://www.sts.org/sites/default/files/documents/pdf/annmtg/STS51_MonJan26.pdf

54. Meyer CG, Frick M, Lotfi S, et al. Regional left ventricular function after transapical vs. transfemoral transcatheter aortic valve implantation analysed by cardiac magnetic resonance feature tracking. Eur Heart J Cardiovasc Imaging. 2014;15(10):1168–76.

55. Bleiziffer S, Ruge H, Mazzitelli D, et al. Survival after transapical and transfemoral aortic valve implantation: talking about two different patient populations. J Thorac Cardiovasc Surg. 2009;138:1073–80.

56. Reynolds MR, Magnuson EA, Wang K, et al. Health-related quality of life after transcatheter or surgical aortic valve replacement in high-risk patients with severe aortic stenosis: results from the PARTNER (Placement of AoRTic TraNscathetER Valve) Trial (Cohort A). J Am Coll Cardiol. 2012;60:548–58.

57. Tamburino C, Capodanno D, Ramondo A, et al. Incidence and predictors of early and late mortality after transcatheter aortic valve implantation in 663 patients with severe aortic stenosis. Circulation. 2011;123:299–308.

58. Sinning JM, Vasa-Nicotera M, Chin D, et al. Evaluation and management of paravalvular aortic regurgitation after transcatheter aortic valve replacement. J Am Coll Cardiol. 2013;62:11–20.

59. Martinez CA, Singh V, O'Neill BP, et al. Management of paravalvular regurgitation after Edwards SAPIEN transcatheter aortic valve replacement: management of paravalvular regurgitation after TAVR. Catheter Cardiovasc Interv. 2013;82:300–11.

60. Vasques F, Messori A, Lucenteforte E, Biancari F. Immediate and late outcome of patients aged 80 years and older undergoing isolated aortic valve replacement: a systematic review and meta-analysis of 48 studies. Am Heart J. 2012;163:477–85.

61. Webb JG, Pasupati S, Humphries K, et al. Percutaneous transarterial aortic valve replacement in selected high-risk patients with aortic stenosis. Circulation. 2007;116:755–63.

62. Walther T, Simon P, Dewey T, et al. Transapical minimally invasive aortic valve implantation: multicenter experience. Circulation. 2007;116:I240–5.

63. Rodes-Cabau J, Dumont E, Boone RH, et al. Cerebral embolism following transcatheter aortic valve implantation: comparison of transfemoral and transapical approaches. J Am Coll Cardiol. 2011;57:18–28.

64. Webb JG, Altwegg L, Boone RH, et al. Transcatheter aortic valve implantation: impact on clinical and valve-related outcomes. Circulation. 2009;119:3009–16.

65. Fanning JP, Wesley AJ, Platts DG, et al. The silent and apparent neurological injury in transcatheter aortic valve implantation study (SANITY): concept, design and rationale. BMC Cardiovasc Disord. 2014;14:45.

Chapter 8
Cost-Effectiveness of Transcatheter Aortic Valve Replacement

Jeffrey B. Rich

Introduction

Advancing technology typically brings advancing costs to the healthcare system. The question always posed is whether these technologies add value. This is a multifaceted question since the answer must be posed in the context of the patient (medical benefit and patient costs) and the healthcare payment system. This book describes many highly advanced technologies that carry with them high and sometimes seemingly extraordinary costs. However, they also carry potential substantial benefit to patient care. We are currently in a period of time where there are significant economic strains on the healthcare payment systems, both public and private, with the potential for insolvency if injudicious application of costly technologies occurs, especially when the cost-effectiveness on an individual patient and a collective population is questionable. To be entirely fair, the pressure on the healthcare payment system is also multifaceted and does not solely lie on the shoulders of technology. Costly drugs, inappropriate and excessive care, poor quality of care leading to costly complications, lack of care coordination leading to duplicated services, and inefficiently designed healthcare delivery models are only a few. The most important determinant for the healthcare economic crisis that we now face is a payment system that is designed to reward the volume of services delivered and not their value.

The focus of this chapter is on the cost-effectiveness or more precisely the value of transcatheter-based repair and replacement of cardiac valves as compared to traditional surgical approaches with particular emphasis on transcatheter aortic valve replacement (TAVR). It is clear that this disruptive successful technology has broadened our ability to treat inoperable and extremely high-risk patients with aortic

J.B. Rich, MD (✉)
Virginia Cardiac Surgery, Quality Initiative, 1325 N. Bay Shore Dr,
Virginia Beach, VA 23451, USA
e-mail: jeffrich2014@cox.net

© Springer Science+Business Media New York 2016
G. Ailawadi, I.L. Kron (eds.), *Catheter Based Valve and Aortic Surgery*,
DOI 10.1007/978-1-4939-3432-4_8

stenosis (AS) who otherwise would go untreated. The clinical value of the application of this technology is unquestionable. The harder question to answer is when the treatment of these patients moves from clinical utility to clinical futility. In this extreme the value of this technology arguably approaches zero. With current extensive clinical experience identification of these futile patients has been clarified. The value debate now centers on whether TAVR will provide meaningful long-term results in these patients with multiple comorbidities, fraility and advanced AS, a question that will eventually be answered by the transcatheter valve therapy (TVT) registry. Continued implantation in qualified medical centers participating in the TVT registry will clarify clinical effectiveness in these patients and help determine their cost-effectiveness and the overall impact on the payment systems. When using this technology in intermediate-risk patients, the intensity of the debate regarding the cost/benefit of this expensive technology versus open surgical aortic valve replacement (SAVR) intensifies. There has been much written on this topic, and results from Europe where commercialization has a much longer time frame have produced meaningful information. In the USA, most of our collective data on these lower-risk populations is only now becoming available. While economic data from the PARTNER 1 clinical trial has provided cost/benefit data on highly selected patient populations post-commercialization data is only gradually entering the literature. These areas of interest are truly the focus of this chapter with a look at the value of TAVR as downward risk for implantation is introduced into patients with severe AS. A rigorous debate will ensue as we compare the clinical and economic results of TAVR versus SAVR in lower-risk patients. This debate must consider not only the economics but also the long-term clinical results addressing valve durability especially in younger patients.

Processes for Approval, Coverage, and Payment

To fully understand this debate, one must fully understand how technologies come to market and eventually enter the payment system. The three major steps for the introduction of new technologies into the market revolve around Food and Drug Administration (FDA) approval, a coverage decision, and eventually a payment decision. The FDA's primary objective is to review all available evidence from clinical trials and decide whether the device is "safe and effective." Once so determined a label for use is created. The next two steps occur at the Centers for Medicare and Medicaid Services (CMS). CMS is the largest federal agency under the umbrella of the Department of Health and Human Services (HHS). Annual expenditures exceeded 1 trillion dollars in 2013 split between Medicare ($585 billion) and Medicaid ($450 billion) [1]. CMS has two major jobs: to determine coverage and payment.

At CMS the Coverage and Analysis Group (CAG) makes coverage decisions. CAG determines if the technology is "reasonable and necessary." For example, a coronary artery stent may be deemed "safe and effective" by the FDA, but CAG must decide if it is "reasonable and necessary" to implant stents in Medicare beneficiaries.

As an extreme example, the FDA makes its decision leaving CAG to opine on whether implanting 17 stents in a patient is reasonable and necessary. In the case of TAVR, CAG struggled with "reasonable and necessary" based on the outcome data from the PARTNER trial. Was it reasonable and necessary to expose an elderly Medicare beneficiary to a procedure with a device that has a high major vascular complication rate possibly leading to limb amputation and a high stroke rate despite the fact that mortality was acceptable? More importantly, was post-op quality of life (QOL) acceptable in these elderly patients who had moderate to severe disability and frailty pre-op and specifically in those patients having a major vascular complication or stroke? In general, when making a coverage decision regarding the use of advanced high technology in elderly Medicare beneficiaries, issues revolving around QOL often trump mortality associated with the procedure. Once a coverage decision is made the technology moves on to a payment decision.

Payment decisions at CMS are made by the Center for Medicare (formerly the Center for Medicare Management). Understanding the following concepts will be critical to engaging in any debate regarding the cost/benefit of TAVR. The first decision is whether there is an existing benefit category for the new technology. For example, a biventricular pacer, although ostensibly different than a standard pacemaker, would fit into the general benefit category for pacemakers. A thoracic aortic stent graft for the arch would fall into the general benefit category for aortic stent grafts. When mechanical circulatory support first came to the market, a new benefit category needed to be created. So does all new technology fit easily into an existing benefit category? The answer is no and often requires some revisions to the benefit category but more often to terminology related to the device. TAVR and the transcatheter mitral repair technology, MitraClip, are two excellent and pertinent examples.

Controversy in Payment Decisions

Transcatheter approaches to the aortic valve came to the US regulatory system as transcatheter aortic valve *insertion* (TAVI) rather than as transcatheter aortic valve *replacement* (TAVR). What is the difference and does it matter? CMS struggled with insertion versus replacement. In their evaluations and based on internal recommendations, replacement (as in AVR) meant removal on the valve and *replacing* it with a prosthetic valve. In this procedure they reasoned that the benefit category was therefore not replacement but was insertion as named. This meant that the benefit category would be replacement rather than valvuloplasty, which described a procedure where the valve was manipulated with a balloon (a described part of this procedure) but not removed. However, it was not quite a valvuloplasty as something was left behind: a new valve! Much debate ensued and to the credit of the efforts of Edwards Lifesciences, the procedure was relegated to the AVR benefit category and not the valvuloplasty category, and the name was changed from TAVI to TAVR. Was that important?

It was incredibly important. Recall that benefit category designation places new technology and all medical procedures into procedural categories known as diagnosis-related groups (DRGs). DRGs are the ways hospitals get reimbursed for the care they deliver. Coronary artery bypass grafting has its own group of DRGs based on the presence or absence of comorbidities and complications as does AVR, mitral valve replacement (MVR), and thoracic aortic reconstruction. Each DRG and the groups within it are assigned a fixed dollar amount of reimbursement to the hospital (with exception for cost outliers as defined by CMS). This payment is inclusive of all aspects of the care for that in-hospital procedure and stay, including the cost of any implanted technology (valves, pacemakers, etc.). For example, a hospital may receive $50,000 for an SAVR (that includes the price of the valve) and $18,000 for a catheter based valvuloplasty. The importance of DRG designation is obvious. And the importance of the price of the valve is obvious as well even when the DRG designation is correct.

A more poignant example is transcatheter mitral valve repair using MitraClip technology. Unfortunately, that technology was placed in the mitral valvuloplasty DRG. This pays on average 1/3 of a mitral valve repair DRG. The DRG payment does not even cover the cost of the technology. This conundrum will drive much of the discussion later when determining whether based on the cost of the device an hospital can adopt a new technology economically, be it TAVR or mitral transcatheter therapies.

Cost-Effectiveness: TAVR

The *clinical* effectiveness for TAVR in inoperable and high-risk patients has been demonstrated in the Edwards Lifesciences PARTNER 1 trial and the Medtronic CoreValve trial [4, 5]. Clinical effectiveness in intermediate-risk patients is the focus of the PARTNER 2 and SURTAVI trials. The focus of this chapter is to examine the cost-effectiveness of TAVR in all risk categories of patients versus conventional medical therapy or SAVR. The analyses will vary depending on the surgical risk category of the patient population, and as risk falls, there is more focus on the cost of the valve itself. In addition, cost-effectiveness in clinical trials where patient selection is tightly controlled will be different than that seen in post-commercialization patient populations.

Clinical effectiveness as defined by mortality and major morbidities is relatively easy to define and identify across clinical trials, real-life use of devices, and health-care systems (USA, Canada, and Europe). *Cost*-effective analyses are not as simple to define across those domains.

Clinical trials enroll a tightly defined population, whereas post-commercialization real-life use of these devices will have a very different profile of patients. Clinical trials generally omit patients with certain and excessive comorbidities for treatment. Only 12 % of screened patients were ultimately randomized in the PARTNER 1 trial resulting in limited generalizability of both clinical and economic outcomes [6]. In a large statewide database in Virginia, costs of treating patients with severe AS by a standard surgical approach were stratified by STS predicted risk of mortality (STS PROM) scores. The costs of SAVR for high-risk patients were $20,000 less than the high-risk category in the PARTNER trial underscoring the caution needed in understanding the cost-effectiveness analysis from the trial [6]. Also, device costs within a clinical trial are different and generally lower than post-commercialization sales price (e.g., the SAPIEN valve was discounted in the PARTNER 1 trial). These two factors therefore would generally skew the cost-effective analyses generated from this trial. This also underscores the need to look at real-life observational data generated after commercialization as a complement to data from clinical trials. "The final answer on the comparative cost-effectiveness of TAVR will be provided by ongoing registries with TAVR cost data from everyday practice" [6, 7]. Such is the value of the transcatheter valve therapy (TVT) registry which did show 1-year results from TAVR with clinical outcomes as seen in the clinical trial (www.ACC.org/STS-ACC-TVT-registry) but has yet to provide an economic analysis.

Cost-effective analyses will also vary depending on site of service. Costs for care vary tremendously not only across nations, making European economic data difficult to compare to US data, but also geographically in the USA. Recall the discussion above regarding DRG payments for new technology and in particular transcatheter approaches to valvular heart disease. All DRG payments are adjusted geographically across the USA. For example, the DRG payment for left ventricular assist devices (LVAD) may be $250,000 in New York based on local economic conditions, but $150,000 in Virginia. Similar discrepancies exist for TAVR. Why is that important? With a fixed sales price across the USA for a transcatheter aortic valve, the cost of the valve becomes a proportionately lower percentage of the DRG payment. Therefore, in New York, a cost-effective analysis may have different results based on this higher DRG payment. The PARTNER 1 trial demonstrated cost-effectiveness for inoperable patients and arguably so for high-risk patients [2, 3] across all geographies, but did the high enrollment of patients in New York skew the results?

Cost-effectiveness for TAVR will also vary according to the access route. The PARTNER A trial conclusively demonstrated cost-effectiveness in inoperable patients, but for transapical TAVR (TA-TAVR) patients, there was no clear clinical benefit as noted by the absence of measurable improvements in quality of life, survival or LOS, and therefore cost-effectiveness [8, 9]. Again, this represents limited data from the clinical trials. Hopefully, the TVT and other registries will provide more clarity on this issue. It is clear that a transfemoral approach (TF-TAVR), if possible, lends itself to reductions in resource utilization and LOS and therefore is likely cost-effective [10] depending on the cost of the valve.

Types of modeling (e.g., Markov modeling) will also lend variation to the conclusions of cost-effective analyses not only when looking at the procedure itself but also whether the analysis takes into account future healthcare costs. Most cost-effective analyses do add future costs of related illness (e.g., readmissions for heart failure and device-related complications) but do not include future costs of unrelated illness (e.g., costs of treating dementia) [11]. Using this as a baseline or standard of analysis for cost-effectiveness, the current data remains at times difficult to interpret. In an extensive literature review, Iannconne [12] analyzed data from 16 studies that included cost-effectiveness data for TAVR versus medical management or SAVR. They concluded that "The quality of the cost-effectiveness analyses (CEAs) were generally sufficient. In contrast, we found an extreme heterogeneity of input assumptions with consequent difficulties to generalize the conclusions." Despite these input difficulties, this analysis supported TAVR in inoperable patients but did not in high-risk patients. "In AS patients with high (but not prohibitive) surgical risk, the choice between TAVR and SAVR is still debatable. Both procedures are comparable in terms of efficacy and safety but the evidence is inconclusive from an economic point of view" [12]. This issue of data coming from multiple nonharmonized data sources and modeling techniques and then reaching conclusions based on it is highlighted by Falk [13] in his point/counterpoint debate with Haussig in Circulation. He states that "Although TAVR is cost-effective in inoperable patients, conflicting results exist with regard to its cost-effectiveness compared with surgery in high-risk operable patients. For high-risk operable patients in the PARTNER trial, the incremental cost-effectiveness ratios were well beyond the generally accepted maximum threshold. The currently available data do not conclusively demonstrate that TAVR is incrementally cost-effective compared with SAVR for high risk surgical candidates…." This, of course, is based on the European perspective where there is "wide variability of incremental cost-effectiveness ratio values….in different countries and reimbursement systems" [13]. Others have supported the conclusion that overall data demonstrated an economic advantage for inoperable patients but that the other data was inconclusive for high-risk patients due to the nonharmonized economic and reimbursement systems in Europe [14]. More recently, Osnabrugge [15] and colleagues added more debate to the issue of modeling in the current ongoing trials for intermediate-risk patients (PARTNER 2). They questioned Van Brabandt's criticism of the methodology of the continuing access PARTNER trial and suggestions for improvement [16]. Obviously, this data will be extremely important to making future recommendations for intermediate-risk patients, and the analyses should be done so that conclusions for use of TAVR in these patients are accurate and meaningful. Despite all these issues, the data from the clinical trials as well as the large European and US experience both before and after commercialization should be used as conclusive evidence for TAVR's cost-effectiveness in inoperable patients and highly suggestive for the high-risk populations primarily when the transfemoral approach is used.

The challenge in moving on from here is the expansion of the use of TAVR in intermediate-risk patients. The PARTNER 2 and the SURTAVI trials are designed to answer that question. Early results for *clinical* effectiveness are encouraging. Cost-effectiveness is yet to be addressed. In a propensity-matched study from Europe, Osnabrugge and colleagues looked at the costs of TAVR versus SAVR in intermediate-risk patients [17]. They concluded that the costs of TAVR that included the index hospitalization are significantly more expensive than TAVR at 1 year. TAVR had shorter LOS and lower blood utilization than SAVR, but the biggest cost driver for TAVR was the cost of materials, i.e., the valve. The transcatheter valve was priced at US $20,052 while the surgical valve was US $3078. They calculated that the price of the valve would have to drop to $7847 in order to make TAVR cost-effective. The higher predicted cost of the transcatheter valve versus the surgical valve ($7847 versus $3078) for equivalency is explained by the increased costs of hospitalization and resource utilization (e.g., blood) in SAVR than for TAVR. These results were supported by data from Neyt [18] in Belgium and Ribera [19] in Spain. Specifically, Ribera confirmed that the biggest driver of costs in TAVR is the cost of the valve and that a price reduction of 30 % would make TAVR a more cost-effective option.

In a recent presentation at the STS annual meeting, Ailawadi and LaPar [20] described the "real-world" costs associated with TAVR. This was the data from the Virginia Cardiac Surgery database and was a propensity-matched study of TAVR and SAVR clinical outcomes and costs in intermediate-risk (STS PRO 4–8 %) and high-risk patients (STS PROM > 8 %) in the post-commercialization era. This study is invaluable because it describes the results of the true experiences in the use of TAVR, thereby addressing the criticisms of the strict inclusion criteria in clinical trial for high-risk patients and the vagaries of data from European countries that have different economies and healthcare systems with substantially different material and labor costs. Iannconne highlighted the need for these results: "the cost effectiveness of this procedure in the real world, particularly in patients with high healthcare costs from other comorbid conditions, may be less favorable…and that the details of risk evaluation and patient selection will be critical in understanding how improvements in survival can be used to target the use of TAVR to ensure the cost-effective and sustainable use of resources" [12].

The results show that while TAVR had reduced LOS and blood utilization versus SAVR, there was an increase in mortality and total overall costs in both the intermediate- and high-risk patients. TAVR had two times the median costs of SAVR ($69,921 vs. $39,075, $p < 0.001$) largely driven by the cost of the valve ($32,500 vs. $5592, $p < 0.001$) with the cost differential most pronounced in the intermediate-risk population. Transfemoral TAVR did have lower mortality than transapical (%6 vs. %15) and lower overall costs (%68,223 vs. $72,568). They summarized that TAVR in the "real-world" use of the device was associated with higher costs and mortality in both risk classes but did have lower major morbidity and resource utilization. The cost differential of the valve was the single biggest driver for the lack of cost-effectiveness for TAVR, but the opportunity to continue to lower costs through improved care delivery models focusing on reduction in LOS, resource utilization, and complications will make a difference [21–24]. However improved these care delivery model becomes the largest cost-savings opportunity for TAVR is lowering the cost of the valve. This will make TAVR unquestionably cost-effective in all categories of risk and in particular lower-risk patients.

Despite all the vagaries with the current cost-effectiveness data, we must recognize that these are rapidly evolving technologies and this data may be skewed because of its age and clinical and financial outcomes using outdated delivery platforms. Therefore, we must accept the challenge that cost-effectiveness can be achieved for certain populations of patients. We as providers must work with industry to make this disruptive technology available to Medicare beneficiaries as well as all patients. We as physicians must work with our hospital to create new care delivery pathways that reduce costs for this and all transcatheter technologies. Industry must recognize that the cost of the valve currently is prohibitive to widespread adoption. We must all recognize that the National Coverage Determination (NCD) is here to stay and that we can work together to possibly reopen it and create physician and institutional criteria to expand the use of all of these technologies, be it TAVR or mitral valve therapies. We must, however, pay attention to appropriate use of these technologies not only in patients with advanced age and multiple comorbidities but most importantly in younger patients. The risk of multiple TAVR procedures in younger patients when the durability of the device is not completely known should be part of a ongoing discussion. Do we need to use cost-effectiveness models to include not only the cost of the procedure and future-related costs but also unrelated future costs? Are we doing a patient with moderate dementia a favor by performing a TAVR only for the patient to forget who he or she is afterwards? Our obligation should always be: what is the societal value in performing life-extending procedures when the quality of life following it cannot be determined or does not improve? As TAVR moves farther away from these questionable patients and into expanded lower risk populations, clinical-effectiveness and cost-effectiveness must be demonstrated through the methods outlined above. If that can be accomplished we will have given our patients enormous clinical benefit and payers the security of knowing that value can be obtained through the use of all transcatheter technologies.

References

1. 2014 Medicare Trustees Report at www.CMS.gov
2. Reynolds MR, Magnuson EA, Lei Y, et al. Cost-effectiveness of transcatheter aortic valve replacement compared with surgical aortic valve replacement in high-risk patients with severe aortic stenosis: results of the PARTNER (Placement of Aortic Transcatheter Valves) trial (Cohort A). J Am Coll Cardiol. 2012;60(25):2683–92.
3. Reynolds MR, Magnuson EA, Wang K, et al. Cost-effectiveness of transcatheter aortic valve replacement compared with standard care among inoperable patients with severe aortic stenosis: results from the placement of aortic transcatheter valves (partner) trial (Cohort B). Circulation. 2012;125(9):1102–9.
4. Leon MB, Smith CR, Mack M, et al. Transcatheter aortic-valve implantation for aortic stenosis in patients who cannot undergo surgery. N Engl J Med. 2010;363(17):1597–607.
5. Smith CR, Leon MB, Mack M. Transcatheter versus surgical aortic-valve replacement in high-risk patients. N Engl J Med. 2011;364(23):2187–98.
6. Osnabrugge RL, Speir AM, Head SJ, Fonner CE, Fonner Jr E, Ailawadi G, Kappetein AP, Rich JB. Costs for surgical aortic valve replacement according to pre-operative risk categories. Ann Thorac Surg. 2013;96:500–6.
7. d'Arcy J, Prendergast B, et al. Valvular heart disease: the next cardiac epidemic. Heart. 2011;97:91–3.
8. Reynols MR, Magnuson EA, et al. Health related quality of life after transcatheter or surgical aortic valve replacement in high-risk with severe AS: results from the Partner Trial (Cohort A). J Am Coll Cardiol. 2012;60:548–58.
9. Osnabrugge RL, Kappetein AP, Reynolds MR, Cohen DJ. Cost-effectiveness of transcatheter valvular interventions: economic challenges. EuroIntervention. 2013;9(Suppl):S48–54.
10. Gada H, Kapadia SR, et al. Markov model for selection of aortic valve replacement implantation versus transcatheter aortic valve implantation (without replacement) in high risk patients. Am J Cardiol. 2012;109:1326–33.

11. Van Baal PH, et al. Future costs, fixed healthcare budgets, and the decision rules of cost-effective analysis. Health Economics (2014). Wiley Online Library (wileyonline library. com). doi:10.1002/hec.3138.
12. Iannconne A, et al. Cost-effectiveness of transcatheter aortic valve replacement compared with medical management or surgery for patients with aortic stenosis. Appl Health Econ Health Policy. 2015;13(1):29–45.
13. Falk V. Should transcatheter aortic valve replacement be expanded to lower-risk and younger patients. Circulation. 2014;130:2332–42.
14. Indranatna P, Ang SC, et al. Systematic review of the cost-effectiveness of transcatheter aortic valve implantation. J Thorac Cardiovasc Surg. 2014;148:509–14.
15. Osnabrugge RL, Head SJ, Kappentein AP. Transcatheter aortic valve implantation (TAVI): risky and costly or challenging and promising? BMJ. Letter to the Editor. August 2012.
16. Van Brabandt H, Neyt M, et al. Transcatheter aortic valve implantation (TAVI): risky and costly. BMJ. 2012;345, e4710.
17. Osnabrugge RL, Head SJ, et al. Costs of transcatheter versus surgical aortic valve replacement in intermediate-risk patients. Ann Thoac Surg. 2012;94:1954–60.
18. Neyt M, Van Brabandt H, et al. A cost-utility analysis of transcatheter aortic valve implantation in Belgium: focusing on a well-defined and identifiable population. BMJ Open 2012;2(3).
19. Ribera A, Slof J, Andrea R, et al. Transfemoral transcatheter aortic valve replacement compared with surgical replacement in patients with severe aortic stenosis and comparable risk: cost-utility and its determinants. Int J Cardiol. 2014;182C:321–8.
20. Ailawadi G, LaPar D, et al. Establishing the "RealWorld" costs associated with transcatheter aortic valve replacement: a propensity matched-cost analysis. Presented at the society of thoracic surgeons annual meeting, Jan 27, 2015.
21. LaPar DJ, Crosby IK, Ailawadi G, et al. Blood product conservation is associated with improved outcomes and reduced costs after cardiac surgery. J Thorac Cardiovasc Surg. 2013;145(3):796–803. discussion 45–6.
22. Arnold SV, Lei Y, et al. Costs of peri-procedural complications in patients treated with transcatheter aortic valve replacement: results from placement of aortic transcatheter valve trial. Circ Cardiovasc Interv. 2014;7(6):829–36.
23. Rich JB, Speir AM, Fonner Jr E. Virginia cardiac surgery quality initiative. Making a business case for quality by regional information sharing involving cardiothoracic surgery. Am Heart Hosp J. 2006;4:142–7.
24. Speir AM, Kasirajan V, Barnett SD, et al. Additive costs of post-operative complications for isolated coronary bypass grafting patients in Virginia. Ann Thorac Surg. 2009;88(1):40–5. discussion 45–6.

Chapter 9
Challenges in Valve-in-Valve Therapy for Aortic Valves

Vinnie (Vinayak) Bapat, Rizwan Attia, Waqar Aziz, Rahee Radia, and Francesco Prione

Introduction

Transcatheter aortic valve replacement (TAVR) has recently established itself as the treatment of choice in inoperable and high-risk patients with aortic stenosis [1–5]. Experience in this field has led to its usage for novel indications such as its use in the treatment of a degenerative biological surgical heart valve (SHV). Although the early data on valve-in-valve (VIV) is promising, the data from the Global VIV registry demonstrates that the procedure is not without risks [6–9]. High residual gradients, i.e. >20 mmHg were not uncommon, especially in smaller-sized SHVs, the reported incidence of coronary occlusion was 3.5 % and device malpositioning was 15.3 % [9]. Incidences of embolization, dislodgment, and thrombosis have also been reported [10–13].

There are at least 16 stented SHVs and 6 stentless SHVs implanted in the last two decades. Similarly, there are 8 different transcatheter heart valves (THV) currently available, namely, Sapien® and its newer generations (Edwards Lifesciences),

V. Bapat, MBBS, MS, FCRS, FRCSCTh (✉) • R. Attia, BMedSci, MBChB, MRCS, PhD
Department of Cardiothoracic Surgery, Guys and St. Thomas' Hospital,
6th floor, East Wing, St. Thomas' Hospital, London SE1 7EH, UK
e-mail: vnbapat@yahoo.com; rizwanattia@doctors.org.uk

W. Aziz, MB, BCh, BAO, MSc, MRCPI, MRCP
Department of Cardiology, Guys and St. Thomas' Hospital,
Westminster Bridge Road, London SE1 7EH, UK
e-mail: wkhan5@gmail.com

R. Radia
Department of Cardiology, Guys and St. Thomas' Hospital,
Chorleywood Road, Rickmansworth, Herts WD3 ER, UK
e-mail: raheeradia@icloud.com

F. Prione, MD
St. Thomas Hospital, Westminster Bridge Road, London SE17EH, UK
e-mail: pironef@virgilio.it

© Springer Science+Business Media New York 2016   119
G. Ailawadi, I.L. Kron (eds.), *Catheter Based Valve and Aortic Surgery*,
DOI 10.1007/978-1-4939-3432-4_9

CoreValve® and its newer generation (Medtronic Inc., USA), Portico® (St Jude Medical, USA), Lotus® valve (Boston Scientific, USA), Engager® (Medtronic), JenaValve (JenaValve, Germany), ACURATE TA® (Symetis SA, Switzerland), and Direct Flow ® (Direct Flow Medical, USA) [14]. Of these, the largest experience with VIV has been reported with the use of Sapien valve and CoreValve [9]. To optimize the result following a VIV procedure, it is important to understand the structure of the SHV being treated, the THV being used, and the interaction between them. This is important to avoid three main complications—embolization (as a result of incorrect placement and/or under sizing), high gradients (due to oversizing and/or lower placement), and coronary obstruction. We aim to discuss relevant features of the different devices (SHV and THV) and discuss the optimal strategy to avoid these complications after a VIV procedure. We aim to outline:

1. The design features of THV relevant to VIV

   Sizing
   Positioning

2. The design features of the stented SHVs relevant to VIV

   Classification
   Features that impact sizing
   Features that impact positioning

3. The design features of the stentless SHVs relevant to VIV

   Classification
   Features that impact sizing
   Features that impact positioning

4. Coronary obstruction and VIV
5. Patient selection

The Design Features: THV

At the time of writing there are eight THVs available for implantation in Europe. The most experience in the aortic position is with the balloon-expandable Edward Sapien® valve (this includes the first-generation Sapien, the second-generation Sapien XT, and the third-generation Sapien 3) (Edwards Lifesciences, Irvine, CA, USA) and the self-expanding Medtronic CoreValve and Evolute (Medtronic Inc, Minneapolis, MN, USA) [6–10]. Other THVs that have also been used for a VIV procedure but in limited numbers are St. Jude Portico® valve (St. Jude Medical, St. Paul, MN, USA), JenaValve® (JenaValve, Munich, Germany), Lotus® (Boston Scientific, USA), Engager® aortic valve bioprosthesis (Medtronic Inc., IS), and Symetis ACURATE TA® valve (Symetis, Ecublens, Switzerland) [15–17]. The similarities and differences in between the prostheses are highlighted in Table 9.1.

Table 9.1 Differences between various transcatheter heart valves

	Frame	Leaflets	Expandable	Aortic fixation	Reposition allowed	Treatable annulus diameter (mm)	Suitability for valve-in-valve	Access	FDA	CE mark
Edward Sapien/XT/ES3	Cobalt-chromium	Bovine pericardium	Balloon expandable	No	No	16–28	All four valve positions	Transapical/transaortic/transaxillary/transfemoral	2012	2007/2012/2014
Medtronic CoreValve	Nitinol	Porcine pericardium	Self-expanding	Yes	Yes	18–29	Aortic only	Transaortic/transaxillary/transfemoral	2014	2007
St. Jude Portico	Nitinol	Bovine pericardium	Self-expanding	Yes	Yes	19–27	Aortic only	Transfemoral	No	2012
JenaValve	Nitinol	Porcine root valve	Self-expanding	Yes	Yes	21–27	Aortic only	Transapical	No	2011 for AS and 2013 for AR
Lotus	Nitinol	Bovine pericardium	Self-expanding	Yes	Yes	20–27	Aortic only	Transfemoral	No	2013
Engager	Nitinol	Bovine pericardium	Self-expanding	Yes	Yes	21–27	Aortic only	Transapical	No	2013
Symetis ACURATE TA	Nitinol	Porcine Pericardium	Self-expanding	Yes	No	21–27	Aortic only	Transapical	No	2014

AS aortic stenosis, *AR* aortic regurgitations, *FDA* food and drug administration, *CE* Conformité Europeéne

All THVs have leaflet tissue (bovine or porcine) mounted into a frame. While leaflets are not visible, the stent frame of all THV (part or complete) is visible under fluoroscopy.

Two important features relevant to VIV procedure are:

1. Size range: dictates the internal diameter (ID) that can be treated
2. Structure under fluoroscopy with reference to the "nadir" of the leaflets and percentage of THV stent covered at its inflow

Majority of the published VIV data is for the Sapien valve and CoreValve prosthesis and hence these are discussed in detail regarding the sizing and positioning of device.

THV Size Range

Sapien and Sapien XT balloon-expandable valves are available in three sizes with 3 mm increments in diameter, i.e., 23, 26, and 29 mm (Fig. 9.1a, b). These can be used to treat an annulus size from 18 to 27 mm and hence can also be used to treat degenerated SHVs with ID of 18 to 27 mm [6–9, 18–20].

CoreValve is a self-expanding nitinol-based THV, which is also available in three sizes, i.e., 26, 29, and 31 mm (Fig. 9.1c), and can be used to treat SHVs with ID between 20 and 29 mm. Recently, 23 mm Evolute has been added to this line of devices (Fig. 9.1d) and it can be used to treat a smaller ID from 18 to 20 mm [9, 19–21].

Hence, SHVs with an ID less than 18 mm and larger than 27 mm may not be suitable for a VIV procedure with currently available Sapien and CoreValve.

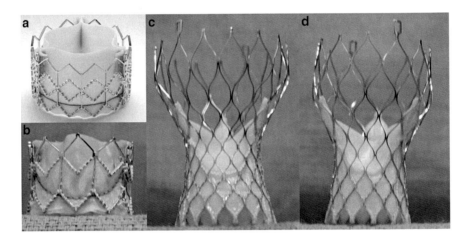

Fig. 9.1 First- and second-generation transcatheter valves. (**a**) First-generation balloon-expandable Sapien valve. Frame made of steel. (**b**) Second-generation balloon-expandable Sapien XT valve. Frame made of cobalt-chromium. (**c**) First-generation self-expandable CoreValve. Nitinol frame. (**d**) Second-generation Evolute valve. Compact nitinol frame

This also explains the higher residual gradients reported in the Global VIV registry when SHVs with label sizes of 23 or below were treated [9]. This is because of an incomplete and/or uneven expansion of the THV in a relatively smaller-sized SHV.

For detailed description of THV and SHV sizes and description of dimensions for Edwards Sapien XT, Evolute/CoreValve, Portico, and JenaValve, readers are referred to an interactive portal available as an app: https://itunes.apple.com/gb/app/valve-in-valve/id655683780?mt=8.

THV Structure Under Fluoroscopy

To place a THV in an ideal position within an SHV, it is important to know how to identify the "nadir" of the leaflets and covered portion of its inflow. Position of the "nadir" may decide intra- or supra-annular placement, which can influence hemodynamics. Similarly, the relationship between the covered part of the inflow and SHV can influence the presence of an intravalvular leak.

Sapien XT Size 23 and 26 mm are composed of two rows of cells, whereas the 29 mm device is composed of three rows of cells (Fig. 9.2a, b) with the 1st node marking the nadir of the leaflets. Only the top row is not covered with cloth. Hence, placement of the top row below the annular level will result in an intravalvular leak.

Evolute and CoreValve The third node marks the nadir of the leaflets and is an important anatomical landmark for supravalvular placement of this THV. The inflow is covered to the third node at the nadir and rises up to the outflow at its commissures (Fig. 9.2c).

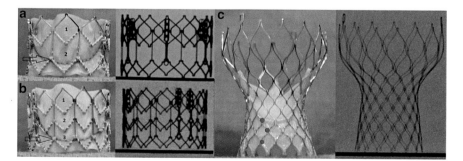

Fig. 9.2 Fluoroscopic correlation of Sapien XT and CoreValve. (**a**) Sapien XT device has a cobalt-chromium frame where the 23 and 26 mm valves are composed of two rows of cells. Row 2 is cloth covered. *Arrow* pointing to the nadir of the leaflets. (**b**) Sapien XT 29 mm device has three rows of cells. Row 2 and 3 are cloth covered. *Arrow* points to the nadir of the leaflets. (**c**) CoreValve, the inflow is covered up to the third node at the nadir and rises up to the outflow at its commissures (nodes marked with *red dots*)

The Design Features: Stented SHV

Although different in size, shape and components, all SHVs are composed of three different constituent parts. They are the stent frame, leaflets, and sewing ring. The stent frame with three posts or struts supports the leaflet tissue. The stent is made of titanium, polypropylene, or other polymers such as Elgiloy or Delrin and covered in a fabric or pericardium. The leaflets are sewn to the stent frame either inside or outside and are made of either porcine aortic leaflets or bovine pericardial tissue (Fig. 9.3). The sewing ring is made of cloth and is situated outside the stent frame at the level of the inflow of a SHV. This is sewn to the native aortic valve annulus after excising the aortic valve. Level of the sewing ring is the narrowest part of the SHV [17] (Fig. 9.4).

Classification or Types of SHVs

Stented valves can be further classified according to:

1. The type and arrangement of their leaflets, which may be:

    (a) Porcine aortic leaflets and sutured inside the stent (e.g., Mosaic) (Fig. 9.5a)
    (b) Bovine pericardial and sutured inside the stent (e.g., Perimount) (Fig. 9.5b)
    (c) Bovine pericardial and sutured outside the stent (e.g., Mitroflow) (Fig. 9.5c)

2. Their fluoroscopic appearances, which can include:

    (a) A visible sewing ring (e.g., Medtronic Hancock valve) (Fig. 9.6a)
    (b) A visible frame or (e.g., CE porcine valve) (Fig. 9.6b)
    (c) No radiopaque part (e.g., Vaskutek Aspire) (Fig. 9.6c)
    (d) A visible tip of the stent post (e.g., Medtronic Mosaic valve) (Fig. 9.6d)

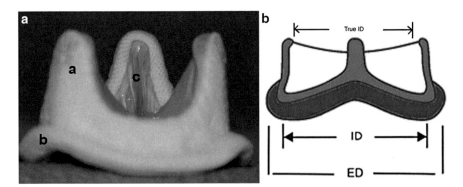

Fig. 9.3 Structure of a stented surgical heart valve. (**A**) Example of a bioprosthetic heart valve to highlight three parts, i.e., (a) stent frame, (b) sewing ring, and (c) leaflets. (**B**) Diagrammatic representation highlighting three important dimensions, which should be considered. ED: external diameter, which reflects usually the label size. ID: stent frame internal diameter without leaflet tissue. True ID: most relevant dimension for VIV procedure as it reflects ID with leaflet tissue mounted inside the stent frame

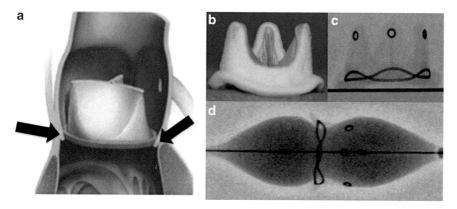

Fig. 9.4 Neo-annulus of a stented surgical heart valve. (**a**) Diagrammatic representation of a surgical heart valve implantation. *Arrows* point to the level where the sewing ring is sutured to the aortic valve annulus. (**b**) Hancock 2 porcine stented surgical valve. (**c**) Fluoroscopic appearance of Hancock 2 with visible markers at the sewing ring and three dots at the tip of the stent posts. (**d**) The neo-annulus of the Hancock 2 valve is the narrowest portion at the level of the sewing ring as seen by the waist in the balloon filled with contrast

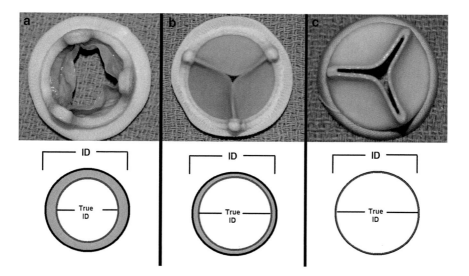

Fig. 9.5 Effect of valve type of the internal diameter of surgical heart valves—true ID (**a**) porcine valves where leaflets are mounted inside the stent frame (e.g., Mosaic). Stent ID is reduced by at least 2 mm. (**b**) Pericardial valves with leaflets inside the stent posts (e.g., Perimount 2700). Stent ID is reduced by at least 1 mm. (**c**) Pericardial valves with leaflets outside the stent posts (e.g., Mitroflow). Stent ID remains the same as the leaflets are mounted outside the frame

3. Their intended function or position after implantation:

    (a) Intra-annular (e.g., Edwards porcine CE Standard valve) (Fig. 9.7a)

    (b) Supra-annular (e.g., Edwards porcine CE SAV valve) (Fig. 9.7b)

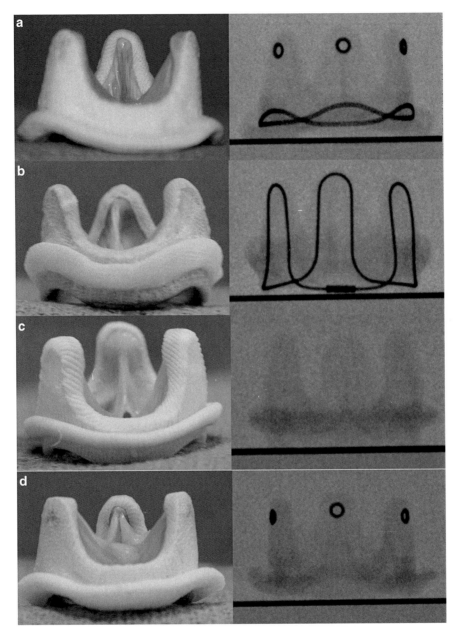

Fig. 9.6 Classification of stented surgical heart valves according to fluoroscopic appearance. (**a**) Sewing ring is visible: a visible fluoroscopic marker usually in the form of a ring is visible. Example shown is Hancock 2 porcine valve. (**b**) Stent frame is visible: Part or entire stent frame is visible under fluoroscopy. Example shown is CE porcine standard valve. (**c**) Not visible: although stented in structure, none of the valve parts are visible. Example shown is Aspire valve. (**d**) Mosaic valve: only tip of the three stent posts are visible

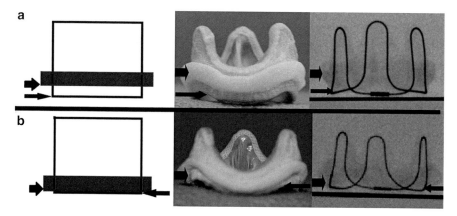

Fig. 9.7 Classification of surgical heart valves according to function. (**a**) Intra-annular design: Sewing ring (*short arrow*) is few mm above the base of the stent frame (*long arrow*). Once sutured, the base of the stent frame is within the left ventricular outflow tract. Example shown is CE porcine standard. (**b**) Supra-annular design: Sewing ring (*short arrow*) and the base of the stent frame (*long arrow*) are at the same level. Once sutured, no part of the stent frame is within the left ventricular outflow tract and valve sits supra-annularly. Example shown is CE porcine SAV

SHV Features that Influence THV Sizing

SHV label size usually reflects the external diameter (ED) of the SHV. But it is well known that SHVs of similar label size have different stent ID (Table 9.2). The stent ID is the diameter of the stent frame with cloth or pericardium but without leaflets. Hence, it may not reflect the true ID of a SHV after mounting of the leaflet material [22–24]. The degree of reduction in the stent ID depends on the type of leaflet (porcine or pericardium) and the way they are mounted (inside or outside) (Fig. 9.5). Table 9.2 highlights the differences between the label size 25 of four types of SHVs, their stent ID, and true ID.

Correct sizing is essential as undersizing increases the risk of paravalvular regurgitation or valve migration whereas oversizing leads to incomplete and/or uneven expansion of the THV with associated risk of leaflet distortion. This would determine immediate, gradients, and long-term, durability, results [25]. Hence, the true ID rather than the stent ID should be used to choose an appropriate THV (https://itunes.apple.com/gb/app/valve-in-valve/id655683780?mt=8).

SHV Features that Influence THV Positioning

An ideal level of implant within the SHV is where the THV is secure and has optimum function. During a TAVR within a calcified native aortic valve, the level of the annulus is used as a reference level [7]. During VIV, the level of the sewing ring is taken as the

Table 9.2 Table highlighting the differences between the label size 25 for four dufferent SHVs

Valve	Labeled size = Outer stent diameter	Stent Internal diameter	True internal diameter	Projected valve	Preferred valve
CE Standard (Edwards Lifesciences, Irvine, CA;aortic)	25	23	21	21	ES23, CV26, PV23, JV23
Mitroflow (Sorin, Milan, Italy; aortic)	25	21	21	21	ES23, CV26, PV23, JV23
Perimount (Edwards Lifesciences, Irvine, CA; aortic)	25	24	23	23	ES26, CV26, PV25, JV25
Magna (St. Jude Medical, St. Paul, MN; mitral)	25	25	24	23	ES26, CV26, PV25, JV25
Mosaic (Medronic Inc.; mitral)	25	21	21	21	ES23, CV23, PV23, JV23

ES Edward Sapien, *CV* Core Valve, *PV* Portico, *JV* Jena valve

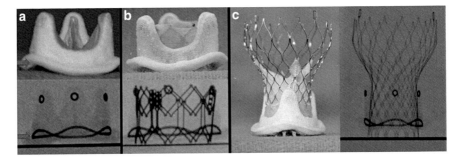

Fig. 9.8 Ideal position for implantation with relation to the neo-annulus or level of the sewing ring of a stented surgical valve. (**a**) Example shown is Hancock 2 valve. *Red arrow* point to the level for the sewing ring, which is its neo-annulus. (**b**) Fluoroscopic image of Hancock 2 to demonstrate level of neo-annulus is at the level of the sewing ring marker (*red arrow*). (**c**) Sapien XT ideal position: 15 % below the sewing ring marker to achieve secure anchoring and optimal function. (**d**) CoreValve ideal position: 4 mm below the sewing ring marker

reference level and is referred to as the "neo-annulus" [22, 23]. This is because it is the level of the inflow and is also the narrowest portion of the SHV (Fig. 9.4).

Thus, positioning of THV must be below this level. Higher placement may result in embolization. Thus, for the Sapien valve, the ideal implant level is 15 % below the sewing ring and for the CoreValve it is 4 mm below the sewing ring (Fig. 9.8). Too low a placement may still secure the THV but may result in suboptimal expansion and/or intravalvular leak as discussed earlier.

As most of the stented SHVs are visible on fluoroscopy, it is important to know how the level of the sewing ring relates to the fluoroscopic appearance of the SHV. This is explained below (Fig. 9.6):

(a) When part of the sewing ring is radiopaque: it identifies the level of the sewing ring, i.e., the neo-annulus and can be used to position the THV. There is no difference in the position of the neo-annulus between intra- and supra-annular valves. For example, the Sapien valve should be placed 15 % below the visible sewing ring marker for both Biocor (intra-annular design; Fig. 9.9a) and Biocor Supra (supra-annular design) to achieve an ideal position (Fig. 9.9b).

(b) When the stent frame is visible: it is important to differentiate between supra- and intra-annular models of the SHVs. When the design is supra-annular, as with the Trifecta, Perimount Magna Ease, and CE SAV valves, the lowest part of the stent is at the level of the sewing ring. Here, the Edwards Sapien valve should be placed 15 % below the fluoroscopically visible frame (Fig. 9.9c).

But, when the design is intra-annular, as with the Perimount and CE Standard valves, the sewing ring is 15 % above the lowest part of the visible stent. Here, the Edwards Sapien valve should be placed level with the fluoroscopically visible frame and not 15 % below to avoid low implantation (Fig. 9.9d).

(c) The Mosaic SHV is unique in its design as it has only three eyelets visible on the tip of the stent posts. An ideal position in this case is challenging and malposition has been reported with greater frequency [21]. Bench testing has now provided useful guidance in using these markers for ideal placement (https://itunes.apple.com/gb/app/valve-in-valve/id655683780?mt=8) [24]. Placement of the Sapien valve just below the eyelets and placement of the fourth node of CoreValve at the level of the eyelets results in an ideal and secure position (Fig. 9.10).

(d) When the SHV is not in radiopaque, use of contrast injections, echocardiographic and/or a balloon valvuloplasty to identify the neo-annulus is essential for correct placement (Fig. 9.11).

The Design Features: Stentless SHVs

There are eight different stentless SHVs that have been implanted in the last two decades. There are numerous challenges specific to stentless prostheses:

1. Stentless valves are not radiopaque.
2. The mechanism of valve failure is predominantly regurgitation.
3. The ID is affected by the method of implantation (supra- vs. intra-annular).
4. Risk of coronary obstruction may be high.

Classification

Stentless SHVs can be stentless valves or stentless roots. Stentless valves are either pericardium (bovine or equine) sutured to mimic an aortic valve or porcine aortic valves minus excessive sinus tissue (Fig. 9.12a). Stentless roots on the other hand

Fig. 9.9 Ideal implantation depending on the supra- and intra-annular design and visible fluoroscopic part. (**a**) Biocor intra-annular design: sewing ring visible and hence CoreValve is placed 4 mm below its level. (**b**) Biocor supra supra-annular design: sewing ring visible and hence CoreValve is placed 4 mm below its level. (**c**) Perimount 2800 intra-annular design: the level of the sewing ring is few mm higher to the base of the stent frame and hence CoreValve implanted to match the level of base of the stent frame. (**d**) Magna Ease supra-annular design: the level of the sewing ring is same as level of the base of the stent frame and hence CoreValve implanted 4 mm below the stent frame

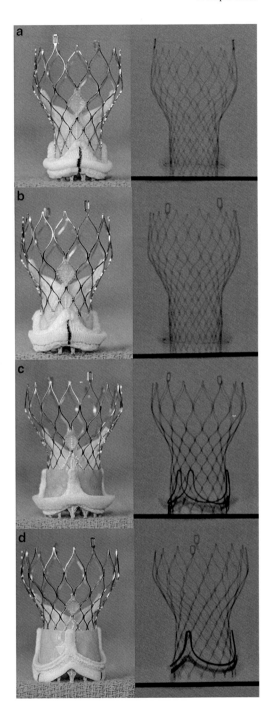

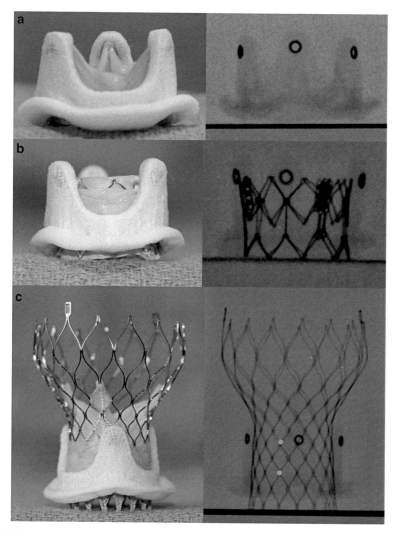

Fig. 9.10 Mosaic valve positioning (**a**) Only the stent post tips are visible on fluoroscopy (**b**) Sapien XT ideal position: For each combination of Mosaic and Sapien XT the ideal position is to place top margin just below the eyelets on the stent post tips. This confirms 15 % below the sewing ring level. (**c**) CoreValve ideal position: By placing the 4th node just below the eyelets on the stent post tips secures 4 mm of CoreValve below the sewing ring

are intact porcine roots with a part of the ascending aorta (Fig. 9.12b). Table 9.3 provides the different ways of implanting various stentless valves. Mini-root replacement is seldom done and few of the stentless models have been discontinued for more than a decade.

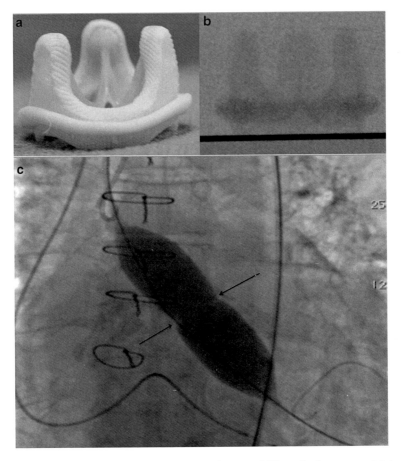

Fig. 9.11 Ideal position for stented surgical heart valves not visible under fluoroscopy. (**a**) Aspire valve by Vascutek is a stented porcine valve. (**b**) Aspire valve is not visible under fluoroscopy. (**c**) Balloon valvuloplasty if feasible can be used to delineate the level for the neo-annulus, which can be then used for the correct placement of the transcatheter valve

Stentless SHV Features that Influence THV Sizing

When stentless valves are implanted within an aortic root, it results in reduction in the ID of the native root. This should be measured by echocardiography, MSCT, and/or BAV as in performing TAVR in a native aortic root.

When treating a stentless root, the ID, also referred to as tissue annulus diameter (TAD) and true ID should be used as in the stented SHV (https://itunes.apple.com/gb/app/valve-in-valve/id655683780?mt=8).

As there is no frame and thick sewing ring, the neo-annulus lacks the rigidity of the stented SHV and hence it may be important to choose a larger THV in borderline cases for secure implantation [26].

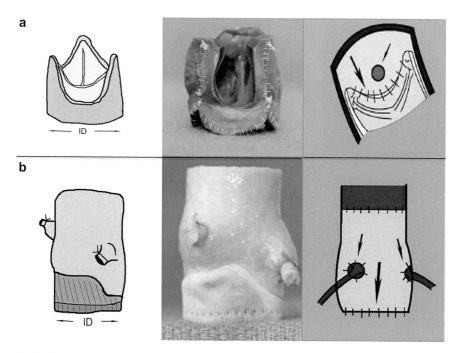

Fig. 9.12 Stentless porcine heart valves. Panel (**a**) demonstrates the subtype, i.e., "stentless valve." Example shown is the Cryolife O'Brien valve made of three porcine leaflets sutured together and is implanted in the subcoronary position within native aortic root (*long arrow* points to the suture line and *short arrow* to the coronary ostia). Panel (**b**) demonstrated the second subtype, i.e., "stentless root." Example shown is freestyle porcine root. It is an intact porcine root. Implantation is usually as a root replacement (*long arrow* points to the suture line at the level of the aortic annulus and *short arrow* to the site of reimplantation of the coronary arteries)

Table 9.3 Stentless valve types and aortic root replacement bioprostheses with placement details

Valve type and manufacturer	Root placement
Homograft	Full root, mini-root, subcoronary
Prima Plus (Edward Lifesciences)	Full root, mini-root, subcoronary
Freestyle (Medtronic)	Full root, mini-root, subcoronary
Toronto Root (St. Jude Medical)	Full root, mini-root
Shelhigh BioConduit (Shelhigh)	Full root
Shelhigh SuperStentless (Shelhigh)	Subcoronary
CryoLife-O'Brien (CryoLife)	Subcoronary
Elan (AorTech)	Subcoronary
Biocor PSB/SJM (St. Jude Medical)	Subcoronary
3 F Aortic Bioprosthesis (3 F Therapeutics)	Subcoronary
Pericarbon Freedom (Sorin)	Subcoronary
Toronto SPV (St. Jude Medical)	Subcoronary

Stentless SHV Features that Influence THV Positioning

As none of the stentless SHVs are visible under fluoroscopy, the following adjunct methods could be used for correct THV placement:

(a) Placement of a pigtail catheter in the aortic root with intermittent IV contrast injections to locate the level of the neo-annulus
(b) Slow two-stage inflation of the THV with aortic root injection of contrast with fine manipulation of the THV device during deployment
(c) Placement of a guide-wire in the left and/or right coronary ostia not only to protect the ostia from coronary obstruction but to act as a distal landmark during the slow inflation of the device (Fig. 9.13)
(d) Echocardiography

Use of the above methods is critical to avoid complications such as malpositioning and embolization. Risks and prevention of coronary obstruction are discussed in the following section.

Performing VIV in a stentless root may be easier than for stentless valves. VIV in a stentless root has lesser chance of coronary obstruction than VIV in stentless valves as in the former the coronary arteries are reimplanted and the anatomy is similar to native aortic root, while in the latter the suture line of the implanted valve is in close proximity to the coronary ostia (Fig. 9.12a) and hence there is a lower risk of coronary obstruction for root replacements. Additionally sizing is more straightforward as the ID is the same as the tissue internal diameter.

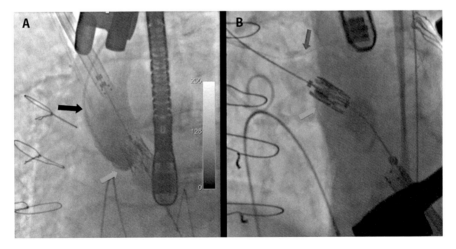

Fig. 9.13 Useful tricks for VIV procedure in a stentless valve. (**a**) Slow deployment of the device with contrast injection through a pigtail catheter (*black arrow*) to delineate the level of the annulus (*green arrow*). (**b**) Placement of a guide-wire (*red arrow*) in the left main stent not only helps to provide another landmark. *Green arrow* is at the level of the annulus

Coronary Obstruction

Coronary obstruction is a unique complication following an aortic VIV procedure. The reported incidence is 3.5 % and the etiology is multifactorial.

1. Risk is higher with stented SHVs with leaflets wrapped outside the stent (Fig. 9.5c) as seen in Mitroflow (Sorin) and Trifecta (St. Jude). The most likely reason is the outward displacement of the SHV leaflets toward coronary ostia.
2. Narrow aortic root.
3. Excessive oversizing of the THV, which leads to displacement of stent posts as well as leaflets.
4. Stentless valves but not stentless root, because of the proximity of the suture line to the coronary ostia (Fig. 9.12a).

Anticipation and treatment is the key for a positive outcome. Thus:

1. When in doubt and when feasible, one should use BAV with aortic root injection.
2. Use recently available smaller THV sizes, e.g., Sapien XT 20 mm and Evolute 23 mm.
3. Use third-generation THV devices such as JenaValve/Evolute/Portico/Lotus (Fig. 9.14), which are either retrievable after complete/near complete deployment or preventing outward displacement of the SHV leaflets [15–17].
4. Protect the coronary ostia with guide-wires for rapid access if necessary.
5. Availability of CPB and peripheral cannulae with extra guide-wires in the right atrium and femoral artery for rapid peripheral cannulation.

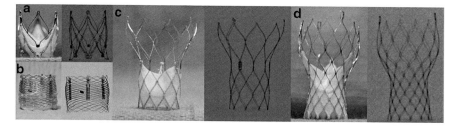

Fig. 9.14 Third-generation transcatheter heart valves. (**a**) Jenavalve: self-expandable device with unique-leaflet clipping mechanism. (**b**) Lotus: self-expanding valve made of a single nitinol wire. Repositionable and retrievable after complete deployment. (**c**) Portico: self-expanding device, which is retrievable after 80 % deployment. (**d**) Evolute: self-expanding second-generation CoreValve. Retrievable after 80 % deployment

Patient Selection: Current Recommendations

There are no guidelines available for patient selection specific to VIV. Although an attractive alternative, which is well suited for THV implantation, one should be aware of its limitations [27]. Hence, VIV should be considered only if:

1. A surgical option is considered prohibitive or high-risk.
2. A correct size of THV can be implanted to avoid high residual gradients.
3. Life expectancy of the patient is considered less than the predicted durability of the VIV combination.

Thus, small-size SHVs such as a 19-label size should be avoided when possible as they not only have a small true ID but are also implanted within narrow aortic root anatomy. Other important questions such as need and duration of anticoagulation and intermediate/long-term durability of unevenly expanded THV are yet to be answered. Ongoing work such as Global VIV registry, TCT VIV registry, and SOURCE VIV registry will help us shed light on these important issues and till then it is prudent to restrict the use of this therapy to a select group of patients.

References

1. Leon MB, Smith CR, Mack M, Miller DC, Moses JW, Svensson LG, Tuzcu EM, Webb JG, Fontana GP, Makkar RR, Brown DL, Block PC, Guyton RA, Pichard AD, Bavaria JE, Herrmann HC, Douglas PS, Petersen JL, Akin JJ, Anderson WN, Wang D, Pocock S, PARTNER Trial Investigators. Transcatheter aortic-valve implantation for aortic stenosis in patients who cannot undergo surgery. N Engl J Med. 2010;363:1597–607.
2. Smith CR, Leon MB, Mack MJ, Miller DC, Moses JW, Svensson LG, Tuzcu EM, Webb JG, Fontana GP, Makkar RR, Williams M, Dewey T, Kapadia S, Babaliaros V, Thourani VH, Corso P, Pichard AD, Bavaria JE, Herrmann HC, Akin JJ, Anderson WN, Wang D, Pocock SJ, PARTNER Trial Investigators. Transcatheter versus surgical aortic-valve replacement in high-risk patients. N Engl J Med. 2011;364:2187–98.
3. Reynolds MR, Magnuson EA, Wang K, Lei Y, Vilain K, Walczak J, Kodali SK, Lasala JM, O'Neil WW, Davidson CJ, Smith CR, Leon MB, Cohen DJ. Cost-effectiveness of transcatheter aortic valve replacement compared with standard care among inoperable patients with severe aortic stenosis: results from the Placement of Aortic Transcatheter Valves (PARTNER) trial (cohort B). Circulation. 2012;125:1102–9.
4. Kodali SK, Williams MR, Smith CR, Svensson LG, Webb JG, Makkar RR, Fontana GP, Dewey TM, Thourani VH, Pichard AD, Fischbein M, Szeto WY, Lim S, Greason KL, Teirstein PS, Malaisrie SC, Douglas PS, Hahn RT, Whisenant B, Zajarias A, Wang D, Akin JJ, Anderson WN, Leon MB, PARTNER Trial Investigators. Two-year outcomes after transcatheter or surgical aortic-valve replacement. N Engl J Med. 2012;366:1686–95.
5. Di Mario C, Eltchaninoff H, Moat N, Goicolea J, Ussia GP, Kala P, Wenaweser P, Zembala M, Nickenig G, Alegria Barrero E, Snow T, Iung B, Zamorano P, Schuler G, Corti R, Alfieri O, Prendergast B, Ludman P, Windecker S, Sabate M, Gilard M, Witowski A, Danenberg H, Schroeder E, Romeo F, Macaya C, Derumeaux G, Maggioni A, Tavazzi L, Transcatheter Valve Treatment Sentinel Registry (TCVT) Investigators of the EURObservational Research Programme (EORP) of the European Society of Cardiology. The 2011-12 pilot European Sentinel Registry of Transcatheter Aortic Valve Implantation: in-hospital results in 4,571 patients. EuroIntervention. 2013;22(8):1362–71.

6. Eggebrecht H, Schäfer U, Treede H, Boekstegers P, Babin-Ebell J, Ferrari M, Möllmann H, Baumgartner H, Carrel T, Kahlert P, Lange P, Walther T, Erbel R, Mehta RH, Thielmann M. Valve-in-valve transcatheter aortic valve implantation for degenerated bioprosthetic heart valves. JACC Cardiovasc Interv. 2011;4:1218–27.
7. Makkar RR, Jilaihawi H, Chakravarty T, Fontana GP, Kapadia S, Babaliaros V, Cheng W, Thourani VH, Bavaria J, Svensson L, Kodali S, Shiota T, Siegel R, Tuzcu EM, Xu K, Hahn RT, Herrmann HC, Reisman M, Whisenant B, Lim S, Beohar N, Mack M, Teirstein P, Rihal C, Douglas PS, Blackstone E, Pichard A, Webb JG, Leon MB. Determinants and outcomes of acute transcatheter valve-in-valve therapy or embolization: a study of multiple valve implants in the U.S. PARTNER trial (Placement of AoRTic TraNscathetER Valve Trial Edwards SAPIEN Transcatheter Heart Valve). J Am Coll Cardiol. 2013;62:418–30.
8. Ihlberg L, Nissen H, Nielsen NE, Rück A, Busund R, Klaarborg KE, Soendergaard L, Harnek J, Miettinen H, Eskola M, Wahba A, Laine M. Early clinical outcome of aortic transcatheter valve-in-valve implantation in the Nordic countries. J Thorac Cardiovasc Surg. 2013;146:1047–54.
9. Dvir D, Webb J, Brecker S, Bleiziffer S, Hildick-Smith D, Colombo A, Descoutures F, Hengstenberg C, Moat NE, Bekeredjian R, Napodano M, Testa L, Lefevre T, Guetta V, Nissen H, Hernández JM, Roy D, Teles RC, Segev A, Dumonteil N, Fiorina C, Gotzmann M, Tchetche D, Abdel-Wahab M, De Marco F, Baumbach A, Laborde JC, Kornowski R. Transcatheter aortic valve replacement for degenerative bioprosthetic surgical valves: results from the global valve-in-valve registry. Circulation. 2012;126:2335–44.
10. Eggebrecht H, Schmermund A, Kahlert P, Erbel R, Voigtländer T, Mehta RH. Emergent cardiac surgery during transcatheter aortic valve implantation (TAVI): a weighted meta-analysis of 9,251 patients from 46 studies. EuroIntervention. 2013;8:1072–80.
11. Tay EL, Gurvitch R, Wijeysinghe N, Nietlispach F, Leipsic J, Wood DA, Yong G, Cheung A, Ye J, Lichtenstein SV, Carere R, Thompson C, Webb JG. Outcome of patients after transcatheter aortic valve embolization. JACC Cardiovasc Interv. 2011;4:228–34.
12. Cota L, Stabile E, Agrusta M, Sorropago G, Pucciarelli A, Ambrosini V, Mottola G, Esposito G, Rubino P. Bioprostheses "thrombosis" after transcatheter aortic valve replacement. J Am Coll Cardiol. 2013;61:789–91.
13. Mylotte D, Andalib A, Thériault-Lauzier P, Dorfmeister M, Girgis M, Alharbi W, Chetrit M, Galatas C, Mamane S, Sebag I, Buithieu J, Bilodeau L, de Varennes B, Lachapelle K, Lange R, Martucci G, Virmani R, Piazza N. Transcatheter heart valve failure: a systematic review. Eur Heart J. 2015;36(21):1306–27.
14. Taramasso M, Pozzoli A, Latib A, La Canna G, Colombo A, Maisano F, Alfieri O. New devices for TAVI: technologies and initial clinical experiences. Nat Rev Cardiol. 2014;11:157–67.
15. Kim WK, Kempfert J, Walther T, Möllmann H. Transfemoral valve-in-valve implantation of a St. Jude Medical Portico in a failing trifecta bioprosthesis: a case report. Clin Res Cardiol. 2015;104(4):363–5.
16. Van Linden A, Blumenstein J, Möllmann H, Kim WK, Walther T, Kempfert J. Image-based decision-making treatment of degenerated mitroflow and trifecta prostheses. Ann Thorac Surg. 2014;98:1809–13.
17. Kemfert J, Mollmann H, Walther T. Symetis ACURATE TA valve. Eurointervention. 2012;8(Suppl Q):Q102–9. doi:10.4244/EIJV8SQA19.
18. Piazza N, Bleiziffer S, Brockmann G, Hendrick R, Deutsch MA, Opitz A, Mazzitelli D, Tassani-Prell P, Schreiber C, Lange R. Transcatheter aortic valve implantation for failing surgical aortic bioprosthetic valve: from concept to clinical application and evaluation (part 2). J Am Coll Cardiol Cardiovasc Interv. 2011;4:733–42.
19. Pasic M, Unbehaun A, Dreysse S, Buz S, Drews T, Kukucka M, Hetzer R. Transapical aortic valve implantation after previous aortic valve replacement: clinical proof of the "valve-in-valve" concept. J Thorac Cardiovasc Surg. 2011;142:270–7.
20. Kempfert J, Van Linden A, Linke A, Borger MA, Rastan A, Mukherjee C, Ender J, Schuler G, Mohr FW, Walther T. Transapical off-pump valve-in-valve implantation in patients with degenerated aortic xenografts. Ann Thorac Surg. 2010;89:1934–41.

21. Khawaja MZ, Haworth P, Ghuran A, Lee L, de Belder A, Hutchinson N, Trivedi U, Laborde JC, Hildick-Smith D. Transcatheter aortic valve implantation for stenosed and regurgitant aortic valve bioprostheses CoreValve for failed bioprosthetic aortic valve replacements. J Am Coll Cardiol. 2010;55:97–101.
22. Bapat V, Mydin I, Chadalavada S, Tehrani H, Attia R, Thomas M. A guide to fluoroscopic identification and design of bioprosthetic valves: a reference for valve-in-valve procedure. Catheter Cardiovasc Interv. 2013;81:853–61.
23. Noorani A, Attia R, Bapat V. Valve-in-valve procedure: importance of the anatomy of surgical bioprostheses. Multimed Man Cardiothorac Surg. 2014. doi:10.1093/mmcts/mmu020.
24. Christakis GT, Buth KJ, Goldman BS, Fremes SE, Rao V, Cohen G. Inaccurate and misleading valve sizing: a proposed standard for valve size nomenclature. Ann Thorac Surg. 1998;66:1198–203.
25. Milburn K, Bapat V, Thomas M. Valve-in-valve implantations: is this the new standard for degenerated bioprostheses? Review of the literature. Clin Res Cardiol. 2014;103:417–29.
26. Bapat V, Davies W, Attia R, Hancock J, Bolter K, Young C, Redwood S, Thomas M. Use of balloon expandable transcatheter valves for valve-in-valve implantation in patients with degenerative stentless aortic bioprostheses: technical considerations and results. J Thorac Cardiovasc Surg. 2014;148:917–22.
27. Bapat V, Attia R, Redwood S, Hancock J, Wilson K, Young C, et al. Use of transcatheter heart valves for a valve-in-valve implantation in patients with degenerated aortic bioprosthesis: technical considerations and results. J Thorac Cardiovasc Surg. 2012;144:1372–9.

Chapter 10
Anatomy and Pathophysiology of Mitral Valve

Leora T. Yarboro and Stephen W. Davies

Mitral Valve Anatomy

Leaflets

The mitral valve is comprised of the anterior ("aortic") and posterior ("mural") leaflets. The anterior leaflet is trapezoidal and has a greater surface area than the crescentic posterior leaflet. At the level of coaptation, however, it is the posterior leaflet which occupies two-thirds of the valve orifice. The posterior leaflet is often scalloped with each of the three scallops individually named, P1 (lateral), P2 (middle), and P3 (medial). The corresponding regions of the anterior leaflet where the valve coapts are identified as A1–3 [1–3] (Fig. 10.1).

The leaflets are composed of three distinct layers: atrialis, spongiosa, and fibrosa/ventricularis [2–4]. Each layer has a unique composition of collagen and proteins which are responsible for leaflet remodeling and mechanical stability. The normal leaflet is 3–5 mm in thickness and has three functional zones. The rough zone is the free edge of the leaflet where the main chordal attachments exist. The clear zone is the area between the rough zone and the basal zone where the leaflet connects to the annulus [3] (Fig. 10.2).

L.T. Yarboro, MD (✉)
Department of Surgery, University of Virginia, PO Box 800679,
Charlottesville, VA 22908, USA
e-mail: LJT9R@Virginia.edu

S.W. Davies, MD, MPH
Department of Surgery, University of Virginia Medical Center, 1215 Lee Street,
Room 4067, Charlottesville, VA 22903, USA
e-mail: SD2WF@virginia.edu

© Springer Science+Business Media New York 2016
G. Ailawadi, I.L. Kron (eds.), *Catheter Based Valve and Aortic Surgery*,
DOI 10.1007/978-1-4939-3432-4_10

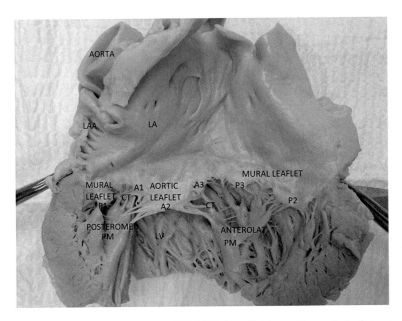

Fig. 10.1 Normal mitral valve anatomy. A1/A2/A3, three divisions of the aortic leaflet; anterolat PM, anterolateral papillary muscle; CT, chordae tendineae; LA, left atrium; LAA, left atrial appendage; LV, left ventricle; P1/P2/P3, three divisions of the mural leaflet; posteromed PM, posteromedial papillary muscle

Fig. 10.2 Mitral valve leaflet zones. LA, left atria; LV, left ventricle

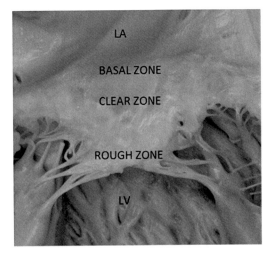

Annulus

The mitral valve leaflets are supported at their rough zone by a dynamic fibrous annulus with firm anchored attachments located at the trigones [1–3]. The average mitral annular orifice ranges between 4 and 6 cm², and the average leaflet to annulus area ratio is approximately 1.5–2.0 [2]. The anterior portion of the mitral valve annulus is in direct continuity with the fibrous skeleton of the heart which limits the degree of remodeling of the anterior leaflet. In contradistinction, the posterior annulus is comprised of muscular attachments in the intraventricular septum. This makes the posterior leaflet more dynamic and subject to dilation in cases of severe cardiomyopathy.

Chordae Tendineae

Tethering the leaflets to the left ventricle are the chordae tendineae [1–3] (see Fig. 10.1). These fibrocollagenous structures are classified by the location of their attachment upon the leaflet. Primary chordae are thin, originate from the papillary muscles, and insert upon the free edge of the leaflet, thus preventing prolapse. Secondary chordae also originate from the papillary muscles but insert upon the body of the leaflet to prevent billowing. Finally, tertiary chordae are the thickest of the chordae and anchor the posterior leaflet to the ventricular, thus serving to reinforce and maintain ventricular shape.

Papillary Muscles

The papillary muscle bundles arise from the apical one-third of the left ventricle [1–3] (see Fig. 10.1). They are grouped into the anterolateral and posteromedial positions. Anatomic variability exists among the papillary muscle bundles both in regard to the number of muscle heads and their blood supply. Most commonly, the anterolateral muscle is single headed and derives a dual blood supply from both the circumflex and left anterior descending artery. The posteromedial muscle is most commonly dual headed and has a singular blood supply from either the circumflex or right coronary artery. The papillary muscles contract during systole, maintaining the mitral valve in the closed position against systemic pressure.

Mitral Valve Apparatus

The normal mitral valve apparatus (leaflets, annulus, chordae, and papillary muscles) is saddle shaped in three-dimensional appearance owing to the previously mentioned disparate annular composition [2, 4]. This configuration allows for maximum patency and coaptation at the annular level during diastole and systole, respectively. Maintaining this configuration is important to off-load strain from the leaflets and reduce leaflet tear and chordae rupture.

Surrounding Structures

The mitral valve is centrally located within the heart and surrounded by many vital structures [1]. Lying within the posterior atrioventricular groove near the posterior leaflet are the circumflex artery and coronary sinus. The anterior leaflet of the mitral valve abuts the left and noncoronary annuli of the aortic valve. At the area of the right trigone lies the bundle of His as it passes through the intraventricular septum. Awareness of these structures is important as they may be affected by the underlying pathology or may be at risk during repair.

Pathophysiology of the Mitral Valve

Mitral valve dysfunction can result from a disturbance in any aspect of the mitral valve apparatus and is broadly grouped into the functional categories of stenosis or insufficiency. The clinical presentation of both advanced mitral stenosis and insufficiency is similar. The timing and method of treatment, however, depends on the mechanism of failure.

Mitral Stenosis

Mitral stenosis (MS) is largely prevalent in developing countries and often associated with rheumatic fever from group A beta-hemolytic *Streptococcus* [5–7]. It is estimated that nearly 30 million people, worldwide, have chronic rheumatic heart disease and that one-third of these have mitral stenosis. Rheumatic fever stimulates persistent inflammation and hemodynamic injury, which over time may result in fibrosis, calcification, and fusion of the valve leaflets, annulus, and chordae (Fig. 10.3). In developed countries, stenosis is more commonly caused by calcification secondary to old age, poorly controlled diabetes, or end-stage renal disease [5]. Rarely, congenital deformities, metabolic disorders, systemic lupus erythematosus, and rheumatoid arthritis may also result in stenosis. Severe MS is defined as a mean valve area less than 1.0 cm^2 and a mean transvalvular gradient more than 10 mmHg. If left untreated, restricted blood flow into the left ventricle may result in left atrial enlargement, dysrhythmia, pulmonary hypertension, and right-sided heart failure. Clinical symptoms typically include dyspnea, which most prominently occurs

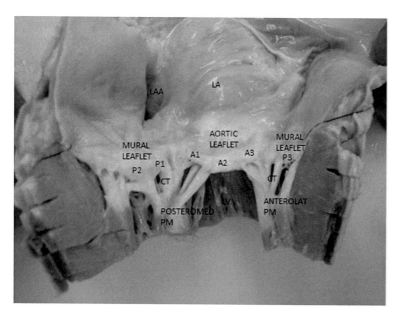

Fig. 10.3 Rheumatic mitral valve anatomy. A1/A2/A3, three divisions of the aortic leaflet; antero-lat PM, anterolateral papillary muscle; CT, chordae tendineae; LA, left atrium; LAA, left atrial appendage; LV, left ventricle; P1/P2/P3, three divisions of the mural leaflet; posteromed PM, posteromedial papillary muscle

during activity. Current treatment guidelines recommend percutaneous mitral balloon commissurotomy (Class of recommendation I, Level of evidence A) for symptomatic patients with severe MS (<1.5 cm²) and favorable valve morphology [8].

Mitral Insufficiency

Mitral insufficiency (MI) can result from primary leaflet pathology or secondary to ventricular dysfunction and dilation [2, 3, 9–12]. Carpentier's functional classification is often used to describe mitral insufficiency as the relationship of leaflet motion to the annular plane [3]. Type I refers to regurgitation resulting from isolated leaflet perforation (as seen in endocarditis) or annular dilation (Fig. 10.4). Type II refers to leaflet motion above the annular plane (e.g., degenerative MI). Finally, type III refers to restriction of leaflet function secondary to either ischemic cardiomyopathy or rheumatic heart disease. The following are subcategories of mitral insufficiency listed in order of prevalence.

Degenerative mitral valve disease is the most common etiology of mitral valve insufficiency. Characteristics of this process include chordal elongation/rupture, leaflet elongation, dilated and flattened mitral annulus, and leaflet coaptation at or superior to the annulus [2]. Degenerative mitral valve disease is often associated with other connective tissue disorders such as Marfan's or Ehlers-Danlos.

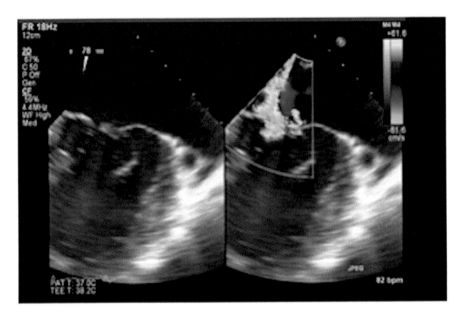

Fig. 10.4 Echo image of mitral regurgitation

Degenerative valve disease can affect a single segment of one leaflet (P2 prolapse) or involve the entire valve as seen with the billowing leaflets of Barlow's disease.

Ischemic mitral valve disease is the second most common etiology of mitral valve insufficiency. Disruption in the coronary blood supply can result in an acute presentation of mitral valve insufficiency as in papillary muscle rupture, or it can be insidious with progressive ventricular dilation resulting in annular dilation and restricted posterior leaflet function [11].

Rheumatic disease as discussed in relation to mitral stenosis can also result in mitral insufficiency. The thickened leaflets are unable to coapt appropriately resulting in valve insufficiency [3, 12]. In developing countries, this is the primary presentation of mitral insufficiency.

Finally, infectious endocarditis can result in mitral insufficiency [3, 12]. *Streptococcus* and *Staphylococcus* are the most common organisms identified in this disease process. The bacteria can cause insufficiency through acute leaflet perforation, large obstructive vegetation, and/or annular abscesses.

Catheter-Based Approach

Restoring mitral valve competence was once strictly performed via an open surgical approach [13, 14]. Increasingly, percutaneous techniques are being offered to "high-risk" patients (i.e., Society for Thoracic Surgeons Predicted Risk of Mortality >12 % and those with three or greater established the Society for Thoracic Surgeons high-risk criteria) as an alternative approach [13–20]. Mitral valve repair as well as replacement has been performed percutaneously. For these procedures, the mitral valve may be accessed via a venous atrial transseptal approach and retrograde arterial approach through the aortic valve or directly through the left ventricular apex. Each approach carries a unique risk profile, and access is often subject to patient-specific factors.

For mitral valve repair, the MitraClip (Abbott Vascular, Santa Clara, California System) is currently the most widely studied transcatheter-based mitral valve repair system [21, 22]. Access is obtained via the venous atrial transseptal approach using transesophageal echocardiographic guidance. The clip is positioned over the regurgitant jet, opened, advanced into the left ventricle, retracted to grasp the free edges of the mitral leaflets, closed, and then deployed (Fig. 10.5). This edge-to-edge repair corrects the regurgitation by coapting the leaflets and creating a double-orifice valve (Fig. 10.6). Multiple clips may be deployed to decrease the regurgitant jet. Additional transcatheter-based mitral valve repair modalities currently being evaluated include chordal repair and both direct and indirect annuloplasty.

Techniques for replacing the mitral valve are also being developed and optimized [21, 22]. Mitral valve anatomy is less suitable for implantation when compared to the aortic valve. As previously discussed, the mitral annulus is asymmetrical. Formfitting prosthesis to this while minimizing leak, left ventricular outflow obstruction, and aortic valve deformation has proven challenging. Initial success has been observed in those patients who undergo a valve-in-valve procedure where a new transcatheter-based valve is positioned inside of an old surgically placed valve. Valve migration, thromboembolism, and vascular injury are among the potential complications of these transcatheter-based procedures.

Fig. 10.5 Echo image of mitral clip deployment for mitral regurgitation

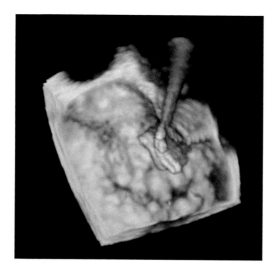

Fig. 10.6 Echo image of
mitral valve following
mitral clip deployment

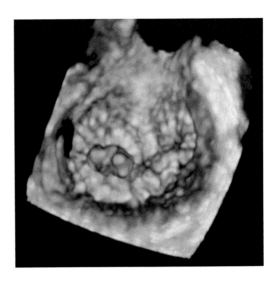

Summary

The mitral valve apparatus is a complex, multifaceted unit integral to normal heart function. Dysfunction in any of the components can result in valve incompetence and symptoms of heart failure. Restoring mitral valve competence was once strictly performed via an open surgical approach [13, 14]. Increasingly, percutaneous techniques are being used to access the valve. These approaches may have some benefit among patients who are high risk for open surgery. As the options for mitral valve repair and replacement continue to evolve, a precise understanding of anatomy and pathophysiology is as important as ever. Using this approach, the appropriate procedure can then be tailored for patient-specific needs.

References

1. Van Mieghem NM, Piazza N, Anderson RH, Tzikas A, Nieman K, De Laat LE, et al. Anatomy of the mitral valvular complex and its implications for transcatheter interventions for mitral regurgitation. J Am Coll Cardiol. 2010;56(8):617–26.
2. Dal-Bianco JP, Levine RA. Anatomy of the mitral valve apparatus: role of 2D and 3D echocardiography. Cardiol Clin. 2013;31(2):151–64.
3. McCarthy KP, Ring L, Rana BS. Anatomy of the mitral valve: understanding the mitral valve complex in mitral regurgitation. Eur J Echocardiogr. 2010;11(10):i3–9.
4. Schoen FJ. Evolving concepts of cardiac valve dynamics: the continuum of development, functional structure, pathobiology, and tissue engineering. Circulation. 2008;118(18):1864–80.
5. Chandrashekhar Y, Westaby S, Narula J. Mitral stenosis. Lancet. 2009;374(9697):1271–83.

6. Messika-Zeitoun D, Iung B, Brochet E, Himbert D, Serfaty JM, Laissy JP, et al. Evaluation of mitral stenosis in 2008. Arch Cardiovasc Dis. 2008;101(10):653–63.
7. Tani LY. Echocardiographic screening for rheumatic heart disease. Circulation. 2014;129(19):1912–3.
8. Nishimura RA, Otto CM, Bonow RO, Carabello BA, Erwin III JP, Guyton RA, et al. 2014 AHA/ACC guideline for the management of patients with valvular heart disease: a report of the American College of Cardiology/American Heart Association Task Force on Practice Guidelines. J Am Coll Cardiol. 2014;63(22):e57–185.
9. Adams DH, Rosenhek R, Falk V. Degenerative mitral valve regurgitation: best practice revolution. Eur Heart J. 2010;31(16):1958–66.
10. Grayburn PA, Weissman NJ, Zamorano JL. Quantitation of mitral regurgitation. Circulation. 2012;126(16):2005–17.
11. Boyd JH. Ischemic mitral regurgitation. Circ J. 2013;77(8):1952–6.
12. Madesis A, Tsakiridis K, Zarogoulidis P, Katsikogiannis N, Machairiotis N, Kougioumtzi I, et al. Review of mitral valve insufficiency: repair or replacement. Journal of Thorac Dis. 2014;6 Suppl 1:S39–51.
13. Glower DD. Surgical approaches to mitral regurgitation. J Am Coll Cardiol. 2012;60(15):1315–22.
14. Kaneko T, Cohn LH. Mitral valve repair. Circ J. 2014;78(3):560–6.
15. LaPar DJ, Isbell JM, Crosby IK, Kern J, Lim DS, Fonner Jr E, et al. Multicenter evaluation of high-risk mitral valve operations: implications for novel transcatheter valve therapies. Ann Thorac Surg. 2014;98(6):2032–7. discussion 7–8.
16. Chiam PT, Ruiz CE. Percutaneous transcatheter mitral valve repair: a classification of the technology. J Am Coll Cardiol Intv. 2011;4(1):1–13.
17. Wong RH, Lee AP, Ng CS, Wan IY, Wan S, Underwood MJ. Mitral valve repair: past, present, and future. Asian Cardiovasc Thorac Ann. 2010;18(6):586–95.
18. Mauri L, Foster E, Glower DD, Apruzzese P, Massaro JM, Herrmann HC, et al. 4-year results of a randomized controlled trial of percutaneous repair versus surgery for mitral regurgitation. J Am Coll Cardiol. 2013;62(4):317–28.
19. Glower DD, Kar S, Trento A, Lim DS, Bajwa T, Quesada R, et al. Percutaneous mitral valve repair for mitral regurgitation in high-risk patients: results of the EVEREST II study. J Am Coll Cardiol. 2014;64(2):172–81.
20. Feldman T, Young A. Percutaneous approaches to valve repair for mitral regurgitation. J Am Coll Cardiol. 2014;63(20):2057–68.
21. Grasso C, Capodanno D, Tamburino C, Ohno Y. Current status and clinical development of transcatheter approaches for severe mitral regurgitation. Circ J. 2015.
22. Maisano F, Alfieri O, Banai S, Buchbinder M, Colombo A, Falk V, et al. The future of transcatheter mitral valve interventions: competitive or complementary role of repair vs. replacement? Eur Heart J. 2015.

Chapter 11
Percutaneous Balloon Valvuloplasty for Mitral Stenosis

Michael Ragosta

Mitral stenosis is almost exclusively caused by rheumatic heart disease, a condition that has essentially disappeared from industrialized nations. In the United States, rheumatic mitral stenosis has become very rare but may still be seen in immigrants from countries where the condition remains prevalent or where medical care is underserved such as in rural populations or among Native Americans.

Worldwide, however, rheumatic heart disease remains a significant global health problem in impoverished and developing nations and the prevalence appears to be increasing [1]. It is estimated that 15 million individuals have rheumatic heart disease worldwide with 282,000 new cases each year [2]. The prevalence of rheumatic heart disease varies widely with the highest prevalence (>10 cases/1000 persons) in India, Pakistan, Southeast Asia, some African nations, the South Pacific, and in Central America. Patients with rheumatic heart disease living in developing countries suffer severely, not only due to the symptoms of their disease but also because the condition propagates their impoverished state as it leaves them unable to work or care for their families.

Pathophysiology of Mitral Stenosis The immune-mediated, inflammatory process triggered by untreated group A beta-hemolytic streptococcal pharyngitis damages the mitral valve causing thickening and fibrosis of the valve leaflets, commissural fusion and scarring, and shortening of the chordae and subvalvular apparatus resulting in mitral stenosis and creating the stenotic "fish mouth" orifice characteristic of rheumatic mitral valve disease and "hockey stick" deformity seen on echocardiography (Fig. 11.1) [3]. Other causes of mitral stenosis are very rare and include lupus, radiation heart disease, carcinoid heart disease, rheumatoid arthritis, endocarditis, and mitral annular calcification.

M. Ragosta, MD (✉)
Cardiovascular Division, Cardiac Catheterization Laboratory, University of Virginia Health System, Lee Street, Box 800158, Charlottesville, VA 22909, USA
e-mail: mr8b@virginia.edu

© Springer Science+Business Media New York 2016
G. Ailawadi, I.L. Kron (eds.), *Catheter Based Valve and Aortic Surgery*,
DOI 10.1007/978-1-4939-3432-4_11

149

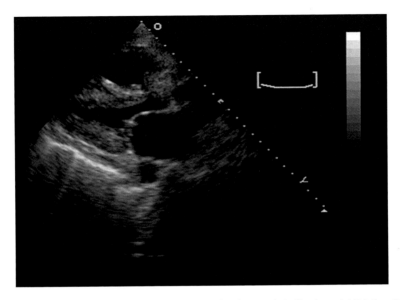

Fig. 11.1 Parasternal long axis view demonstrating the characteristic "hockey stick" deformity of rheumatic mitral stenosis. There is also thickening and calcification of the valve and thickening of the subvalvular apparatus

The normal mitral valve orifice is 4–6 cm². Symptoms generally occur with the development of severe stenosis, defined when the orifice area is < 1.5 cm². This usually correlates with left atrial to left ventricular diastolic gradients of 5–10 mmHg. Normally, a small pressure gradient exists between the left atrium and left ventricle only in early diastole; pressures rapidly equilibrate and there is normally no pressure gradient by mid to end diastole. As the valve area narrows, the left atrium cannot empty adequately during the time allotted for ventricular diastole and left atrial pressure rises. This causes a pressure gradient between the left atrium and the left ventricle to persist throughout diastole (Fig. 11.2). As stenosis severity worsens, the pressure gradient increases. In addition to stenosis severity, the pressure gradient is also influenced by the cardiac output and the heart rate. Patients with low cardiac output or hypovolemia may have low gradients despite severe stenosis. Importantly, since left atrial emptying is dependent upon the diastolic filling period, bradycardia allows more emptying time and will reduce the gradient while tachycardia shortens the diastolic filling period and increases the gradient (Fig. 11.3).

Mitral stenosis causes elevated left atrial pressure and this pressure is passively transmitted to the pulmonary veins, pulmonary capillaries, and the pulmonary arteries; thus, pulmonary hypertension is commonly seen in patients with severe mitral stenosis. If untreated, chronic elevation of pulmonary artery pressure may lead to permanent changes in the pulmonary vasculature and increase pulmonary vascular resistance. With long-standing, severe mitral stenosis, there may be severe and irreversible pulmonary hypertension with marked elevation of the pulmonary vascular resistance leading to right heart failure and end-stage mitral stenosis.

Fig. 11.2 This is a recording of simultaneous left ventricular and left atrial pressure obtained in a patient with mitral stenosis. Note the presence of a pressure gradient at end diastole (*arrow*)

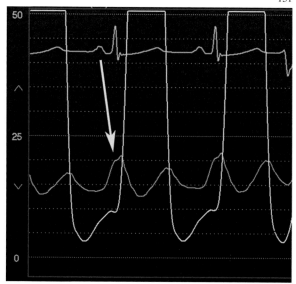

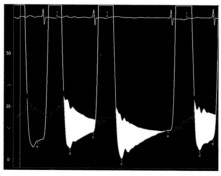

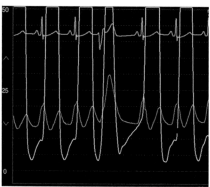

Fig. 11.3 This figure demonstrates the effect of the diastolic filling period on the transmitral pressure gradient. The panel on the *left* shows simultaneous left ventricular and pulmonary capillary wedge pressure in a patient with mitral stenosis and atrial fibrillation. The shorter cardiac cycles have a shorter diastolic filling period resulting in a greater pressure gradient while the longer cycles have a longer diastolic filling period and subsequently less pressure gradient. The panel on the *right* demonstrates the same phenomenon in a patient with mitral stenosis and sinus rhythm with a premature ventricular contraction. The prolonged filling period associated with the premature ventricular contraction resulted in a smaller transmitral pressure gradient

The symptoms of mitral stenosis reflect the underlying pathophysiology. Dyspnea syndromes, including dyspnea on exertion, paroxysmal nocturnal dyspnea, and orthopnea, are all familiar manifestations of mitral stenosis and are due to elevation of the left atrial pressure and from pulmonary hypertension. Wheezing and cough are common; mitral stenosis is not infrequently misdiagnosed as asthma. Mitral stenosis is associated with low cardiac output, and this causes profound fatigue and exercise intolerance. Additional symptoms include palpitations from atrial arrhythmias, hemoptysis from pulmonary congestion, and pulmonary hypertension and hoarseness from enlargement of the left atrium with compression of the recurrent laryngeal nerve. Edema and ascites are seen in the presence of right heart failure and are late signs of mitral stenosis.

Mitral stenosis generally has a long latent period and a slow progressive course; however, the disease may progress more rapidly in children. The rate of progression for moderate mitral stenosis is variable with some patients showing steady progression and others demonstrating no change over long periods of time [4]. Natural history studies have shown that, if untreated, long-term survival is good for asymptomatic patients but is poor when symptoms develop and prognosis is particularly poor when there are severe symptoms and/or there is severe pulmonary hypertension and right heart failure [5, 6]. Thus, it seems prudent to intervene prior to the development of pulmonary hypertension to prevent late and irreversible right heart failure. Complications of the condition include atrial arrhythmias and embolic events such as stroke, endocarditis, progressive biventricular heart failure, and increased risk of infections.

Therapy for Mitral Stenosis For patients with minimal or no symptoms and mild to moderate stenosis, medical therapy is the mainstay of treatment for rheumatic mitral stenosis [6]. Beta-blockers allow increased diastolic filling time, and diuretics are used to manage volume status and edema. Warfarin is strongly indicated for thromboembolic protection in patients with atrial fibrillation.

Symptomatic patients benefit from relief of valve obstruction either surgically or by balloon valvuloplasty. The surgical options of open commissurotomy and mitral valve replacement are effective; however, percutaneous mitral balloon valvuloplasty (PMBV) is less invasive and generally recommended as a first-line approach in patients with appropriate valvular anatomy [7].

Percutaneous Mitral Balloon Valvuloplasty (PMBV) Mitral stenosis was one of the first cardiac conditions approached surgically. The first closed commissurotomy was performed in 1925 by Henry Souttar, and this remained the only option for management of severe mitral stenosis for about 30 years until the introduction of cardiopulmonary bypass allowed direct visualization of the mitral valve and the development of open commissurotomy techniques. In 1982, the first percutaneous mitral commissurotomy was performed in Japan by Dr. Kanji Inoue using a clever balloon design that inflated differentially in the left ventricle, the left atrium, and finally the mitral valve orifice [8]. This device would not become available elsewhere until later. Other centers performed percutaneous mitral valvuloplasty initially with a single-balloon technique with some success [9]. This technique was subsequently replaced by the

Table 11.1 Indications for mitral balloon valvuloplasty

Class I indications
1. Symptomatic patients with severe mitral stenosis (mitral valve area ≤ 1.5 cm^2) and favorable valve morphology in the absence of left atrial thrombus or moderate-to-severe mitral regurgitation
Class IIa indications
1. Asymptomatic patients with very severe mitral stenosis (mitral valve area ≤ 1.0 cm^2) and favorable valve morphology in the absence of left atrial thrombus or moderate-to-severe mitral regurgitation
Class IIb indications
1. Asymptomatic patients with severe mitral stenosis (mitral valve area ≤ 1.5 cm^2) and valve morphology favorable for percutaneous mitral balloon commissurotomy in the absence of left atrial thrombus or moderate-to-severe mitral regurgitation who have new onset of atrial fibrillation
2. Symptomatic patients with mitral valve area greater than 1.5 cm^2 if there is evidence of hemodynamically significant mitral stenosis based on pulmonary artery wedge pressure greater than 25 mmHg or mean mitral valve gradient greater than 15 mmHg during exercise
3. Severely symptomatic patients (NYHA class III to IV) with severe mitral stenosis (mitral valve area ≤ 1.5 cm^2) who have a suboptimal valve anatomy for valvuloplasty but who are not candidates for surgery or who are at high risk for surgery

double-balloon technique [10]. These methods were effective but associated with a high complication rate including acute mitral regurgitation or cardiac perforation from balloon slippage. Eventually, in the early 1990s, the Inoue balloon became available. A comparison between the double-balloon and Inoue techniques found similar efficacy but less complications and shorter procedure time with the Inoue technique [11]. Specifically, the risk of cardiac perforation was less with the Inoue balloon, primarily because the balloon inflates in a more stable and predictable manner. The Inoue balloon is currently the preferred device for PMBV [12].

Recent guidelines for the management of valvular heart disease provide the indications for treating mitral stenosis with PMBV and are listed in Table 11.1 [7]. To summarize, PMBV is recommended in patients with severe mitral stenosis (valve area > 1.5 cm^2) and symptoms who have favorable anatomy (described below) and are without left atrial thrombus or significant degrees of mitral regurgitation. It is reasonable to perform PMBV in asymptomatic patients with very severe mitral stenosis (valve area < 1.0 cm^2) as long as they have favorable anatomy and no contraindications. Finally, valvuloplasty may also be considered in the following scenarios: (1) asymptomatic patients with severe mitral stenosis, favorable anatomy, and no contraindications who have new-onset atrial fibrillation; (2) symptomatic patients with lesser degrees of stenosis (valve area > 1.5 cm^2) but elevated wedge pressure or valve gradient > 15 mmHg during exercise; and (3) severely symptomatic patients with severe mitral stenosis and suboptimal valve anatomy but who are not good candidates for surgery.

Mitral balloon valvuloplasty works similar to surgical closed or open commissurotomy by separating the leaflets along the plane of commissural fusion. Therefore, this procedure is most effective when stenosis is caused primarily by commissural

Table 11.2 Echocardiographic scoring system used to predict success of mitral valvuloplasty [14]

Score	Leaflet mobility	Leaflet thickening	Leaflet calcification	Subvalvular thickening
1	Highly mobile, only tips restricted	Normal (4–5 mm)	Single area of echo brightness	Minimal thickening below mitral leaflets
2	Mid and base have normal mobility	Mid-leaflet normal, thick at margins (5–8 mm)	Scattered areas of brightness confined to leaflet margins	Thickened chordal structures up to 1/3 chordal length
3	Valve moves forward in diastole only from base	Entire leaflet thickened 5–8 mm	Brightness extends to mid-portion of leaflets	Thickening extending to distal 2/3 of chords
4	No movement of leaflets in diastole	Marked thickening (>8–10 mm)	Extensive brightness throughout	Extensive thickening and shortening of chordal structures to papillary muscles

fusion and when there is no heavy calcification of the leaflets or thickening and fibrosis of the subvalvular apparatus.

Echocardiography has proven extremely helpful in guiding the performance of PMBV [13]. During the planning stages, transthoracic echocardiography determines severity of mitral stenosis and provides valuable information regarding valve anatomy and suitability for balloon valvuloplasty. Several scoring systems have been developed to guide the operator in patient selection [13]. The Wilkins score is the most popular and takes into consideration several important pathologic features predicting success (Table 11.2) [14]. A score of 1–4, ranging from mild to severe abnormalities, is used to describe 4 variables: leaflet mobility, leaflet thickening, leaflet calcification, and subvalvular thickening. A Wilkins score < 8 is considered favorable for PMBV. Although the acute hemodynamic results and complication rates are higher in patients with scores > 8, patients with significant symptoms who are poor operative candidates may still derive benefit from mitral valvuloplasty, and PMBV is considered a reasonable option in those patients.

The degree of commissural and valve calcification is also an important predictor of outcome with PMBV. The greater the extent and severity of commissural calcification, the less likely PMBV will be successful and the more likely that significant mitral regurgitation will result [13, 15]. Heavy commissural calcification is a particularly important predictor in patients with low Wilkins score. Additional studies have found that the presence of a calcified valve leads to higher post-procedure gradients and worse long-term results [16]. Other scoring systems have been proposed but are somewhat more cumbersome to apply and have not yet been fully embraced by practitioners [13, 17].

The procedure is contraindicated in the presence of significant (more than 2+) mitral regurgitation and in the presence of a left atrial thrombus. As noted earlier, heavy commissural calcification may also be considered a contraindication since the balloon is more likely to tear the leaflets and cause mitral regurgitation instead of cleaving the fused commissures. Transesophageal echocardiography is recommended prior to the procedure to exclude left atrial thrombus; if present, the patient can be treated with anticoagulation until there is resolution of the clot.

Description of the Inoue Balloon Technique for Performance of PMBV Mitral balloon valvuloplasty is a technically demanding procedure [12]. It requires skill in transseptal puncture, a thorough understanding of the hemodynamics of mitral stenosis, skill in catheter manipulation, and skill in decision-making regarding the balance between the hemodynamic effect achieved with valve dilation and the potential for creating a greater degree of mitral regurgitation. This decision regarding "when to stop" is perhaps the most challenging aspect of the procedure and requires careful judgment and experience.

Once a transesophageal echo has been performed to exclude left atrial thrombus, the procedure is begun by performing a right and left heart catheterization from the femoral artery and vein. Right and left heart chamber pressures along with simultaneous left ventricular and pulmonary capillary wedge pressures are recorded at baseline along with determination of the cardiac output by Fick and/or thermodilution techniques. Mitral valve area at baseline is calculated by the Gorlin formula [18]. A left ventriculogram is usually performed to assess the presence and degree of mitral regurgitation prior to valvuloplasty.

Following the collection of baseline hemodynamics, a transseptal puncture is performed and a transseptal sheath inserted into the left atrium. The transseptal puncture is an important part of the procedure and is associated with one of the greatest risks of the procedure (perforation and tamponade). The transseptal puncture may be performed using fluoroscopic guidance or may be guided by intracardiac or transesophageal echocardiography during the procedure. The operator records simultaneous left atrial and left ventricular pressures and calculates mitral valve area at baseline. At this point, heparin is typically administered (50–70 U/kg intravenous bolus) to prevent thrombus formation on the catheters and wires.

A coiled-tip guide wire is then advanced through the sheath and positioned in the left atrium. Over this wire, a 14 F tapered dilator is carefully advanced across the atrial septum to allow easier passage of the balloon catheter. Next, the Inoue balloon (Toray Industries, Inc., Tokyo, Japan) is selected from one of the three available sizes (26, 28, and 30 mm). The appropriate balloon size is chosen based on the following formula: (patient height (in cm) divided by 10) + 10. For example, a 26 mm balloon would be chosen for a patient measuring 160 cm tall. For each balloon size, the initial inflation begins 4 mm less than the stated size. An additional 1 cc of saline can then be added to the balloon to incrementally increase its size during the procedure. Thus, the initial inflation size for a 26 mm balloon is 22 mm, but this can be increased to 23, 24, 25, and finally 26 mm by incrementally adding 1 cc of saline until the desired hemodynamic effect is achieved. This allows for a wide range of balloon inflation diameters during the procedure.

The Inoue balloon is prepared outside the body and inflated under saline to test that there are no leaks and to calibrate the inflation syringe to the balloon diameter.

A straightening tube is inserted to facilitate passage of the balloon. The tapered dilator is withdrawn, and the Inoue balloon with the straightening tube is advanced over the coiled-tip guide wire across the septum to about 12 o'clock. The straightening tool is pulled back about 2–3 cm and the catheter system carefully advanced to the 3 o'clock position. At this point, the inner tube is unlocked and pulled back and the catheter advanced to the 6 o'clock position. The guide wire and stretching tube are removed at this point. A stylet is then advanced within the balloon catheter to allow the catheter tip to be manipulated across the mitral valve orifice. Gentle counterclockwise turns while pulling back on the stylet guides the balloon catheter across the mitral orifice. This part of the procedure may be quite challenging and difficult to accomplish. Slight inflation of the balloon may facilitate its passage across the mitral valve.

There is usually ectopy when the balloon catheter crosses the mitral valve and enters the left ventricle. Care should be taken not to entangle the balloon in the chordae tendineae. Starting with the smallest balloon inflation for the chosen balloon catheter, the assistant begins to inflate the balloon. When the ventricular side is inflated, the operator gently snugs the balloon back against the mitral valve (Fig. 11.4). The assistant continues to inflate the balloon thereby inflating the atrial side and creating the characteristic dumbbell shape (Fig. 11.5). When the balloon is fully inflated, the middle and less compliant portion inflates exerting force on the mitral valve (Fig. 11.6).

The entire inflation process should take just a few seconds, and the balloon is then rapidly deflated. The steering wire is then removed and simultaneous left ventricular and left atrial pressure measured to assess the residual transmitral gradient (Figs. 11.7 and 11.8). Transthoracic echocardiography is performed to determine the presence or severity of mitral regurgitation.

Success is typically defined as a residual gradient < 5 mmHg or valve area > 1.5 cm^2 and no more than 1+ or 2+ mitral regurgitation. If the initial balloon dilatation fails to achieve the desired hemodynamic effect and there is no regurgitation, then additional balloon inflations can be performed by the addition of 1 cc of saline to the balloon (adding 1 mm to the balloon diameter). Following each inflation, hemodynamic measurements and assessment for degree of mitral regurgitation are repeated until a satisfactory result is obtained or mitral regurgitation develops.

Once the operator is satisfied, the straightening tube is reinserted along with the coiled-tip guide wire. The balloon catheter is carefully backed out of the left atrium and removed from the body. Right heart catheterization is repeated to determine cardiac output and pulmonary pressures and ventriculography performed to document the final degree of mitral regurgitation.

Acute Results of PMBV   The clinical results with PMBV have been well described [19–21]. The acute hemodynamic results are very good and are similar to those achieved with closed commissurotomy [19]. Palacios and colleagues describe the acute and long-term results in a carefully described cohort of 879 patients undergoing PMBV during the 1990s [20]. Overall, the investigators found that the average mitral valve area increased from 0.9±0.3 cm^2 to 1.9±0.7 cm^2 following

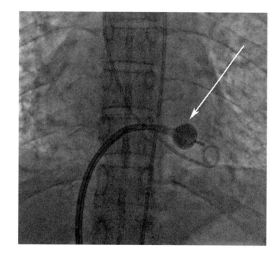

Fig. 11.4 The Inoue balloon is positioned from a transseptal approach across the mitral valve and is inflated. The balloon first inflates on the left ventricular side as shown here

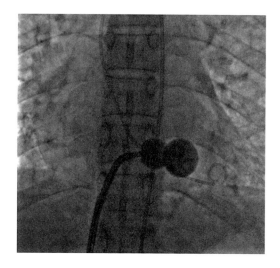

Fig. 11.5 With the ventricular portion expanded, the Inoue balloon is then pulled against the mitral annulus; further inflation results in inflation of the left atrial side of the balloon

PMBV. Similarly, the transmitral gradient decreased from an average of 14 ± 6 mmHg to 6 ± 3 mmHg. Immediately after PMBV, cardiac output increased, and both left atrial and pulmonary artery systolic pressures decreased significantly. Patients with Wilkins score ≤ 8 had better acute results with PMBV (valve area increased from 1.0 ± 0.3 cm^2 to 2.0 ± 0.6 cm^2) as compared to those with Wilkins score >8 (valve area increased from 0.8 ± 0.3 cm^2 to 1.6 ± 0.6 cm^2). Overall, 9.4 % of patients developed severe mitral regurgitation, 8.3 % of patients with Wilkins score ≤ 8, and 11.6 % of patients with Wilkins score >8. The overall procedural success is defined as achieving a valve area >1.5 cm^2 and no significant regurgitation occurred in 79 % of patients with Wilkins score ≤ 8 and 56.4 % of patients with Wilkins score>8. In

Fig. 11.6 The Inoue
balloon is then fully
inflated resulting in
dilatation of the mitral
valve orifice

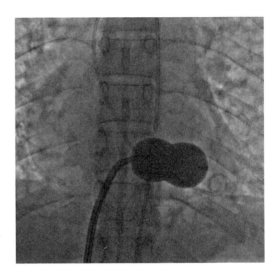

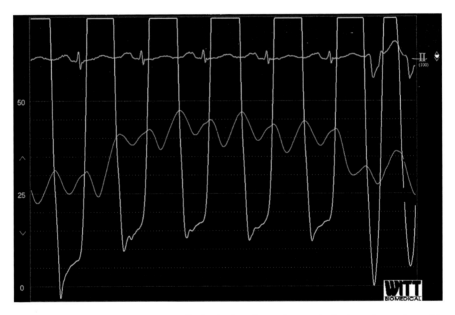

Fig. 11.7 Example of hemodynamics obtained at baseline, prior to valvuloplasty, in a patient with severe mitral stenosis. Simultaneous recording of left ventricular and left atrial pressure prevalvuloplasty shows a large diastolic gradient of approximately 25 mmHg

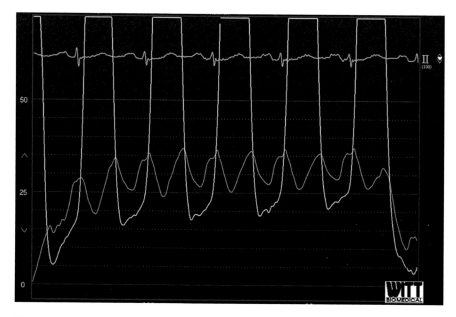

Fig. 11.8 Hemodynamics obtained post valvuloplasty in the same patient show that the gradient was reduced to about 5–6 mmHg

this series, complications were significant and included procedural-related death (0.6 %), tamponade (1 %), stroke (1.8 %), and significant mitral regurgitation (9.4 %). The need for acute mitral valve replacement was 3.3 % and the presence of a significant left to right shunt (Qp/Qs > 1.5) was 5 %.

Another series of 4850 patients from India with very severe mitral stenosis showed similar acute hemodynamic results of PMBV [21]. In this cohort consisting primarily of younger individuals (mean age of 27 years), the mean valve area increased from 0.7 ± 0.2 cm^2 to 1.9 ± 0.3 cm^2 ($p < 0.001$) and mean gradient decreased from increased from 29.5 ± 7.0 mmHg to 6.09 ± 2.1 mmHg ($p < 0.001$). The complication rate was substantially lower in this cohort with tamponade seen in only 0.2 %, an embolic event in only 0.1 %, and the development of severe mitral regurgitation in only 1.4 %.

Long-Term Results of PMBV and Comparison with Surgical Commissurotomy
The beneficial hemodynamic effects of PMBV are sustained over several years. In general, cardiac event and restenosis rates are very low for the first 5 years following PMBV [20, 22]. Younger patients with favorable valve anatomy and low (<8) echo scores do better than older patients with high (>8) echo scores and more calcified valves [20–22]. Importantly, it is clear that the greater the final valve area achieved immediately after PMBV, the better the long-term outcome [23]. Table 11.3 summarizes some of the larger series reporting the long-term outcomes after PMBV [20–22, 24, 25]. By about 10–12 years, roughly half of patients treated with PMBV will have developed restenosis and require repeat procedures or heart surgery.

Table 11.3 Long-term outcome after percutaneous mitral balloon valvuloplasty

Author (citation)	Number of patients	Mean age	Mean follow-up	Outcome
Palacios et al. [20]	879	55 ± 15	4.2 years	12-year event-free survival 38 % for echo score ≤8 and 22 % for echo score >8
Arora et al. [21]	4850	27 ± 11	7.8 years	Restenosis rate 4.8 %
Fawzy et al. [22]	531	31 ± 11	8.5 years	77 % 10-year survival free from restenosis
Iung et al. [24]	1024	49 ± 14	4 years	61 % 10-year survival free of surgery or repeat dilatation
Chen et al. [25]	4832	37 ± 12	2.7 years	Restenosis rate 5.2 %

Several randomized trials have compared outcomes between PMBV and both closed and open surgical commissurotomy [19, 26–28]. These studies demonstrate that the hemodynamic effect and long-term outcomes of PMBV are comparable to those achieved surgically. Patients with high echo scores, however, appear to do better with open surgical commissurotomy [29].

Role of PMBV in Specific Patient Subsets Patients with mitral stenosis living in industrialized nations tend to be significantly older than those from developing nations and the outcome of PMBV in elderly patients is less well established. Several investigators have shown that, while the success rates and long-term outcomes are clearly better in younger patients, outcomes are still good in elderly patients with mitral stenosis and are related primarily to the echo score [30–33].

Mitral stenosis is common in young women and may first manifest during pregnancy. Symptoms may greatly exacerbate and culminate in decompensated heart failure due to the detrimental effects caused by the increases in heart rate, cardiac output, and blood volume associated with pregnancy. In such circumstances, the performance of PMBV may be necessary during pregnancy. Several studies have found PMBV safe and effective during pregnancy with low morbidity and mortality for the mother and infant, improved conditions for labor and delivery, and favorable long-term outcomes [34, 35].

Patients with atrial fibrillation tend to be older and have more complex valve pathology with greater degrees of calcification and higher proportion of unfavorable characteristics for PMBV. Not surprisingly, valvuloplasty results in worse short- and long-term outcomes as compared to patients without atrial fibrillation [36, 37]. However, atrial fibrillation by itself is not an unfavorable characteristic but, instead, is a marker for features that are associated with worse outcomes with PMBV [37].

Severe pulmonary hypertension is another interesting subgroup. A recent study found PMBV safe and effective in this group [38]. Although the long-term results were not as good as compared to patients without severe pulmonary hypertension, PMBV resulted in a reduction in pulmonary pressure (79 ± 14 to 36 ± 7.5 mmHg; $p < 0.001$) and improvement in tricuspid regurgitation over 12 months.

Balloon valvuloplasty can be repeated in patients who have had prior balloon valvuloplasty (i.e., mitral valve restenosis) and appears safe and effective in patients who have had prior open, surgical commissurotomy, although the results are less favorable as compared to an initial procedure [39–42]. In general, patients with bioprosthetic valve stenosis are not appropriate candidates for PMBV; however, case reports have been published describing successful PMBV procedures in patients deemed inoperable [43].

Finally, PMBV is sometimes contemplated in the rare patient with severe mitral stenosis from conditions other than rheumatic heart disease. These include radiation-induced mitral stenosis and severe mitral annular calcification. In these conditions, PMBV is unlikely to be safe or effective because stenosis is not due to commissural fusion, and the procedure is more likely to tear the valve and create regurgitation. Thus, PMBV should not be offered in these conditions.

Summary

Rheumatic mitral stenosis is increasingly rare in developed countries but remains a problem in developing nations. Percutaneous mitral balloon valvuloplasty (PMBV) is the procedure of choice for symptomatic patients with severe mitral stenosis, suitable valve anatomy, and no contraindications. Echocardiography is an extremely useful tool for planning and guiding the procedure. The procedure is technically demanding and requires great skill and careful judgment for optimal results. The acute results are very good and similar to those obtained with open commissurotomy; optimal results are obtained in young patients with noncalcified, pliable valves with low echo scores. Event rates are low for the first 5 years after PMBV. However, by 10–15 years, about 50 % of patients develop restenosis and need either another valvuloplasty or surgery.

References

1. Seckeler MD, Hoke TR. The worldwide epidemiology of acute rheumatic fever and rheumatic heart disease. Clin Epidemiol. 2011;3:67–84.
2. Carapetis JR, Steer AC, Mulholland EK, Weber M. The global burden of group A streptococcal diseases. Lancet Infect Dis. 2005;5:685–94.
3. Selzer A, Cohn KE. Natural history of mitral stenosis: a review. Circulation. 1972;45:878–90.
4. Rinkevich D, Lessick J, Mutlak D, Markiewicz W, Reisner SA. Natural history of moderate mitral valve stenosis. IMAJ. 2003;5:15–8.
5. Chandrashekhar Y, Westaby S, Narula J. Mitral stenosis. Lancet. 2009;374:1271–83.
6. Carabello BA. Modern management of mitral stenosis. Circulation. 2005;112:432–7.
7. Nishimura RA, Otto CM, Bonow RO, Carabello BA, Erwin III JP, Guyton RA, O'Gara PT, Ruiz CE, Skubas NJ, Sorajja P, Sundt III TM, Thomas JD. 2014 AHA/ACC guideline for the management of patients with valvular heart disease: executive summary: a report of the

American College of Cardiology/American Heart Association Task Force on Practice Guidelines. Circulation. 2014;129:e521–643.

8. Inoue K, Owaki T, Nakamura T, Kitamura F, Miyamoto N. Clinical application of transvenous mitral commissurotomy by a new balloon catheter. J Thorac Cardiovasc Surg. 1984;87:394–402.

9. Lock JE, Khalilullah M, Shrivastava S, Bahl V, Keane JF. Percutaneous catheter commissurotomy in rheumatic mitral stenosis. N Engl J Med. 1985;313:1515–8.

10. Al Zaibag M, Ribeiro PA, Al Kasab S, Al Fagih MR. Percutaneous double-balloon mitral valvotomy for rheumatic mitral-valve stenosis. Lancet. 1986;327:757–61.

11. Bassand JP, Schiele F, Bernard Y, Anguenot T, Payet M, Abdou S, Daspet JP, Maurat JP. The double balloon and Inoue techniques in percutaneous mitral valvuloplasty: comparative results in a series of 232 cases. J Am Coll Cardiol. 1991;18:982–9.

12. Nobuyoshi M, Arita T, Shirai S, Hamasaki N, Yokoi H, Iwabuchi M, Yasumoto H, Nosaka H. Percutaneous balloon mitral valvuloplasty: a review. Circulation. 2009;119:e211–9.

13. Wunderlich NC, Beigel R, Siegel RJ. Management of mitral stenosis using 2D and 3D echo-Doppler imaging. JACC Cardiovasc Imaging. 2013;6:1191–205.

14. Wilkins GT, Weyman AE, Abascal VM, Block PC, Palacios IF. Percutaneous balloon dilatation of the mitral valve: an analysis of echocardiographic variables related to outcome and the mechanism of dilatation. Br Heart J. 1988;60:299–308.

15. Cannan CR, Nishimura RA, Reeder GS, et al. Echocardiographic assessment of commissural calcium: a simple predictor of outcome after percutaneous mitral balloon valvotomy. J Am Coll Cardiol. 1997;29:175–80.

16. Bouleti C, Iung B, Himbert D, Messika-Zeitoun D, Brochet E, Garbarz E, Cormier B, Vahanian A. Relationship between valve calcification and long-term results of percutaneous mitral commissurotomy for rheumatic mitral stenosis. Circ Cardiovasc Interv. 2014;7:381–9.

17. Nunes MCP, Tan TC, Elmariah S, do Lago R, Margey R, Cruz-Gonzalez I, Zheng H, Handschumacher MD, Inglessis I, Palacios IF, Weyman AE, Hung J. The Echo Score Revisited. Impact of incorporating commissural morphology and leaflet displacement to the prediction of outcome for patients undergoing percutaneous mitral valvuloplasty. Circulation. 2014;129:886–95.

18. Gorlin WB, Gorlin R. A generalized formulation of the Gorlin formula for calculating the area of the stenotic mitral valve and other stenotic cardiac valves. J Am Coll Cardiol. 1990;15:246–7.

19. Turi ZG, Reyes VP, Raju BS, Raju AR, Kumar DN, Rajagopal P, Sathyanarayana PV, Rao DP, Srinath K, Peters P. Percutaneous balloon versus surgical closed commissurotomy for mitral stenosis: a prospective, randomized trial. Circulation. 1991;83:1179–85.

20. Palacios IF, Sanchez PL, Harrell LC, Weyman AE, Block PC. Which patients benefit from percutaneous mitral balloon valvuloplasty? Prevalvuloplasty and postvalvuloplasty variables that predict long-term outcome. Circulation. 2002;105:1465–71.

21. Arora R, Kalra GS, Singh S, Mukhopadhyay S, Kumar A, Mohan JC, Nigam M. Percutaneous transvenous mitral commissurotomy: immediate and long-term follow-up results. Catheter Cardiovasc Interv. 2002;55:450–6.

22. Fawzy ME, Shoukri M, Fadel B, Badr A, Al Ghamdi A, Canver C. Long-term (up to 18 years) clinical and echocardiographic results of mitral balloon valvuloplasty in 531 consecutive patients and predictors of outcome. Cardiology. 2009;113:213–21.

23. Song JK, Song JM, Kang DH, Yun SC, Park DW, Lee SW, Kim YH, Lee CW, Hong MK, Kim JJ, Park SW, Park SJ. Restenosis and adverse clinical events after successful percutaneous mitral valvuloplasty: immediate post-procedural mitral area as an important prognosticator. Eur Heart J. 2009;30:1254–62.

24. Iung B, Garbarz E, Michaud P, Helou S, Farah B, Berdah P, Michel PL, Cormier B, Vahanian A. Late results of percutaneous mitral commissurotomy in a series of 1024 patients: analysis of late clinical deterioration: frequency, anatomic findings, and predictive factors. Circulation. 1999;99:3272–8.

25. Chen CR, Cheng TO. Percutaneous balloon mitral valvuloplasty by the Inoue technique: a multicenter study of 4832 patients in China. Am Heart J. 1995;129:1197–203.

26. Arora R, Nair M, Kalra GS, Nigam M, Khalilullah M. Immediate and long-term results of balloon and surgical closed mitral valvotomy: a randomized comparative study. Am Heart J. 1993;125:1091–4.
27. Reyes VP, Raju BS, Wynne J, Stephenson LW, Raju R, Fromm BS, Rajagopal P, Mehta P, Singh S, Rao DP. Percutaneous balloon valvuloplasty compared with open surgical commissurotomy for mitral stenosis. N Engl J Med. 1994;331:961–7.
28. Ben Farhat M, Ayari M, Maatouk F, Betbout F, Gamra H, Jarra M, Tiss M, Hammami S, Thaalbi R, Addad F. Percutaneous balloon versus surgical closed and open mitral commissurotomy: seven-year follow-up results of a randomized trial. Circulation. 1998;97:245–50.
29. Song JK, Kim MJ, Yun SC, Choo SJ, Song JM, Song H, Kang DH, Chung CH, Park DW, Lee SW, Kim YH, Lee CW, Hong MK, Kim JJ, Lee JW, Park SW, Park SJ. Long-term outcomes of percutaneous mitral balloon valvuloplasty versus open cardiac surgery. J Thorac Cardiovasc Surg. 2010;139:103–10.
30. Neumayer U, Schmidt HK, Fassbender D, Mannebach H, Bogunovic N, Horstkotte D. Early (three-month) results of percutaneous mitral valvotomy with the Inoue balloon in 1,123 consecutive patients comparing various age groups. Am J Cardiol. 2002;90:190–3.
31. Shapiro LM, Hassanein H, Crowley JJ. Mitral balloon valvuloplasty in patients > 70 years of age with severe mitral stenosis. Am J Cardiol. 1995;75:633–6.
32. Chmielak Z, Klopotowski M, Demkow M, Konka M, Hoffman P, Kukula K, Kruk M, Witkowski A, Ruzyllo W. Percutaneous mitral balloon valvuloplasty beyond 65 years of age. Cardiol J. 2013;20:44–51.
33. Ramondo A, Napodano M, Fraccaro C, Razzolini R, Tarantini G, Iliceto S. Relation of patient age to outcome of percutaneous mitral valvuloplasty. Am J Cardiol. 2006;98:1493–500.
34. Nercolini DC, da Rocha Loures Bueno R, Eduardo Guerios E, Tarastchuk JC, Pacheco AL, Pia de Andrade PM, Pereira da Cunha CL, Germiniani H. Percutaneous mitral balloon valvuloplasty in pregnant women with mitral stenosis. Catheter Cardiovasc Interv. 2002;57:318–22.
35. Esteves CA, Munoz JS, Braga S, Andrade J, Meneghelo Z, Gomes N, Maldonado M, Esteves V, Sepetiba R, Sousa JE, Palacios IF. Immediate and long-term follow-up of percutaneous balloon mitral valvuloplasty in pregnant patients with rheumatic mitral stenosis. Am J Cardiol. 2006;98:812–6.
36. Fawzy ME, Shoukri M, Osman A, El Amraoui S, Shah S, Nowayhed O, Canver C. Impact of atrial fibrillation on immediate and long-term results of mitral balloon valvuloplasty in 531 consecutive patients. J Heart Valve Dis. 2008;17:141–8.
37. Leon MN, Harrell LC, Simosa HF, Mahdi NA, Pathan A, Lopez-Cuellar J, Inglessis I, Moreno P, Palacios IF. Mitral balloon valvotomy for patients with mitral stenosis in atrial fibrillation: immediate and long-term results. J Am Coll Cardiol. 1999;34:1145–52.
38. Fawzy ME, Osman A, Nambiar V, Nowayhed O, El DA, Badr A, Canver CC. Immediate and long-term results of mitral balloon valvuloplasty in patients with severe pulmonary hypertension. J Heart Valve Dis. 2008;17:485–91.
39. Pathan AZ, Mahdi NA, Leon MN, Lopez-Cuellar J, Simosa H, Block PC, Harrell L, Palacios IF. Is redo percutaneous mitral balloon valvuloplasty (PMV) indicated in patients with post-PMV mitral restenosis? J Am Coll Cardiol. 1999;34:49–54.
40. Chmielak Z, Klopotowski M, Kruk M, Demkow M, Konka M, Chojnowska L, Hoffman P, Witkowski A, Ruzyllo W. Repeat percutaneous mitral balloon valvuloplasty for patients with mitral valve restenosis. Catheter Cardiovasc Interv. 2010;76:986–92.
41. Bouleti C, Iung B, Himbert D, Brochet E, Messika-Zeitoun D, Detaint D, Garbarz E, Cormier B, Vahanian A. Reinterventions after percutaneous mitral commissurotomy during long-term follow-up, up to 20 years: the role of repeat percutaneous mitral commissurotomy. Eur Heart J. 2013;34:1923–30.
42. Chatterjee SS, Uddin MJ, Rahman AK, Hussain KS, Rahman MS, Hossain MA, Mitra KK, Saha J, Siddiqui KN, Agarwal D. Percutaneous mitral balloon valvuloplasty in patients with post surgical mitral restenosis: result of 70 cases. Indian Heart J. 2010;62:17–20.
43. Hamatani Y, Saito N, Tazaki J, Natsuaki M, Nakai K, Makiyama T, Sasaki Y, Imai M, Watanabe S, Shioi T, Kimura T, Inoue K. Percutaneous balloon valvuloplasty for bioprosthetic mitral valve stenosis. Heart Vessel. 2013;28:667–71.

Chapter 12
Edge-to-Edge Repair with MitraClip for Functional Mitral Regurgitation

Emily Downs and Gorav Ailawadi

Functional Mitral Regurgitation

Functional mitral regurgitation (FMR) presents a challenge in decision-making as the clinical indications for repair are less compelling than the indications for degenerative MR (DMR). MitraClip is now available in the United States for treatment of DMR in patients at prohibitive risk for surgery. Most MitraClip trials and registries collect data with attention to the etiology of mitral dysfunction, but FMR has been less comprehensively studied with respect to the ideal management strategy. While controversy exists regarding the optimal role of MitraClip in FMR treatment, the device has been successfully used in patients with FMR, and ongoing trials should clarify the proper indications and timing of MitraClip application for such patients (Table 12.1).

Anatomy and Physiology

FMR encompasses mitral disease stemming not from pathologic lesions of the valve structures but from underlying dysfunction of the left heart structures. One major category of FMR is ischemic mitral regurgitation. Wall motion abnormalities and remodeling displace the papillary muscles, causing tethering of the posterior leaflet and poor coaptation with an eccentric regurgitant jet. With additional left ventricular

E. Downs, MD
Department of Surgery, Thoracic Surgery Resident, University of Virginia,
PO Box 800679, Charlottesville, VA 22908, USA
e-mail: ead6m@virginia.edu

G. Ailawadi, MD (✉)
Section of Adult Cardiac Surgery, Department of Surgery, Advanced Cardiac Valve Center,
University of Virginia, 1215 Lee Street, Charlottesville, VA 22903, USA

© Springer Science+Business Media New York 2016
G. Ailawadi, I.L. Kron (eds.), *Catheter Based Valve and Aortic Surgery*,
DOI 10.1007/978-1-4939-3432-4_12

165

Table 12.1 Results of published trials of MitraClip in FMR

Author	Date	Study population	Procedural success	Mortality	Outcomes at follow-up
Franzen et al. [1]	2011	50 MitraClip patients with EF ≤ 25 %	48 of 50 patients with successful clip placement; MR grade 2+ or less in 92 % of successful procedures	6 % 30-day mortality (both in-hospital after initial procedure)	• 8 deaths during follow-up 6-month outcomes in 32 patients with clinical and TTE follow-up: • 13 % with MR 3+ and 0 % 4+ • 72 % NYHA class I or II
Taramasso et al. [2]	2012	52 MitraClip and 91 mitral surgical (including concomitant) patients	9.6 % of MitraClip patients with residual MR $\geq 3+$ (0 % in surgical group)	0 % in-hospital mortality (6.6 % in surgical patients)	1-year outcomes: • 87.5 % actuarial survival • 79.1 % freedom from MR $\geq 3+$ • 84.1 % of patients with NYHA class I–II
Conradi et al. [3]	2013	95 MitraClip and 76 isolated surgical mitral patients	4.7 % of MitraClip patients with residual MR $\geq 3+$ (1.3 % in surgical group)	4.2 % 30-day mortality in MitraClip patients (2.6 % in surgical patients)	6-month outcomes: • 87 % actuarial survival • 88 % freedom from MR > grade 2
Braun et al. [4]	2014	47 FMR patients and 72 DMR patients undergoing MitraClip	89.4 % of FMR patients with MR reduction by 1 grade or more. Composite endpoint of freedom from MR 3+ to 4+, mitral valve reintervention, or death at 12 months achieved in 63.8 % of FMR patients	No procedural deaths; 30-day mortality not reported	1-year outcomes: • 80.9 % survival for FMR patients (93.1 % for DMR patients) • 72.2 % of FMR patients with MR $\leq 2+$ • 70 % of FMR patients with NYHA class I or II symptoms
Nickenig et al. [5]	2014	628 MitraClip patients in the European Transcatheter Valve Treatment Sentinel Pilot Registry, 452 with FMR	98 % of FMR patients with none/mild or moderate MR after clip placement	2.0 % in-hospital mortality for FMR group	• Median follow-up 346 days with data available in 552 of 628 patients overall • 1-year mortality 15 % for FMR patients

(continued)

Table 12.1 (continued)

Author	Date	Study population	Procedural success	Mortality	Outcomes at follow-up
Taramasso et al. [6]	2015	109 consecutive patients with FMR undergoing MitraClip	108 of 109 patients with successful clip placement; 13 % with residual MR ≥ 3+	1.8 % 30-day mortality	• Median follow-up 13 months • Actuarial survival 74.5 % at 3 years • EF improvement 27 ± 9.8 % to 34.7 ± 10.4 % at 1 year • 86 % of patients with NYHA class I or II symptoms at 1 year

dilation after large myocardial infarction or repeated infarcts, the mitral annulus dilates leading to worsening coaptation and a central regurgitant jet. Similarly, with idiopathic dilated cardiomyopathy, mitral annular dilation produces a central jet from poor coaptation [7]. Long-standing atrial fibrillation can produce similar changes in annular geometry and result in FMR, though atrial fibrillation is also often a consequence of mitral regurgitation [8].

Medical Treatment of FMR

The primary medical therapy for FMR is aimed at improving underlying left ventricular dysfunction. Beta-blockade and angiotensin-converting enzyme inhibitors have both been shown to reduce the severity of FMR. As such, it is recommended to ensure patients receive maximal medical therapy prior to considering mitral intervention, whether surgical or catheter-based [9]. Additionally, the ACC/AHA guidelines for treatment of valvular disease indicate with a class I recommendation that FMR patients receive cardiac resynchronization therapy if indications are met [10].

Surgical Indications for FMR

ACC/AHA guidelines suggest that it is reasonable to perform mitral valve surgery in patients with severe functional MR undergoing coronary artery bypass grafting (CABG) or aortic valve replacement (AVR), with class IIa recommendation. The recommendation is less compelling for patients with sole FMR and no other cardiac surgical indications; in this case, the guidelines provide a class IIb recommendation to consider mitral repair or replacement in the setting of persistent symptoms despite optimal medical therapy. While it is known that severe FMR worsens heart failure physiology and symptoms by contributing to volume overload and progressive dilation, it is as yet unclear whether correcting the mitral regurgitation actually improves survival. This may be due to the trajectory of the underlying ventricular pathology, whether that is ischemic cardiomyopathy, idiopathic dilation, or other form of cardiomyopathy.

Surgical therapy for ischemic mitral regurgitation as a subset of functional mitral regurgitation has been studied in several recent randomized controlled trials (RCTs). The question of how to approach mitral regurgitation with concomitant revascularization is an important clinical concern. A large RCT of 251 patients with severe ischemic MR assigned each patient to undergo mitral valve repair with a complete ring or chordal sparing valve replacement. The authors found that both groups experienced a similar degree of left ventricular reverse remodeling and survival at 12 months. While there was more recurrent mitral regurgitation in the repair group (32.6 % moderate or severe at 1 year, compared to 2.3 % moderate in the replacement group), it is unknown what effect this has on long-term outcomes [11]. The results of this trial have significant implications for the development and adoption of transcatheter devices for mitral valve therapy. Should long-term follow-up demonstrate that mitral valve replacement is in fact a better option for patients with severe mitral regurgitation resulting from ischemic cardiomyopathy, the preferred transcatheter therapy may be a valve replacement. Fortunately several devices for transcatheter mitral valve replacement are in development and should provide new options once more data is available regarding the ideal therapy for this subset of functional mitral regurgitation.

MitraClip for FMR

The initial trials gauging the feasibility and efficacy of MitraClip technology included patients with both functional and degenerative mitral regurgitation. The device gained CE mark approval in 2008 in Europe and FDA approval for commercial use in the United States specifically in high-risk surgical patients with degenerative mitral regurgitation. The experience gathered during initial clinical trials, commercial use in Europe, and ongoing clinical trials in the United States (COAPT) provides a foundation for the appropriate use of the MitraClip in patients with FMR.

Surgical Mitral Repair versus MitraClip for Functional Mitral Regurgitation

In 2012, Taramasso et al. published the experience of a single Italian center performing either surgical mitral repair or MitraClip in patients with FMR between 2000 and 2011. Retrospective review demonstrated that MitraClip patients were in general older than their surgical counterparts, with a lower left ventricular ejection fraction and a higher log EuroSCORE. Despite this discrepancy in baseline status,

MitraClip patients experienced shorter length of stay (5 versus 11 days for the surgical group, $P < 0.0001$). Mortality was 6.6 % in the surgical group and 0 % in the MitraClip group ($P = 0.01$). The authors did find that patients receiving the MitraClip were more likely to have residual MR of 3+ or greater (9.6 % versus 0 % in the surgical group). At 1 year, 79.1 % of MitraClip patients experienced MR less than 3+ compared with 94.2 % of surgical patients. 1-year survival was comparable for both groups at 88.9 % for the surgical group and 87.5 % for the MitraClip group. The authors concluded that MitraClip could provide an option for patients with FMR at high surgical risk [2]. As in other trials, the consequences of recurrent MR are unclear given similar mortality at 1 year in these groups despite more recurrent MR of 3+ or greater in the MitraClip patients.

Conradi et al. in 2013 published their results comparing surgical mitral repair and MitraClip outcomes in 171 total patients with functional MR. This retrospective review similarly demonstrated that the MitraClip patients were on average older, with lower LVEF and higher log EuroSCORE. While Taramasso et al. included surgical patients undergoing mitral repair as well as concomitant procedures, Conradi et al. describe only isolated surgical mitral valve repairs. The group found reduction in MR to 2+ or less in 95.8 % of MitraClip patients and 98.7 % of surgical patients; however, the risk of recurrent MR (3+ or greater) was significantly higher in MitraClip patients at 6 months. At the completion of follow-up (mean 212 days for surgical and 198 for MitraClip patients), there was no significant difference in the percentage of patients with NYHA class I or II symptoms, though rates of rehospitalization up to 180 days post-procedure were significantly higher in MitraClip patients (22.1 % versus 5.5 % in surgical patients) [3]. These authors concluded that MitraClip should be offered to FMR patients at high or prohibitive surgical risk.

These two studies indicate that at present, in patients with FMR, the risk of recurrent MR with MitraClip may outweigh the risks of mitral valve surgery in high-risk patients. The remaining challenge is how to determine which patients will benefit from MitraClip, as it is clear that a substantial portion of patients do experience reduction in MR with lasting symptomatic relief and echocardiographic improvement up to 1 year. Indeed, the same challenge has been discussed with respect to the question of whether to repair or replace the mitral valve in patients with severe ischemic MR. Many patients benefit from repair, but given the risk of recurrence, the major randomized controlled trial to date has suggested replacement as the preferred surgical therapy. The ability to predict which FMR patients will experience durable repair with MitraClip would broaden options for patients, especially those at some increased risk for surgery who wish to avoid an operation.

Midterm Outcomes for MitraClip in Functional Mitral Regurgitation

Taramasso et al. have published midterm results (up to 3 years) of MitraClip use for patients with FMR at high surgical risk. They reported on outcomes of 109 patients receiving MitraClip since 2008 at a single center. The authors reported 74.5 %

actuarial survival at 3 years. Freedom from MR of 3+ or greater was 70 % at 2.5 years. The authors found that a pro-BNP level greater than 1600 pg/mL was an independent predictor of death at follow-up. The authors posit that more advanced heart failure physiology may prevent patients from receiving optimal benefit from the MitraClip and suggest a role for pro-BNP in the patient selection process. Overall the authors noted a significant decrease in LV end-diastolic diameter and systolic pulmonary artery pressure on 1-year echocardiography with significant improvement in quality of life assessments and 6-minute walk test results. The conclusion of these midterm results continues to support the MitraClip as an option in FMR patients at high or prohibitive surgical risk.

MitraClip versus Optimal Medical Management: The COAPT Trial

For patients who are not eligible for surgery, evidence is lacking as to whether MitraClip provides benefit beyond that seen with optimal medical therapy. To answer this question, the Clinical Outcomes Assessment of the MitraClip Percutaneous Therapy (COAPT) trial for extremely high surgical risk patients is currently enrolling patients. A truly multidisciplinary effort including heart failure cardiologists, cardiothoracic surgeons, cardiac imaging specialists, and interventional cardiologists is required. The trial's primary outcomes include a safety endpoint monitoring for adverse events and an effectiveness endpoint of recurrent heart failure hospitalizations [12]. While the success of the MitraClip for FMR patients at high surgical risk has been demonstrated in a substantial portion of patients, this study should clarify the extent of benefit patients might receive with the MitraClip in addition to maximal medical therapy.

Case Example: MitraClip for Severe Ischemic Mitral Regurgitation

A 72-year-old man presented to the valve center clinic with severe mitral regurgitation. History revealed he had undergone two prior CABG surgeries, as well as placement of an internal cardioverter defibrillator for ventricular tachycardia and subsequent upgrade to a biventricular pacing device. He also dealt with atrial fibrillation and NYHA class III symptoms despite medical management with carvedilol, lisinopril, and furosemide. His estimated STS mortality risk for mitral valve replacement was calculated at 6.8 %. Transthoracic echocardiography demonstrated severe mitral regurgitation with central regurgitant jet, left ventricular ejection fraction of 25–30 %, moderate pulmonary hypertension, moderated dilated left ventricle, and severely dilated left atrium. Cardiac catheterization demonstrated patent graft to the dominant

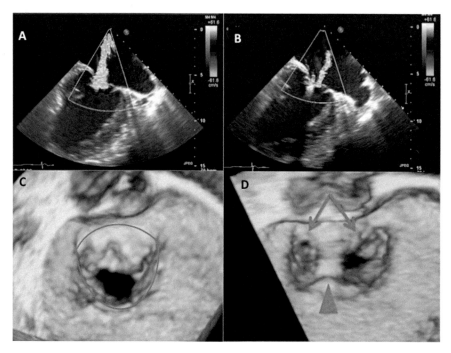

Fig. 12.1 Intraprocedural transesophageal echocardiography images. (**a**) Midesophageal two-chamber view prior to clip placement. (**b**) Midesophageal two-chamber view after clip placement demonstrating 1+ residual regurgitation. (**c**) Three-dimensional view of mitral valve during diastole, with the annulus highlighted (*red line*) to demonstrate dilation in the anteroposterior dimension. (**d**) Post-clip placement (*arrowhead*), three-dimensional view of the double-orifice valve (*arrows*)

right coronary artery, patent left internal mammary to mid-left anterior descending artery, and no other patent vein grafts with no suitable targets for repeat revascularization procedure. Decision was made to proceed with MitraClip placement. He underwent successful MitraClip placement with reduction of mitral regurgitation from 4+ to 1+ (Fig. 12.1). He experienced significant improvement in symptoms on early post-procedure follow-up. At the 2-year post-clip clinic visit, transthoracic echocardiography demonstrated 2+ mitral regurgitation and improvement in left ventricular ejection fraction to 30–35 %. He reported persistent gains in functional capacity with NYHA class I symptoms and was able to play 18 holes of golf without difficulty.

Conclusion

The treatment of functional mitral regurgitation continues to present clinicians with challenges. The benefits of guideline-directed medical therapy for underlying left ventricular dysfunction and appropriate resynchronization therapy are well established. Current evidence suggests valve replacement for severe ischemic mitral regurgitation with concomitant CABG, and transcatheter replacement may one day find a role in severe ischemic MR. The MitraClip has been applied for patients with FMR in the initial clinical trials establishing the safety and efficacy of the device, and at centers outside the United States, it is frequently used for patients with FMR at high or prohibitive surgical risk. In the United States, the COAPT trial continues enrollment to compare MitraClip to optimal medical management, and at present the commercial indications of MitraClip are limited to patients with degenerative mitral regurgitation. Both the COAPT trial results and continuing long-term outcomes from MitraClip use for FMR at centers outside the United States will inform surgeons and cardiologists to the appropriate role of the device in this patient population.

References

1. Franzen O, Van Der Heyden J, Baldus S, Schlüter M, Schillinger W, Butter C, et al. MitraClip® therapy in patients with end-stage systolic heart failure. Eur J Heart Fail. 2011;13:569–76.
2. Taramasso M, Denti P, Buzzatti N, De Bonis M, La Canna G, Colombo A, et al. Mitraclip therapy and surgical mitral repair in patients with moderate to severe left ventricular failure causing functional mitral regurgitation: a single-centre experience. Eur J Cardiothorac Surg. 2012;42:920–6.
3. Conradi L, Treede H, Rudolph V, Graumüller P, Lubos E, Baldus S, et al. Surgical or percutaneous mitral valve repair for secondary mitral regurgitation: comparison of patient characteristics and clinical outcomes. Eur J Cardiothorac Surg. 2013;44:490–6. discussion 496.
4. Braun D, Lesevic H, Orban M, Michalk F, Barthel P, Hoppe K, et al. Percutaneous edge-to-edge repair of the mitral valve in patients with degenerative versus functional mitral regurgitation. Catheter Cardiovasc Interv. 2014;84:137–46.
5. Nickenig G, Estevez-Loureiro R, Franzen O, Tamburino C, Vanderheyden M, Lüscher TF, et al. Percutaneous mitral valve edge-to-edge repair. J Am Coll Cardiol. 2014;64:875–84.
6. Taramasso M, Maisano F, Latib A, Denti P, Buzzatti N, Cioni M, et al. Clinical outcomes of MitraClip for the treatment of functional mitral regurgitation. EuroIntervention. 2014;10(6):746–52.
7. Filsoufi F, Chikwe J, Adams DH. Acquired disease of the mitral valve. In Sabiston and Spencer Surgery of the Chest. Selke F, del Nido PJ, Swanson SJ (eds.). 8th Ed. Elsevier; 1948, pp. 1207–40.
8. Bhamra-Ariza P, Muller DW. The MitraClip experience and future percutaneous mitral valve therapies. Heart Lung Circ. 2014;23(11):1009–19.
9. Enriquez-Sarano M, Akins CW, Vahanian A. Mitral regurgitation. Lancet. 2009;373:1382–94.
10. Nishimura RA, Otto CM, Bonow RO, Carabello BA, Erwin JP, Guyton RA, et al. AHA/ACC guideline for the management of patients with valvular heart disease. J Thorac Cardiovasc Surg. 2014;148:e1–132.
11. Acker MA, Parides MK, Perrault LP, Moskowitz AJ, Gelijns AC, Voisine P, et al. Mitral-valve repair versus replacement for severe ischemic mitral regurgitation. N Engl J Med. 2014;370:23–32.
12. COAPT Clinical Trial, ClinicalTrials.gov. https://clinicaltrials.gov/ct2/show/NCT01626079; n.d.

Chapter 13
Edge-to-Edge Repair (MitraClip), Degenerative

Mohammad Sarraf and Ted Feldman

Introduction

The MitraClip device was conceived of as a percutaneous method to mimic the surgical edge-to-edge or double-orifice mitral repair [1]. A surgical double-orifice repair was initially utilized in patients with degenerative mitral regurgitation (MR), involving prolapse of the middle scallops of the line of mitral coaptation [2]. The first experience with the MitraClip device was in the Phase 1 EVEREST trial, with a target population consisting of a majority of patients with degenerative MR [3]. In fact, the trial enrolled over 3/4 of patients with degenerative MR (DMR) and the remainder with functional MR (FMR), mostly of ischemic origin. The EVEREST II pivotal trial compared MitraClip with any type of surgical mitral repair or replacement, also in a predominantly DMR population. Ultimately, EVEREST 2 demonstrated that surgical repair is more effective at reducing MR than MitraClip, but that the MitraClip device achieved similar levels of clinical efficacy and left ventricular remodeling and is, as was expected, safer than surgical approaches. Subgroup analysis of the trial demonstrated that patients with FMR and high-risk characteristics including older age and diminished left ventricular performance had the greatest likelihood to benefit from MitraClip repair [4].

Since CE mark approval in 2008, the clinical uptake of MitraClip in commercial international practice has reflected findings of the EVEREST 2 subgroup analysis, with 3/4 predominance of use among high-risk patients with FMR. Despite this general practice pattern of preference for utilization of MitraClip in patients with FMR, about 1/4 of treated patients in international commercial use have DMR as the etiology. In addition, subgroup analysis of the EVEREST High-Risk Registry population in 127 patients with DMR showed results similar to the outcomes in

M. Sarraf, MD • T. Feldman, MD, MSCAI, FACC, FESC (✉)
Cardiac Catheterization Laboratory, Cardiology Division, Evanston Hospital, NorthShore University HealthSystem, Walgreen Building 3rd Floor, 2650 Ridge Avenue, Evanston, IL 60201, USA
e-mail: tfeldman@tfeldman.org

© Springer Science+Business Media New York 2016
G. Ailawadi, I.L. Kron (eds.), *Catheter Based Valve and Aortic Surgery*,
DOI 10.1007/978-1-4939-3432-4_13

FMR patients [5]. Interestingly, most comparisons of outcomes of MitraClip therapy in FMR and DMR have shown similar outcomes in reduction in MR severity, left ventricular remodeling, and improvements in descriptors of clinical status such as New York Heart Association class or quality of life questionnaires.

Degenerative Mitral Regurgitation

DMR is a heterogeneous disease that may be the result of degenerative valve disease such as prolapse, myxomatous degeneration, or rupture of the chordae. DMR of any degree is a relatively common valvular disease that occurs in 2 % of the general population [6], while severe MR occurs only in 0.5 % of the population [7]. There is a spectrum of pathology, with variable degrees of leaflet redundancy and chordal elongation. Prolapse may involve one or both leaflets and few or many of the leaflet scallops. MR may be slowly progressive or can present as acute severe MR when chordal rupture occurs. While mitral prolapse typically presents in adults ages 40–60 years, older patients may present with a form of more localized leaflet abnormality, usually involving the middle scallop of the posterior leaflet, fibroelastic deficiency. This latter group is clinically problematic because they are older and often have comorbidities that increase the risk of surgical mitral repair.

The clinical significance of MR centers on the severity of regurgitation and the subsequent impact on symptom status, atrial and ventricular remodeling, and secondary pulmonary hypertension [8].

Medical therapy has little role in the treatment of patients with DMR, since the cause of progression of the disease is due to primary valve pathology. Therefore, mitral repair or replacement surgery has become the standard of care in the management of patients with DMR. Mitral valve repair has better short- and long-term morbidity and mortality compared to mitral valve replacement for DMR [9].

Over the last 4 decades, there has been continuous improvement in surgical techniques for mitral valve repair. Alfieri et al. proposed an "edge-to-edge" approximation of the mitral leaflets as strategy for mitral valve repair [10]. The long-term results of this isolated edge-to-edge repair have been durable for up to 12 years in a selected population [11]. The in-hospital mortality was 3.4 %, with an overall survival of 93 % after a mean follow-up of 6.8 years. The Alfieri technique can be used as a simple approach of "edge-to-edge" repair without an absolute indication to use mitral annular ring.

MitraClip Design and Function

The design of MitraClip recapitulates the "edge-to-edge" repair by mechanical approximation of the mitral valve leaflets. The healing process in animal studies after MitraClip implantation consists of a tissue bridge over the device that results in connection of the two leaflets and long-term anatomic durability [12, 13]. Ladich et al. investigated the pathological healing response in patients receiving MitraClip

[14]. They categorized the healing process into 4 stages: (a) acute <30 days, (b) subacute 31–90 days, (c) chronic 91–300 days, and (d) long-term >300 days. The *acute* healing response consisted of platelet and fibrin deposition. The *subacute* response demonstrates granulation tissue with early fibrous encapsulation, i.e., pannus formation. The *chronic* response was characterized by various degrees of tissue bridging between the device arms. The *long-term* healing response demonstrated type I collagen deposition, incorporating the device components with complete encapsulation by organized, fibrous growth. With the exception of the long-term stage, there is no significant difference between the healing process of DMR and FMR patients after MitraClip implantation. In the *long-term stage*, there is a thicker fibrous capsule and larger atrial tissue bridge area found in FMR compared to DMR. It is theorized that the tissue bridge ultimately stabilizes the mitral annulus and minimizes subsequent annular dilatation.

Procedural Considerations for MitraClip Technique in DMR

The system deployment starts with a venous access via femoral vein. The location of transseptal puncture cannot be overemphasized (Fig. 13.1). The mitral valve orifice is situated anterior and inferior in the left atrium. Therefore, the best location

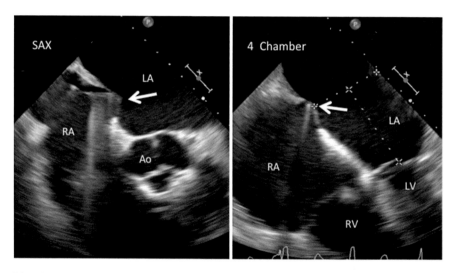

Fig. 13.1 Transseptal puncture for MitraClip requires a posterior and superior entry point into the left atrium. The *white arrow* shows tenting on the *left-hand panel*, a short-axis transesophageal echocardiographic view. The tenting is relatively far away from the aortic valve. Since the aortic valve is anterior, the farther away the puncture point, the more posterior it is. The *right-hand panel* shows a 4-chamber view. The *arrow* indicates point of tenting caused by the transseptal needle. The tenting is far superior to the mitral valve. *Dotted perpendicular lines* have been drawn to delineate the height of the puncture above the mitral valve annulus. *SAX* short axis, *RA* right atrium, *LA* left atrium, *AO* aortic valve, *RV* right ventricle, *LV* left ventricle. Figures 13.1, 13.2, 13.3, 13.4, 13.5, 13.6, and 13.8 are from the same patient and procedure

for transseptal puncture is posterior and superior in fossa ovalis. This approach allows a trajectory toward the mitral line of coaptation from posterior to anterior. This "high" puncture is necessary to have enough distance above the mitral leaflets (ideal height from the annulus should be 3.5–4 cm) to allow for adequate working space for delivery catheter and clip manipulations. If the puncture is placed too low in the fossa, the device may be too close to the annular plane, and subsequent orientation to grasp the leaflets may not be possible because of inadequate space in the LA above the annular plane. Since there is more leaflet excursion in DMR compared to FMR, the puncture can be made at the higher end of the range of 3.5–4 cm above the annular plane. The strategies for clip placement and the need for additional clips are not specific to MR etiology.

After the MitraClip enters the left atrium, the operator carefully navigates the device toward the source of the regurgitant jet (Figs. 13.2 and 13.3). The clip arms are opened and the device oriented perpendicular to the line of coaptation (Fig. 13.4). After the opened clip arms are passed across the mitral valve orifice and into the ventricular side of the leaflets, a gentle pullback on the device will grip the mitral

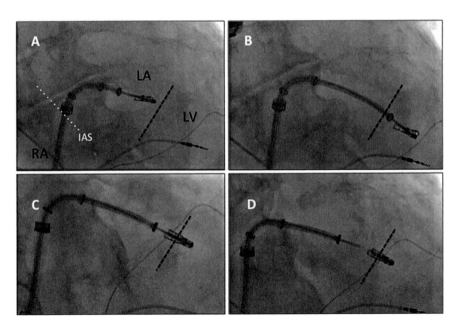

Fig. 13.2 Fluoroscopic images showing the sequence of the MitraClip procedure. Panel (**a**) shows the MitraClip situated above the line of mitral coaptation, indicated by a *dotted black line*. Panel (**b**) shows the open arms of the MitraClip passed beyond the mitral valve into the left ventricle. Panel (**c**) shows that the device has been pulled back and the clip arms closed over the mitral leaflets. In panel (**d**), the clip delivery system has been detached and the MitraClip released after assessment of grasping of the leaflets. Figures 13.1, 13.2, 13.3, 13.4, 13.5, 13.6, and 13.8 are from the same patient and procedure

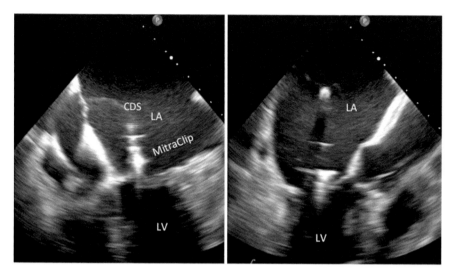

Fig. 13.3 Transesophageal echocardiographic guidance is used to assess the position of the MitraClip during the procedure. In the *left-hand panel*, the clip delivery system and MitraClip can be seen positioned above the central part of the mitral orifice. In the *right-hand panel*, an orthogonal view shows the open clip arms positioned centrally over the mitral valve. *CDS* clip delivery system, *LA* left atrium, *LV* left ventricle. Figures 13.1, 13.2, 13.3, 13.4, 13.5, 13.6, and 13.8 are from the same patient and procedure

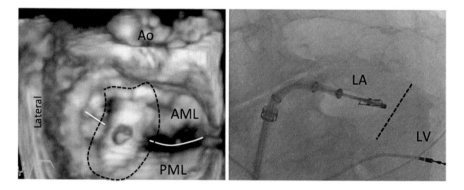

Fig. 13.4 The clip must be oriented with the open arms in the left atrium so that the arms are perpendicular to the line of mitral coaptation. Panel (**a**) is a left atrial view using a three-dimensional display. This 3D echo frame is the so-called surgeon's view. The aortic valve is at the *top* of the picture, and the lateral commissure is on the *left side*. The open clip is seen to be perpendicular to the mitral line of coaptation, which is shown as the *white line*. The MitraClip is highlighted by the *dashed black circle*. *AO* aorta, *AML* anterior mitral leaflet, *PML* posterior mitral leaflet, *LA* left atrium, *LV* left ventricle. Panel (**b**) shows a corresponding fluoroscopic image with the open clip arms above the plane of the mitral valve, shown by the *dotted dash line*. Figures 13.1, 13.2, 13.3, 13.4, 13.5, 13.6, and 13.8 are from the same patient and procedure

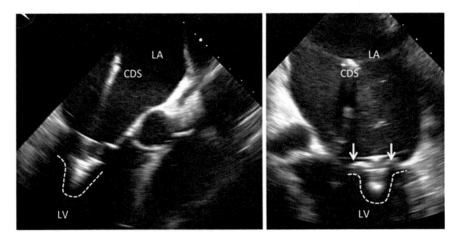

Fig. 13.5 Echocardiographic images showing the clip below the mitral valve on the left with the arms open and on the right pulled back to grasp the mitral leaflets. The clip is highlighted by the *dotted white lines* in both frames. On the *right-hand side*, the mitral leaflets can be seen to drape over the top of the clip and insert into the clip (*white arrows*), indicating that the leaflets have been grasped. *LA* left atrium, *CDS* clip delivery system, *LV* left ventricle. Figures 13.1, 13.2, 13.3, 13.4, 13.5, 13.6, and 13.8 are from the same patient and procedure

valve leaflets (Fig. 13.5). When mitral leaflet grasp is confirmed, careful assessment of the reduction of MR is performed by TEE. If the reduction of the MR jet is not adequate, the grip and the arm of the device are opened and the whole process should be repeated. Sometimes the operator may decide to place a second device. Thus, in addition to TEE assessment of MR severity, simultaneous evaluation of the invasive hemodynamics by right heart catheterization becomes invaluable. These parameters include pulmonary artery pressure, wedge pressure and left atrial V wave pressure, and evaluation of the arterial pressure. The operator must meticulously analyze every hemodynamic component before inserting the second MitraClip device. Careful attention to the simultaneous LV pressure, vasopressor therapy, and analyzing the left atrial V wave and left atrial compliance and other components of hemodynamic assessment is self-evident. After each clip is deployed, it is crucial to assess the gradient after insertion and residual mitral valve area.

Follow-up echocardiogram after completion of each case is essential (Fig. 13.6). The assessment by transthoracic echocardiogram should not be simply limited to assessment of the color Doppler evaluation of the MR jet. Indices of LV remodeling such as LV ejection fraction (LVEF), LV end-diastolic volume (LVEDV), and LV end-systolic volume (LVESV), as well as indices of MR jet such as regurgitant volume, regurgitant fraction, and effective orifice area, must be followed. There is an inherent problem with the conventional approach to quantifying the MR by echocardiography after MitraClip implantation. All of the established indices outlined in the guidelines are validated in native valvular regurgitation, but assessment of MR severity after creation of a double orifice is difficult. Using simple color jet area as an index of MR severity spuriously doubles the appearance of the

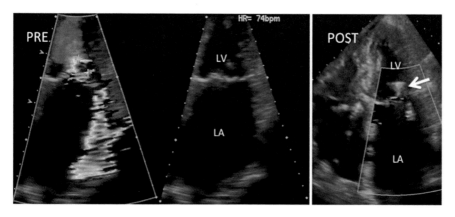

Fig. 13.6 Transthoracic echocardiographic images showing the color Doppler mitral regurgitation jet in the 4-chamber view before and after MitraClip therapy. The jet has a large origin in the baseline image and extends all the way to the roof of the left atrium indicating severe mitral regurgitation. In the post MitraClip image on the right, trivial residual color Doppler MR can be seen. The *white arrow* points at the MitraClip. *LA* left atrium, *LV* left ventricle. Figures 13.1, 13.2, 13.3, 13.4, 13.5, 13.6, and 13.8 are from the same patient and procedure

MR jet area [15]. Ultimately, the clinical response of the patient is of paramount importance; thus, using quality of life questionnaires has been helpful in assessing the clinical response to this therapy.

Evidence-Based Studies and MitraClip

MitraClip has undergone a series of clinical studies and one large randomized clinical trial. We review these studies and focus on the DMR patient population. These studies included mixed patient populations of DMR and FMR; thus, the data on DMR comes from subgroup analyses.

EVEREST I Registry

The EVEREST I registry was the first in-human experience with the device [16]. The study included 107 patients followed for 3 years. Nearly 80 % of patients had DMR and 20 % had FMR in this cohort. The primary efficacy endpoint was defined as freedom from MR >2+, cardiac surgery for valve dysfunction, and death at 12 months. Eleven patients did not receive any clips (10 %) and 29 % of patients received 2 clips. Acute procedural success, defined as placement of at least one clip resulting in MR <2+, was 74 %. After a median follow-up of nearly 23 months, 70 % of patients remained free of surgery. Thirty percent of patients required surgery (23 patients after clip and 9 patients with no clip implantation). The presence of MitraClip did not interfere with subsequent surgical mitral valve repair. There was no clip embolization; however, 9 % of patients had partial detachment of the clip, with attachment to only one of the two mitral leaflets. None of the patients with partial detachment were symptomatic, and they were detected on routine follow-up echocardiograms. These patients were successfully treated with mitral valve surgery. Major adverse events occurred in 9 % of patients with more than half of these events due to receiving more than 2 units of blood transfusion. There was one fatality and one periprocedural stroke that resolved at 12 months. One patient required >3 weeks of ventilation but did not lead to mortality. The acute procedural success results of the patients with DMR and FMR were similar. DMR and FMR patients had substantial and similar improvement in their New York Heart Association Function Class (NYHA-FC). It is noteworthy that this study was the initial experience with a complex and novel technology with a steep learning curve. In spite of these challenges, the results of the EVEREST I trial proved the feasibility and safety of the device upon which the EVEREST II trial was designed.

EVEREST II Trial

The EVEREST II randomized controlled trial was designed to evaluate the safety and effectiveness of the MitraClip compared to mitral valve repair or replacement surgery [17]. Symptomatic patients had LVEF>25 % and LV end-systolic diameter (LVESd)<55 mm. Asymptomatic patients had LVEF between 25 and 60 % or LVESd between 40 and 55 mm, new atrial fibrillation, or pulmonary hypertension. The anatomic inclusion criteria were (a) mitral valve area >4 cm^2, (b) broad flail width <15 mm, (c) flail gap <10 m, (d) deficient coaptation length of >2 mm, and (e) coaptation depth <11 mm (Fig. 13.7). Figure 13.8 shows echo images of the MR jet origin from a patient with DMR, with a central jet along the line of mitral coaptation. This is an ideal MR anatomy for the MitraClip, since the regurgitation arises from the leaflet central chordal free zone.

The primary efficacy endpoint was freedom from death, surgery for mitral valve dysfunction, and grade 3+ or 4+ MR at 12 months. The primary safety endpoint was the rate of major adverse events (MAE) at 30 days. MAE was defined as "the composite of death, myocardial infarction, reoperation for failed mitral valve surgery, nonelective cardiovascular surgery for adverse events, stroke, renal failure, deep wound infection, mechanical ventilation for more than 48 h, gastrointestinal complication requiring surgery, new-onset permanent atrial fibrillation, septicemia, and transfusion of 2 units or more of blood." The premise of the study was that surgery has a superior efficacy by a prespecified margin, but MitraClip has superior safety compared to surgery.

The study randomized patients with a 2:1 ratio for MitraClip implantation and surgical arm (defined as control). Out of 279 patients, 184 patients were randomized to the MitraClip arm and 95 patients to the surgical control. The mean age of the patients was 65 years old and 29 % of patients were older than 75 years. Compared to the Society of Thoracic Surgery database, the patients in this trial were

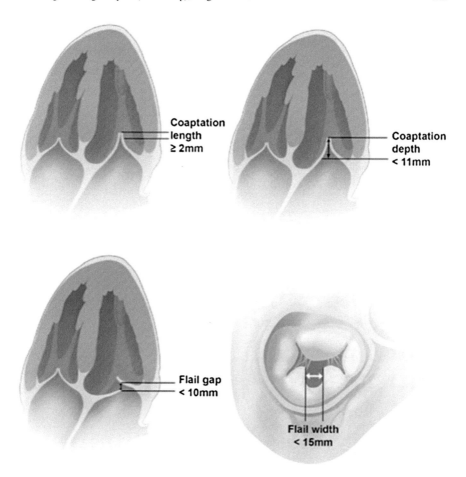

Fig. 13.7 The EVEREST anatomic inclusion criteria. These were designed prior to the treatment and then the patients with the device, reflecting the expected best case mital anatomy for MitraClip use in degenerative MR. Key anatomic inclusion criteria included a regurgitant jet origin associated with the A2 to P2 segments of the mitral valve and, for patients with functional MR, a coaptation length of at least 2 mm, a coaptation depth of no more than 11 mm, and, for patients with leaflet flail, a flail gap <10 mm and a flail width <15 mm. From Feldman et al. [16] with permission

significantly older [18]. Among all the randomized patients, 21 patients (19 %) did not receive therapy, 3 % in MitraClip arm, and 16 % in the surgical arm.

In an intention-to-treat analysis, the primary efficacy endpoint at 1 year occurred in 55 % of patients receiving MitraClip compared to 73 % in the control arm ($p=0.007$). The main difference in the composite endpoint was driven by a higher rate of repeat surgery in the MitraClip arm (20 %) compared to the control (2.2 %). The rates of mortality and MR >3+ were similar in the two groups. In an intention-to-treat analysis, the safety endpoint in the MitraClip arm had a MAE rate of 15 % at 30 days versus 48 % in the surgical arm ($p<0.0001$). On the other hand, there was

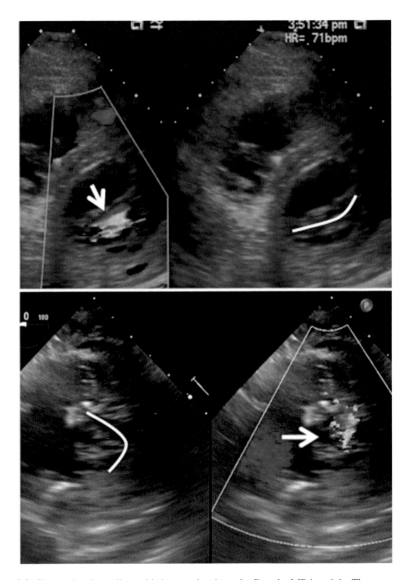

Fig. 13.8 Short-axis echocardiographic images showing color Doppler MR jet origin. The *upper panel* is a transthoracic echo, with the *white arrow* indicating a predominantly central origin of the Doppler jet, along the line of mitral coaptation, shown as a *white line*. The *lower panel* is a transesophageal echocardiographic image, again with the *white arrow* showing the jet origin to be predominantly central along the line of mitral coaptation, again as a *white line*. The most intense color jet is just lateral of central. Figures 13.1, 13.2, 13.3, 13.4, 13.5, 13.6, and 13.8 are from the same patient and procedure

no difference in death, stroke, emergent surgery, or reoperation in patients receiving the MitraClip. Most of the MAE occurred in patients who crossed over to the surgery after a failed MitraClip attempt. Therefore, the MAE rate at 30 days was <10 % when "per protocol" analysis is used. MR reduction to ≤2+ was achieved in 82 % of the MitraClip arm and 96 % of the control (12 % received mitral valve replacement), $p < 0.001$. Despite this marked difference in reduction of MR, there were similar decrease in the indices of LV remodeling, i.e., LV volume and LVEDd/LVESd at up to 24 months. Furthermore, although patients in the control arm had significantly better reduction in MR severity, patients who received MitraClip were more likely to be asymptomatic or minimally symptomatic at 24 months (98 % vs. 88 %). At 30 days the MitraClip patients had better quality of life based on the 36-Item Short Form Health Survey (SF-36) assessment, but at 12 months both arms had similar improved quality of life.

The final conclusion of this study in a predominantly DMR population demonstrates that MitraClip is less effective to reduce MR than conventional surgery, but it has a superior safety. Both arms show similar improvement in clinical outcomes.

The results of the 4-year follow-up have recently been published. At 4 years, the rate of the composite endpoint of freedom from death, surgery, or MR $\geq 3+$ was 39.8 % in the MitraClip arm compared to 53.4 % in the control arm, $p = 0.07$. There was no difference in the rate of death or MR $\geq 3+$ in the overall cohort (see below). However, the rate of surgery for mitral valve dysfunction was significantly higher at 4 years in the MitraClip arm, 24.8 % versus control arm, 5.5 %, $p < 0.001$ [19]. Vast majority of the referral of MitraClip patients to surgery occurred in the first 12 months. Thus, the landmark analysis of the study at 12 months shows similar outcomes between the two groups,

DMR vs. FMR   There were three major interactions observed in the subgroup analysis of the study. Patients who were older than 70 years of age and lower LVEF had better response to MitraClip. When the etiology of MR based on DMR and FMR was analyzed, patients with FMR had similar outcomes to control. Patients with DMR had better outcomes with surgery. These results were consistent at 4-year follow-up. The difference in the composite endpoint was not driven by freedom from death or surgery. The patients with DMR who underwent surgery had a significantly lower rate of MR $\geq 3+$. Thus, among DMR patients who are good candidates for conventional surgery, surgery is likely to result in better MR reduction that MitraClip.

EVEREST High-Risk Registry

The EVEREST II High-Risk Registry (EVEREST II HRR) was a prospective, single-arm study conducted in North America to study nonoperative candidates with severe MR [20]. The study included DMR and FMR (ischemic and nonischemic). Due to the strong support from the surgeons for referring the high-risk patients, the EVEREST II HRR quickly enrolled 78 patients. The qualifying criteria for EVEREST II HRR are summarized in Table 13.1. The prespecified mitral valve anatomic criteria were similar to the EVEREST II pivotal trial. The major efficacy endpoints of the study were defined as freedom from death at 12 months, freedom from death and MR >2+ at 12 months, and clinical measures of benefit at 12 months in surviving patients, defined as NYHA-FC, LV chamber dimensions and volumes, 36-Item Short Form Health Survey (SF-36) quality of life, and rehospitalization for CHF.

Table 13.1 The inclusion criteria used in EVEREST II HRR and REALISM HR identifying eligible patients for the high-risk registry

Enrolling criteria for EVEREST II HRR and REALISM HR
• Calculated STS score ≥12 %
• Surgeon investigator-determined patient risk for mortality ≥12 % owing to the presence of at least 1 of the following:
– Porcelain aorta or mobile ascending aortic atheroma
– Postradiation mediastinum
– Previous mediastinitis
– Functional mitral regurgitation with LVEF<40 %
– Age >75 years with LVEF<40 %
– Prior reoperation with patent grafts
– ≥2 prior chest surgeries
– Hepatic cirrhosis
• ≥3 of the following STS high-risk factors
– Creatinine >2.5 mg/dL
– Prior chest surgery
– Age >75 years
– LVEF<35 %

The average age of the patients was 76 years (vs. 65 years old in EVEREST II trial) and 68 % of patients were older than 75 years of age. The patients had many comorbidities including prior cardiac surgery (62 %), chronic obstructive pulmonary disease (35 %), moderate to severe chronic kidney disease (23 %), and previous myocardial infarction (56 %). Predicted STS risk score was 18.2 ± 8 % and 90 % of patients had NYHA-FC III/IV. As was expected most patients had FMR (59 %), due to their higher risk of morbidity and mortality for surgical repair or replacement.

MitraClip devices were successfully placed in 96 % of patients. Most patients had at least 1+ MR reduction (83 %). MR ≤ 2+ at 30 days, 6 months, and 12 months were 72.9 %, 73.3 %, and 77.8 %, respectively, which represents a statistically significant difference compared to baseline ($p < 0.0001$). Significant improvement in LV dimensions, LV volumes, NYHA-FC, and SF-36 quality of life at 30 days and 1 year was achieved.

The EVEREST II HRR data showed that despite a predicted 30-day mortality of 18 %, the actual mortality was 7.7 %, with 76 % surviving at 1 year. Among the survivors, 79 % of patients had NYHA-FC I/II. The study cohort was compared to a high-risk group that was screened but not treated with MitraClip, who were managed with medical therapy alone. There was a survival advantage at one year with MitraClip compared to the comparator group (73 % vs. 55 %, $p = 0.047$).

DMR vs. FMR   The EVEREST II HRR included 32 patients with DMR and 46 patients with FMR. The mortality was similar between the two groups at 1 year (22 % vs. 26 %, p=NS). At 12 months, 79 % of the FMR and 75 % of the DMR patients had sustained ≤2+ MR by echocardiography. NYHA-FC I/II was achieved similarly in both groups (75 % in DMR and 74 % in FMR patients). Numerically more patients in the DMR group improved by ≥ 1 NYHA-FC at 1 year compared to FMR patients (89 % vs. 80 %). The results of the TTE assessment of LV remodeling such as LVEDV, LVESV, and diastolic and systolic septal-lateral annular dimensions were more interesting. Overall, there was a marked decrease in LVEDV and LVESV, but the results of the study is more granular when fractionated based on the etiology of the MR. DMR patients had a statistically significant 10 % reduction in LEDV at 12 months when compared to baseline with no change in LVESV. FMR patients had a 20 % reduction in LVEDV and 15 % reduction in LVESV. Diastolic and systolic septal-lateral annular dimensions were significantly lower at 1 year in FMR patients, but there was no statistically significant difference in the DMR patient albeit there was a trend toward smaller dimension. Despite better echocardiographic findings in FMR patients, the main finding of this study is similar in clinical endpoint and outcomes, such as NYHA-FC improvement, improved quality of life, and similar survival between DMR and FMR patients.

REALISM Registry

The Real World Expanded Multicenter Study of the MitraClip® System Continued Access study (REALISM) was a prospective, multicenter, continued access registry to collect data on the "real-world" use of the MitraClip device in both high and non-high-surgical risk patients. Enrollment was initiated at the conclusion of the EVEREST II trial to allow patients continued access to the therapy. This study was conducted between 2009 and 2011. Both high-risk and non-high-risk patients were included. All 272 patients completed 1-year follow-up. Although eligibility criteria were similar between the EVEREST II RCT and the non-high-risk arm of the REALISM study, patients enrolled in the registry were older and had more comorbidities. The mean age of patients enrolled in non-high-risk REALISM was 74 ± 11 years vs. 67 ± 13 in EVEREST II trial. DMR was present in 69 % and FMR in 31 % compared to 73 % and 27 %, respectively, in EVEREST II. Freedom from mortality at 12 months was 91.0 % (EVEREST II = 93.7 %). Importantly, freedom from mitral valve surgery at 12 months was 90.1 %, compared to 80 % in the EVEREST II trial. Consistent with the EVEREST II, a majority of patients experienced MR reduction to $\leq 2+$ at 12 months with associated LV remodeling. In addition, 92 % of patients in NYHA-FC I/II at 12 months and scores for the physical and mental components of the SF-36 improved between baseline and 12 months. The results of the non-high-risk REALISM are not yet available. The high-risk REALISM study reported 12-month outcomes [21]. Patients with grades 3 to 4+ MR and a surgical mortality risk of ≥ 12 %, based on the Society of Thoracic Surgeons risk calculator or the estimate of a surgeon coinvestigator following prespecified protocol criteria, were enrolled. 327 of 351 patients completed 12 months of follow-up. Patients were elderly (76 ± 11 years of age), with 70 % having functional MR and 60 % having prior cardiac surgery. The mitral valve device reduced MR to $\leq 2+$ in

86 % of patients at discharge ($p<0.0001$). Major adverse events at 30 days included death in 4.8 %, myocardial infarction in 1.1 %, and stroke in 2.6 %. At 12 months, MR was ≤2+ in 84 % of patients ($p<0.0001$). From baseline to 12 months, LV end-diastolic volume improved from 161 ± 56 ml to 143 ± 53 ml ($p<0.0001$) and LV end-systolic volume improved from 87 ± 47 ml to 79 ± 44 ml ($p<0.0001$). NYHA-FC improved from 82 % in class III/IV at baseline to 83 % in class I/II at 12 months ($p<0.0001$). The 36-item Short Form Health Survey physical and mental quality of life scores improved from baseline to 12 months ($p<0.0001$). Annual hospitalization rate for heart failure fell from 0.79 % pre-procedure to 0.41 % post-procedure ($p<0.0001$). Kaplan–Meier survival estimate at 12 months was 77.2 %. The percutaneous mitral valve device significantly reduced MR, improved clinical symptoms, and decreased LV dimensions at 12 months in this high-surgical-risk cohort.

The results of the High-Risk Registry and REALISM combined prospective registries included predominantly FMR patients.

High-Risk DMR Patients

To define the outcomes for DMR patients, a high-risk DMR subgroup from the High-Risk and REALISM registries was analyzed [5]. A prohibitive-risk DMR cohort was identified by a multidisciplinary heart team that retrospectively evaluated high-risk DMR patients. A group of 127 patients were retrospectively identified as meeting the definition of prohibitive risk and had a median of 1.47 years of follow-up available. Patients were elderly with a mean age of 82.4 years, severely symptomatic with 87 % New York Heart Association class III/IV, and at prohibitive surgical risk with STS score 13.2 ± 7.3 %. MitraClip was successfully performed in 95.3 %. Hospital stay was 2.9 ± 3.1 days. Major adverse events at 30 days included death in 6.3 %, myocardial infarction in 0.8 %, and stroke in 2.4 %. Through 1 year, there were a total of 30 deaths (23.6 %), with no survival difference between patients discharged with MR 1+ or 2+. At 1 year, the majority of surviving patients (82.9 %) remained MR ≤2+ at 1 year, and 86.9 % were in NYHA-FC I or II. Left ventricular end-diastolic volume decreased (from 125.1 ± 40.1 ml to 108.5 ± 37.9 ml ($p<0.0001$). SF-36 quality of life scores improved, and hospitalizations for heart failure were reduced in patients whose MR was reduced. MitraClip in prohibitive surgical risk DMR patients is associated with safety and good clinical outcomes, including decreases in rehospitalization, functional improvements, and favorable ventricular remodeling, at 1 year.

ACCESS-EU Registry

ACCESS-EU study was a two-phased prospective, single-arm, multicenter post-approval observational study of the MitraClip in Europe for the treatment of MR [22]. The primary objective of the ACCESS-EU study was to gain information with respect to health economics and clinical care and to provide further evidence of safety and effectiveness. A total of 567 patients with MR $\geq 3+$ underwent MitraClip implantation at 14 European centers. Mean logistic European System for Cardiac Operative Risk Evaluation (EuroSCORE) at baseline was 23.0 ± 18.3, 84.9 % patients were in NYHA-FC III or IV, and 52.7 % of patients had an LVEF < 40 %. DMR was present in 20 % of the cohort (117/567 patients). Ninety percent of patients with DMR had LVEF > 40 %, while 66 % of patients with FMR had LVEF < 40 %. Cardiogenic shock was present in 5 % of patients at the time of implantation. Logistic EuroSCORE > 20 % was present in 48 % of patients with FMR and 28 % of patients with DMR. Cardiac resynchronization therapy (CRT) and automatic intracardiac defibrillator (AICD) were more common in FMR patients, while the pacemaker rate was similar between DMR and FMR patients.

The MitraClip implant rate was 99.6 %. A total of 19 patients (3.4 %) died within 30 days after the MitraClip procedure. The mortality rate of FMR patients was 2.8 % while that of the DMR patients was 6 %. The survival at 1 year was 81.8 % for the overall cohort with no difference between the FMR and DMR patients. Intensive care unit and hospital length of stay was 2.5 ± 6.5 days and 7.7 ± 8.2 days, respectively. Single leaflet device attachment was reported in 27 patients (4.8 %) with no device embolization. Mitral valve surgery was required in 6.3 % of patients within 12 months after the MitraClip implant procedure. There was improvement in the severity of MR at 12 months, compared with baseline ($p < 0.0001$), with 78.9 % of patients free from MR $> 2+$ at 12 months. There was no difference between FMR and DMR reduction in MR severity at 12 months. At 12 months, 71 % of patients had NYHA-FC I/II. Six-minute walk test improved 59.5 ± 112.4 m, and Minnesota Living With Heart Failure score improved 13.5 ± 20.5 points.

DMR vs. FMR   ACCESS-EU study has meticulously identified patients with DMR vs. FMR. The clinical endpoints of the study are similar between the two groups. The results of the second phase of the study that includes the echocardiographic data of the patients and LV remodeling indices are not yet available. It is important to note, however, that patients in FMR group in this registry have higher comorbidities compared to DMR group. Despite higher rate of congestive heart failure, myocardial infarction, atrial fibrillation, diabetes, and other comorbidities in FMR group, the survival at 12 months are similar between the groups. The clinical outcomes (e.g., 6-minute walk test) and quality of life have certainly improved in both groups of DMR and FMR when MitraClip is implanted.

Indices of LV Reverse Remodeling in DMR and FMR

Grayburn et al. performed an elegant study on the patients who received MitraClip in EVEREST II, EVEREST II HRR, and REALISM studies [23]. A total of 801 patients treated with MitraClip were compared to 80 patients treated with surgery. The study defined reverse remodeling by reduction in LVEDV, LVESV, and

LA volume. These indices were subsequently correlated with MR reduction. They also used a separate model to fit for FMR and DMR at 1 year. Patients with DMR who achieved MR ≤ 2+ at one year had lower LVEDV and LA volume, but LVESV was not different. Patients with FMR and MR ≤ 2+ at one year had a marked reduction in LVEDV, LVESV, and LA volume. These findings recapitulate similar finding observed in EVEREST HRR. MitraClip improves hemodynamic profile and LV reverse remodeling by reducing LV preload and maintains the contractility despite increase in afterload [24].

FDA Approval for MitraClip in High-Risk DMR Patients

MitraClip was approved by FDA on October 24, 2013, for a narrowly defined patient population. The exact language in the instructions for use (IFU) is: "The MitraClip Clip Delivery System is indicated for the percutaneous reduction of significant symptomatic MR (MR ≥ 3+) due to primary abnormality of the mitral apparatus [degenerative MR] in patients who have been determined to be at prohibitive risk for mitral valve surgery by a heart team, which includes a cardiac surgeon experienced in mitral valve surgery and a cardiologist experienced in mitral valve disease, and in whom existing comorbidities would not preclude the expected benefit from reduction of the MR." The IFU warns "DO NOT use MitraClip outside of the labeled indication. Treatment of nonprohibitive-risk DMR patients should be conducted in accordance with standard hospital practices for surgical repair and replacement" and further notes that "the safety and effectiveness of the MitraClip device has not been established in patients with MR due to underlying ventricular pathology (FMR)." The approval specifies the anatomic requirements for treatment (Table 13.2). A multi-society group has proposed operator and institutional requirements for this new procedure (Table 13.3). At the time of this writing, these requirements have not been finalized by CMS. Comment regarding the language of a National Coverage Determination is ongoing.

Table 13.2 Anatomic considerations in the MitraClip IFU

For optimal results, the following anatomic patient characteristics should be considered. The safety and effectiveness of the MitraClip outside of these conditions has not been established. Use outside these conditions may interfere with placement of the MitraClip device or mitral valve leaflet insertion
– The primary regurgitant jet is noncommissural. If a secondary jet exists, it must be considered clinically insignificant
– Mitral valve area ≥4 cm^2
– Minimal calcification in the grasping area
– No leaflet cleft in the grasping area
– Flail width < 15 mm and flail gap < 10 mm

Table 13.3 Proposed institutional and operator requirements for percutaneous mitral repair with MitraClip

Interventional program: 1000 cath/400 PCI per year
– Interventionist: 50 structural procedures per year (including ASD/PFO and transseptal punctures)
– Surgical program: 25 total mitral valve procedures per year, of which at least 10 must be mitral valve repairs
– All cases must be submitted to a single national database
– Existing programs: 15 mitral (total experience)

Conclusion

MitraClip implantation is a novel and viable option in patients with severe MR. The gold standard for patients with DMR remains to be mitral valve repair. However, patients with severe comorbidities resulting in high surgical risk and DMR may benefit from MitraClip therapy. The population for which the device was approved represents high-risk patients for surgery with DMR, for whom results with MitraClip have been clear in terms of improving symptoms and resulting in favorable LF chamber remodeling. These patients represent a population for whom historically there have been no other alternatives for therapy. These are elderly patients, often with fibroelastic deficiency as the etiology of their DMR. Many of these patients have relatively preserved LV systolic function, in contrast to the severely depressed LF ejection fraction seen in the typical patient with ischemic cardiomyopathy and FMR.

References

1. St. Goar F. Development of percutaneous edge-to-edge repair: the MitraClip story. In: Feldman T, St. Goar F, editors. Percutaneous mitral leaflet repair. London: Informa; 2012. p. 31–5. Chapter 6.
2. Alfieri O, Maisano F, De Bonis M, et al. The double-orifice technique in mitral valve repair: a simple solution for complex problems. J Thorac Cardiovasc Surg. 2001;122:674–81.
3. Feldman T, Wasserman HS, Herrmann HC, et al. Percutaneous mitral valve repair using the edge-to-edge technique: six-month results of the EVEREST Phase I Clinical Trial. J Am Coll Cardiol. 2005;46:2134–40.
4. Feldman T, Foster E, Glower D, Kar S, Rinaldi MJ, Fail PS, Smalling RW, Siegel R, Rose GA, Engeron E, Loghin C, Trento A, Skipper ER, Fudge T, Letsou GV, Massaro JM, Mauri L. For the EVEREST II investigators: percutaneous repair or surgery for mitral regurgitation. New Engl J Med. 2011;364:1395–406.
5. Lim DS, Reynolds MR, Feldman T, Kar S, Herrmann HC, Wang A, Whitlow PL, Gray WA, Grayburn P, Mack MJ, Glower D. Improved functional status and quality of life in prohibitive surgical risk patients with degenerative mitral regurgitation following transcatheter mitral valve repair with the MitraClip system. J Am Coll Cardiol. 2014;64:182–92.
6. Enriquez-Sarano M, Akins CW, Vahanian A. Mitral regurgitation. Lancet. 2009;373(9672):1382–94. doi:10.1016/S0140-6736(09)60692-9.

7. Jones EC, Devereux RB, Roman MJ, Liu JE, Fishman D, Lee ET, Welty TK, Fabsitz RR, Howard BV. Prevalence and correlates of mitral regurgitation in a population-based sample (the Strong Heart Study). Am J Cardiol. 2001;87(3):298–304.

8. Carabello BA. The current therapy for mitral regurgitation. J Am Coll Cardiol. 2008;52(5):319–26.

9. Suri RM, Schaff HV, Dearani JA, Sundt III TM, Daly RC, Mullany CJ, Enriquez-Sarano M, Orszulak TA. Survival advantage and improved durability of mitral repair for leaflet prolapse subsets in the current era. Ann Thorac Surg. 2006;82(3):819–26.

10. Fucci C, Sandrelli L, Pardini A, Torracca L, Ferrari M, Alfieri O. Improved results with mitral valve repair using new surgical techniques. Eur J Cardiothorac Surg. 1995;9(11):621–6.

11. Maisano F, Viganò G, Blasio A, Colombo A, Calabrese C, Alfieri O. Surgical isolated edge-to-edge mitral valve repair without annuloplasty: clinical proof of the principle for an endovascular approach. EuroIntervention. 2006;2(2):181–6.

12. St Goar FG, Fann JI, Komtebedde J, Foster E, Oz MC, Fogarty TJ, Feldman T, Block PC. Endovascular edge-to-edge mitral valve repair: short-term results in a porcine model. Circulation. 2003;108(16):1990–3.

13. Fann JI, St Goar FG, Komtebedde J, Oz MC, Block PC, Foster E, Butany J, Feldman T, Burdon TA. Beating heart catheter-based edge-to-edge mitral valve procedure in a porcine model: efficacy and healing response. Circulation. 2004;110(8):988–93.

14. Ladich E, Michaels MB, Jones RM, McDermott E, Coleman L, Komtebedde J, Glower D, Argenziano M, Feldman T, Nakano M, Virmani R, Endovascular Valve Edge-to-Edge Repair Study (EVEREST) Investigators. Pathological healing response of explanted MitraClip devices. Circulation. 2011;123(13):1418–27.

15. Lin BA, Forouhar AS, Pahlevan NM, Anastassiou CA, Grayburn PA, Thomas JD, Gharib M. Color Doppler jet area overestimates regurgitant volume when multiple jets are present. J Am Soc Echocardiogr. 2010;23(9):993–1000.

16. Feldman T, Kar S, Rinaldi M, Fail P, Hermiller J, Smalling R, Whitlow PL, Gray W, Low R, Herrmann HC, Lim S, Foster E, Glower D, EVEREST Investigators. Percutaneous mitral repair with the MitraClip system: safety and midterm durability in the initial EVEREST (Endovascular Valve Edge-to-Edge REpair Study) cohort. J Am Coll Cardiol. 2009;54(8):686–94.

17. Feldman T, Foster E, Glower DD, Kar S, Rinaldi MJ, Fail PS, Smalling RW, Siegel R, Rose GA, Engeron E, Loghin C, Trento A, Skipper ER, Fudge T, Letsou GV, Massaro JM, Mauri L, EVEREST II Investigators. Percutaneous repair or surgery for mitral regurgitation. N Engl J Med. 2011;364(15):1395–406.

18. O'Brien SM, Shahian DM, Filardo G, Ferraris VA, Haan CK, Rich JB, Normand SL, DeLong ER, Shewan CM, Dokholyan RS, Peterson ED, Edwards FH, Anderson RP, Society of Thoracic Surgeons Quality Measurement Task Force. The Society of Thoracic Surgeons 2008 cardiac surgery risk models: part 2--isolated valve surgery. Ann Thorac Surg. 2009;88(1 Suppl):S23–42.

19. Mauri L, Foster E, Glower DD, Apruzzese P, Massaro JM, Herrmann HC, Hermiller J, Gray W, Wang A, Pedersen WR, Bajwa T, Lasala J, Low R, Grayburn P, Feldman T, EVEREST II Investigators. 4-year results of a randomized controlled trial of percutaneous repair versus surgery for mitral regurgitation. J Am Coll Cardiol. 2013;62(4):317–28.

20. Whitlow PL, Feldman T, Pedersen WR, Lim DS, Kipperman R, Smalling R, Bajwa T, Herrmann HC, Lasala J, Maddux JT, Tuzcu M, Kapadia S, Trento A, Siegel RJ, Foster E, Glower D, Mauri L, Kar S, EVEREST II Investigators. Acute and 12-month results with catheter-based mitral valve leaflet repair: the EVEREST II (Endovascular Valve Edge-to-Edge Repair) High Risk Study. J Am Coll Cardiol. 2012;59(2):130–9.

21. Glower D, Kar S, Lim DS, Bajwa T, Quesada R, Whitlow P, Rinaldi MJ, Grayburn P, Mauri L, Feldman T. Percutaneous MitraClip device therapy for mitral regurgitation in 351 patients - high risk subset of the EVEREST II Study. J Am Coll Cardiol. 2014;64:172–81.

22. Maisano F, Franzen O, Baldus S, Schäfer U, Hausleiter J, Butter C, Ussia GP, Sievert H, Richardt G, Widder JD, Moccetti T, Schillinger W. Percutaneous mitral valve interventions in the real world: early and 1-year results from the ACCESS-EU, a prospective, multicenter, nonrandomized post-approval study of the MitraClip therapy in Europe. J Am Coll Cardiol. 2013;62(12):1052–61.
23. Grayburn PA, Foster E, Sangli C, Weissman NJ, Massaro J, Glower DG, Feldman T, Mauri L. Relationship between the magnitude of reduction in mitral regurgitation severity and left ventricular and left atrial reverse remodeling after MitraClip therapy. Circulation. 2013;128(15):1667–74.
24. Gaemperli O, Biaggi P, Gugelmann R, Osranek M, Schreuder JJ, Bühler I, Sürder D, Lüscher TF, Felix C, Bettex D, Grünenfelder J, Corti R. Real-time left ventricular pressure-volume loops during percutaneous mitral valve repair with the MitraClip system. Circulation. 2013;127(9):1018–27.

Chapter 14
Mitral Annular Techniques

Paul A. Grayburn

Mitral annuloplasty has long been a staple of surgical mitral valve repair. In primary MR, annuloplasty is usually an adjunct to leaflet resection, leaflet repair, and chordal replacement. Annuloplasty reduces stress on the leaflets [1, 2] and therefore supports durability of the primary repair. In secondary or functional MR, mitral annuloplasty is usually the primary repair technique, although it can be combined with subvalvular approaches to augment systolic leaflet closure [3, 4]. In secondary MR, mitral valve repair has not been clearly shown to improve survival and accordingly has been generally classified as a IIB indication by the American and European guidelines [5, 6]. Recently, two important randomized clinical trials by the Cardiothoracic Surgery Network (CTSN) have investigated the clinical utility of mitral annuloplasty. In the CSTN Severe MR trial [7], patients with severe functional MR were randomized to chord-sparing MVR or annuloplasty with an undersized complete ring with or without subvalvular procedures. There was no significant difference in the primary endpoint of LV end-systolic volume reduction nor in 30-day or one-year mortality or functional outcomes. However, there was a 32 % recurrence of moderate or greater MR at 1 year in the annuloplasty group. In the CTSN moderate MR trial [8], patients with moderate functional MR undergoing CABG were randomized to CABG alone or CABG plus mitral annuloplasty. There was no significant difference in the primary endpoint of LV end-systolic volume reduction nor in 30-day or 1 year mortality, heart failure hospitalization, or measures of functional capacity. Although the role of mitral annuloplasty as a treatment for functional MR remains unclear, several transcatheter methods have been developed and are in various stages of clinical testing.

P.A. Grayburn, MD (✉)
Department of Cardiology, Baylor University Medical Center, Baylor Heart and Vascular
Institute, 621 North Hall Street, Suite 1-030, Dallas, TX 75093, USA
e-mail: Paul.Grayburn@BSWHealth.org

© Springer Science+Business Media New York 2016
G. Ailawadi, I.L. Kron (eds.), *Catheter Based Valve and Aortic Surgery*,
DOI 10.1007/978-1-4939-3432-4_14

Indirect Annuloplasty via the Coronary Sinus The earliest transcatheter annuloplasty devices attempted to reduce mitral annulus size indirectly via the coronary sinus. The Carillon Mitral Contour System (Cardiac Dimension, Inc., Kirkland, WA) received the CE Mark for clinical use in Europe in 2011. Two studies have been published: AMADEUS, an initial feasibility study of the first generation device [9], and TITAN, an observational study of a second generation device [10]. In AMADEUS, 30 of 48 patients were successfully implanted with a 15 % risk of circumflex coronary artery impingement and one death. In TITAN 36 of 53, enrolled subjects received the device with improved MR grade, LV reverse remodeling, 6-min walk times, and functional class compared to those who did not receive the device.

There are several limitations to the coronary sinus approach. There are anatomical constraints that limit the ability to implant many patients. Chief among these is that the circumflex artery occlusion courses between the coronary sinus and the mitral annulus in a majority of patients [11, 12]. In addition, there can be increased distance between the coronary sinus and the mitral annulus, particularly in dilated cardiomyopathy, limiting the ability of such devices to effectively reduce annulus size [11]. Perhaps more importantly, the coronary sinus does not completely encircle the mitral annulus, so it does not mimic the surgical technique of implanting a complete ring directly over the annulus. Although the Carillon device received the CE Mark in Europe, two other devices (Monarc, Edwards Lifesciences, Irvine, CA and Viacor PTMA, Viacor, Wilmington, MA) are no longer available. Despite initial early success with the Viacor PTMA device [13], two fatal coronary sinus lacerations were reported [14, 15], and the device was taken off the market. It is generally agreed that there is no viable future for mitral annuloplasty via the coronary sinus [16–18].

Direct Annuloplasty: Mitralign The Mitralign System (Mitralign, Inc., Tewksbury, MA) attempts to mimic the Kay annuloplasty [19]. A steerable guiding catheter is placed into the LV via retrograde approach from a femoral artery. An insulated radiofrequency wire is used to cross through the mitral annulus into the LA using TEE guidance. Two pairs of wires are placed in the mitral annulus, two posterior to the posteromedial scallop and two posterior to the posterolateral scallop. The two sets of wires are used as rails to place two pledgets, which are then tightened to reduce MR severity by reducing the anteroposterior annular dimension (Fig. 14.1). A CE Mark trial of 61 patients has been completed, but the results have not been published, yet.

Direct Annuloplasty: Accucinch The Accucinch System (Guided Delivery Systems, Santa Clara, CA) also uses a retrograde approach to the mitral annulus from the LV. A steerable guiding catheter is positioned between the chordae tendineae and the LV wall on the LV side of the anatomic mitral annulus. A series of anchors are placed into the LV myocardium while withdrawing the guiding catheter from the lateral to medial aspect of the posterior mitral annulus (Fig. 14.2). A nitinol wire connected to each anchor is then tightened under TEE guidance until MR reduction is

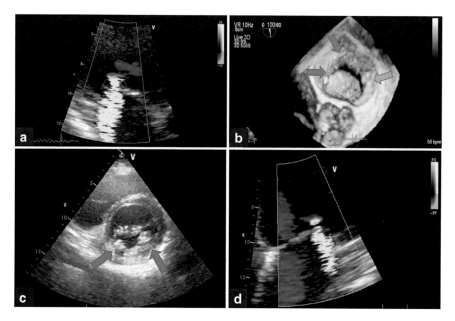

Fig. 14.1 Echocardiographic images of the Mitralign procedure; (**a**) mitral regurgitation before the procedure; (**b**) 3D image of implanted pledget (*orange arrow*) and guiding wires positioned across the annulus (*blue arrows*) before placement of the second implant; (**c**) short axis view, two pledgets implanted (*arrows*); (**d**) reduced mitral regurgitation after the procedure. From Siminiak et al. [19]

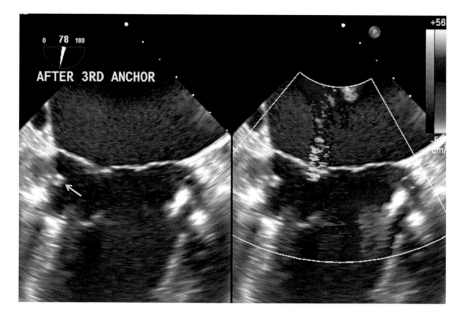

Fig. 14.2 Intraprocedural images during a Accucinch human implant. Mid-commissural TEE images showing a subannular anchor (*yellow arrow*, *left*) behind P3 and the location of the MR jet on color flow imaging (*right*)

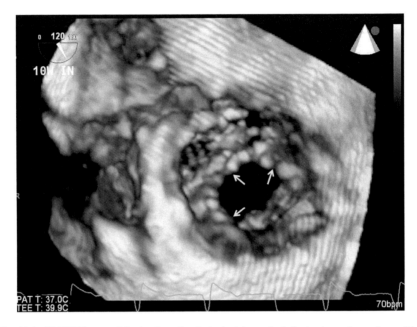

Fig. 14.3 3D TEE image of the implanted and cinched Accucinch device in a subannular position (*yellow arrows*) with reduction of anteroposterior annular dimension. MR was virtually eliminated in this patient on the intraoperative TEE

achieved. This approach offers the theoretical advantage of reducing LV size at the base of the heart, since the anchors are placed in a subannular location in the LV myocardium. MR reduction is observed in a beating heart during cinching of the device. Although initial human implants have been performed successfully (Fig. 14.3), there are no published reports in the medical literature as of this writing.

Direct Annuloplasty: Cardioband The Cardioband device (Valtech Cardio, Inc., Or Yehuda, Israel) is designed to replicate surgical annuloplasty by placing the device directly on the mitral annulus from the left atrium. The device is delivered to the annulus via transseptal puncture using a 25F steerable guiding catheter. A series of 12–16 screw anchors are used to secure the device to the annulus from the anterolateral to the posteromedial commissure. The anchors are placed using TEE guidance (Fig. 14.4) and after all anchors are placed, a cinching tool is used to reduce the anteroposterior dimension of the mitral annulus. The amount of cinching is determined by observing the degree of MR reduction by TEE in the beating heart. The first-in-man use of the transfemoral Cardioband was recently reported [20]. A 30-patient CE Mark study is nearing completion, and results are anticipated soon. Clinical trials in the USA are anticipated to begin in 2015 (Fig. 14.5).

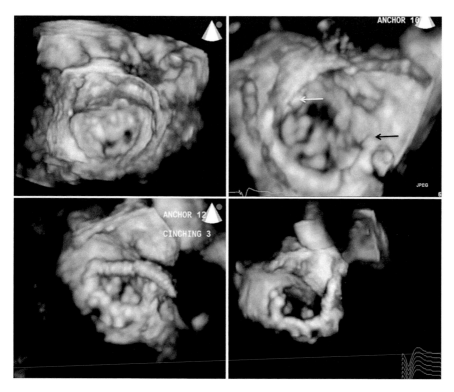

Fig. 14.4 3D TEE images showing the steps in Cardioband placement. (*Top left*) Baseline image at end-systole showing incomplete leaflet closure with two separate regurgitant orifices. (*Top right*) Multiple anchors are placed to fit the device to the annulus from the lateral commissure (*yellow arrow*) to the medial commissure (*black arrow*). (*Bottom left*) The device is cinched to reduce annulus size. Cinching is adjusted using color Doppler to optimize MR reduction. (*Bottom right*) Final result showing the deployed, cinched Cardioband device

Future Devices and Clinical Role for Direct Annuloplasty A number of other devices are currently in preclinical development [16–18]. Given the results of the CTSN trials, it will be important to demonstrate durability of these devices, rate of MR recurrence over time, and whether recurrent MR is due to device dehiscence or progressive LV remodeling and leaflet tethering. Patient selection may play a critical role as such devices would theoretically work better in patients with pure annular dilation and less well in severely restricted posterior leaflets where moving the annulus anteriorly could worsen tethering and therefore MR severity. It is also possible that transcatheter direct annuloplasty may be combined with other transcatheter approaches, such as MitraClip or artificial chords to improve results in individual patients.

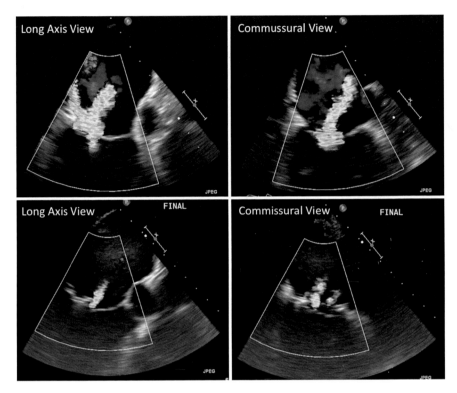

Fig. 14.5 Intraprocedural TEE images showing MR reduction from baseline (*top panels*) to post-Cardioband deployment and cinching (*bottom panels*)

References

1. Kunzelman KS, Reimink MS, Cochran RP. Annular dilatation increases stress in the mitral valve and delays coaptation: a finite element comouter model. Cardiovasc Surg. 1997;5: 427–34.
2. Votta E, Maisano F, Soncini M, Redaelli A, Montevecchi FM, Alfieri O. 3-D computational analysis of the stress distribution on the leafets after edge-to-edge repair of mitral regurgitation. J Heart Valve Dis. 2002;11:810–22.
3. Wagner CE, Kron IL. Subvalvular techniques to optimize surgical repair of ischemic mitral regurgitation. Curr Opin Cardiol. 2014;29:140–4.
4. Fattouch K, Lancellotti P, Castrovinci S, et al. Papillary muscle relocation in conjunction with valve annuloplasty improve repair results in severe ischemic mitral regurgitation. J Thorac Cardiovasc Surg. 2012;143:1352–5.
5. Vahanian A, Baumgartner H, Bax J, et al. Guidelines on the management of valvular heart disease: the Task Force on the Management of Valvular Heart Disease of the European Society of Cardiology. Eur Heart J. 2007;28:230–68.
6. Nishimura RA, Otto CM, Bonow RO, Carabello BA, Erwin III JP, Guyton RA, O'Gara PT, Ruiz CE, Skubas NJ, Sorajja P, Sundt III TM, Thomas JD. 2014 AHA/ACC Guidelines for the Management of Patients With Valvular Heart Disease. J Am Coll Cardiol. 2014;63:e57–185.
7. Acker MA, Parides MK, Perrault LP, et al. Mitral valve repair or replacement for severe ischemic mitral regurgitation. N Engl J Med. 2013;370:23–32.

8. Smith PK, Puskas JD, Ascheim DD, et al. Surgical treatment of moderate ischemic mitral regurgitation. N Engl J Med. 2014;371:2178–88.

9. Schofer J, Siminiak T, Haude M, et al. Percutaneous mitral annuloplasty for functional mitral regurgitation: results of the CARILLON Mitral Annuloplasty Device European Union Study. Circulation. 2009;120:326–33.

10. Siminiak T, Wu JC, Haude M, et al. Treatment of functional mitral regurgitation by percutaneous annuloplasty: results of the TITAN Trial. Eur J Heart Fail. 2012;14:931–8.

11. Choure AJ, Garcia MJ, Hesse B, et al. In vivo analysis of the anatomical relationship of coronary sinus to mitral annulus and left circumflex coronary artery using cardiac multidetector computed tomography: Implications for percutaneous coronary sinus mitral annuloplasty. J Am Coll Cardiol 2006;48:1938–45.

12. Gopal A, Shah A, Shareghi S, et al. The role of cardiovascular computed tomographic angiography for coronary sinus mitral annuloplasty. J Invasive Cardiol. 2010;22:67–73.

13. van Mieghem NM, Schultz CJ, Spencer R, Serruys PW, de Jaegere PP. Transcatheter indirect mitral annuloplasty with the PTMA system: a technical report. EuroIntervention. 2011;7:164-9.

14. Noble S, Vilarino R, Muller H, Sunthorn H, Roffi M. Fatal coronary sinus and aortic erosions following percutaneous transvenous mitral annuloplasty device. EuroIntervention. 2011;7: 148–50.

15. Machaalaney J, St Pierre A, Senechal M, et al. Fatal late migration of Viacore percutaneous transvenous mitral annuloplasty device resulting in distal coronary venous perforation. Can J Cardiol. 2013;29:130.e1–4.

16. Feldman T, Young A. Percutaneous approaches to valve repair for mitral regurgitation. J Am Coll Cardiol. 2014;63:2057–68.

17. Taramasso M, Maisano F. Transcatheter mitral valve repair – transcatheter mitral valve annuloplasty. EuroIntervention. 2014;10:U129–35.

18. Herrmann HC, Maisano F. Transcatheter therapy of mitral regurgitation. Circulation. 2014;130:1712–22.

19. Siminiak T, Dankowski R, Baszko A, Lee C, Firek L, Kałmucki P, Szyszka A, Groothuis A. Percutaneous direct mitral annuloplasty using the Mitralign Bident system: description of the method and a case report. Kardiol Pol. 2013;71(12):1287–92.

20. Maisano F, La Canna G, Latib A, et al. First-in-man transseptal implantation of a "surgical-like" mitral annuloplasty device for functional mitral regurgitation. JACC Cardiovasc Interv. 2014;7:1326–8.

Chapter 15
Interventional Mitral Annular Reduction Techniques

Robert Schueler, Georg Nickenig, and Christoph Hammersting

Mitral regurgitation (MR) is the second most frequent native valve disease, and its prevalence increases with age and cardiac comorbidities [1, 2]. Compared to the aortic valve, the anatomy and function of the mitral valve (MV) and its apparatus is more complex, and there are complicated interactions between the annulus, the leaflets, the subvalvular apparatus, and the left ventricle. There are two entities that should be defined and separated for both diagnosis and treatment: primary MR, with an abnormality of the MV itself being the reason for regurgitation which ultimately can cause left ventricle dysfunction, and secondary MR, where the MV leaflets are more or less normal and impairment and dysfunction of the valvular apparatus is caused by pathological left ventricular remodeling in presence of either ischemic heart disease or other forms of cardiomyopathy (Fig. 15.1) [3, 4]. Patients with secondary MR are often elderly with relevant comorbidities, increasing the risk for interventional or surgical MV therapy [5–8]. Current European and American guidelines recommend cardiac surgery in symptomatic patients with severe MR, as well as in asymptomatic patients with deteriorated left ventricular (LV) function and in asymptomatic patients with normal LV function when there is a high likelihood of successful surgical repair or other risk factors exist such as atrial fibrillation or pulmonary hypertension. Surgery may also be considered in patients with secondary MR in symptomatic patients after optimal medical management if bypass surgery is indicated [3, 4]. Stand-alone surgery in patients with secondary MR remains controversial and is indicated only in exceptional cases. Surgical reconstruction of the regurgitant valve has been considered superior over valve replacement, and restrictive annuloplasty has been the method of choice in most of these patients, although recent data cast doubts on this strategy [9–11].

R. Schueler, MD • G. Nickenig, MD • C. Hammersting, MD (✉)
Department of Cardiology, Pulmonology, Angiology, and Internal Intensive Care, University Hospital, University of Bonn, Sigmund-Freud Str. 25, NRW, Bonn 53127, Germany
e-mail: robert.schueler@ukb.uni-bonn.de; Georg.nickenig@ukb.uni-bonn.de; christoph.hammerstingl@ukb.uni-bonn.de

© Springer Science+Business Media New York 2016
G. Ailawadi, I.L. Kron (eds.), *Catheter Based Valve and Aortic Surgery*,
DOI 10.1007/978-1-4939-3432-4_15

Fig. 15.1 Schematical 2 chamber view of the left ventricle and the mitral apparatus: *1* Dilation and distortion of the mitral annulus, *2* asymmetric or symmetric displacement of the papillary muscles, *3* global dilation and left ventricular dysfunction may lead to dysfunction of the mitral apparatus resulting in secondary mitral regurgitation

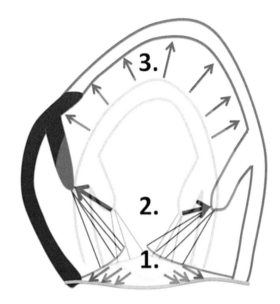

Numerous interventional approaches for the treatment of patients with symptomatic MR at prohibitive surgical risk have been investigated so far (Table 15.1) and up to now only two of them have received CE mark (MitraClip and Carillon systems). A limited number of other MV devices are currently tested in (pre-) clinical studies for use in highly selected patients (Table 15.1).

Currently, the predominantly used interventional technique worldwide is the percutaneous edge-to-edge repair with the MitraClip system with over 16,000 treated patients, interestingly thereof 70 % of patients with secondary MR which is in contrast to the earlier EVEREST studies [12]. Despite its beneficial effects on heart failure related symptoms in such patients, a positive influence on patient's survival has not been proven yet [13]. In general, the durability of the MitraClip system in patients with secondary MR has been discussed vigorously since this technique approaches the MV leaflets and not the underlying pathological annular dilatation [14, 15].

On the other side, in high risk patients surgical mortality rates are suggested to be as high as 17 % with cardiovascular or heart failure related morbidity occurring in more than 30 % of patients [16]. Furthermore, surgery in elderly patients is associated with a rate of re-hospitalization in the first 30 days of greater than 20 % [17]. In both ischemic and non-ischemic secondary MR, age and comorbidities are the most important predictors of survival. In these patients, surgery is indicated for improvement of clinical symptoms [3, 4], such as dyspnea, peripheral edema, and progressive fatigue.

Unlike the extensive toolbox available to the mitral surgeon, transcatheter approaches for mitral annuloplasty are still limited by technical feasibility, the demand for low invasiveness of the procedure, and other aspects such as cost effectiveness. In this chapter, we will give an overview on currently available MV devices and future directions of interventional MV treatment.

Table 15.1 Comparison, details and status of transcatheter direct annuloplasty devices currently in development

Anatomic target	Device	Manufacturer	Approach	Complication rates	Pros/Cons	Data	Development status
Leaflets	MitraClip	Abbott Vascular	transvenous/-septal	Death: Re-surgery: Stroke:	+ Huge experience, low complication rates, device replaceable − Only leaflet grasping might not be "enough" in the context of secondary MR (?)	Multiple single-/multicenter studies; impact on survival and outcome still lacking	CE Mark, FDA approved
Indirect annuloplasty	Carillon XE2 Mitral Contour System	Cardiac dimensions Inc.	Transvenous via coronary sinus	In about 20 % implantation not possible because of crossing RCX	+ Easy to implant, low complication rate, device replaceable − Possible coronary artery interference, no direct complete MR reduction	Two studies available	CE Mark

(continued)

Table 15.1 (continued)

Anatomic target	Device	Manufacturer	Approach	Complication rates	Pros/Cons	Data	Development status
Direct annuloplasty	Mitralign	Mitralign Inc.	transarterial	13 % conversion to surgery: more data lacking	– Technically demanding, results visible not before definite implantations	Phase 1 results awaited	Phase 1
	Accucinch	Guided Delivery Systems	transarterial	28 % conversion to surgery; more data lacking	+ "Complete" annuloplasty – Technically demanding, high invasive	Phase 1 results awaited	Phase 1
	Cardioband	Valtech Cardio	transvenous/-septal	Data lacking	+ "Complete" annuloplasty, mimics surgery, "low risk" because of transvenous approach – Technically demanding	Phase 1 results awaited	Phase 1
	Mitral Restriction Ring	Cardiac Implant Solutions	transvenous/-septal	Data lacking	+ Noninvasive chronic progressive cinching possible	No published data	Preclinical

Indirect Annuloplasty Devices

The coronary sinus (CS) "embraces" the MV and is closely related to the posterior and lateral mitral annulus. Animal models have shown that indirect MV annuloplasty is possible by inserting a dedicated device into the CS, which creates a continuous pressure and tension forces on the MV annulus: Thereby, the annular circumference is decreased and mitral leaflet coaptation, theoretically, improves. Different CS devices have been studied so far in clinical practice; currently, the *Carillon Mitral Contour System* (Cardiac Dimension, Inc., Kirkland, Washington) is the only commercially available system still using this approach. The system is implanted via a 9F sheath that is introduced in the internal jugular vein; thereafter, the CS is entered with a guiding catheter. A sizing catheter is introduced in the CS for determination of device size. The CS device has a proximal and distal nitinol anchor connected by a nitinol wire ribbon. The distal anchor is released deep in the coronary sinus as near as possible to the anterior commissure, whereas the proximal anchor should reside near the coronary sinus ostium (Fig. 15.2). To plicate tissue adjacent to the MV, direct tension is placed on the delivery system. Intraprocedural transesophageal or transthoracic echocardiography is often used for the assessment of acute MR reduction, and the device can be repositioned or removed and replaced, if necessary.

Despite its easy use, very low procedural risk, and a certain reduction in MR in majority of cases, several limitations of the Carillon device have been reported: Noninvasive imaging by cardiac computed tomography has demonstrated that the separation between the coronary sinus and mitral apparatus potentially increases significantly in dilated hearts compared with patients with normal hearts; in such cases indirect MV annuloplasty might be less effective [18]. About 20 % of patients have a coronary vessel, particularly the left circumflex artery, which crosses inferiorly to the coronary sinus. Because of the close regional relationship between the coronary sinus and the circumflex artery, the cinching forces of the device potentially cause myocardial ischemia by compromising of the circumflex artery or its major branches. This problem was observed in the AMADEUS (CARILLON Mitral Annuloplasty Device European Union Study), a prospective, single arm feasibility study, and TITAN (The Transcatheter Implantation of the Carillon Mitral Annuloplasty Device), a prospective, non-randomized study of patients with secondary MR, in which a second-generation device was used. In these studies, 15–17 % of patients did not receive a CS device due to compromising of the left circumflex coronary artery [19]. Another reported limitation of the second generation devices was a relevant proportion of fractures of the nitinol wire ribbon, which were, importantly, not associated with adverse clinical outcomes. In the currently used third-generation devices, wire fractures did not occur when tested in a model that reproduced the fractures seen in earlier versions of the device.

The AMADEUS trial was performed to examine the safety and efficacy of the Carillon device for treatment of secondary MR. Patients undergoing indirect annuloplasty with the Carillon system demonstrated significant reduction in mitral annular diameter and MR by at least 1 grade, as well as a continuous improvement in functional NYHA class and quality of life during the follow-up period of 24 months.

R. Schueler et al.

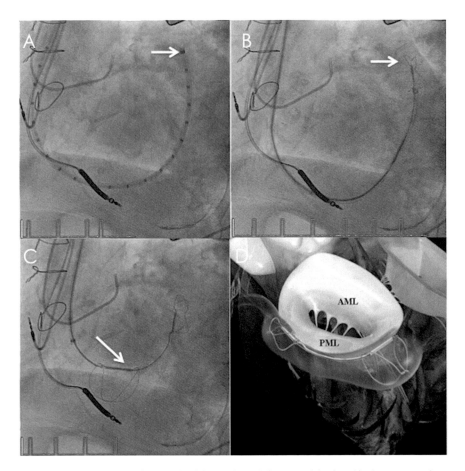

Fig. 15.2 Carillon implantation (**a**) The sizing catheter (*white arrow*) is placed in the coronary sinus for determination of device size. (**b**) Deployment of the distal anchor (*white arrow*) of the device. (**c**) After deployment of the proximal anchor (*white arrow*), the mitral annulus is cinched. (**d**) Schematic illustration of the Carillon device in the coronary sinus and its relation to the mitral annulus

A second-generation device was used in the TITAN trial. Among the 53 enrolled patients, 36 patients underwent successful permanent device implantation [20]. Comparable to results from the AMADEUS study, patients who received the device showed significant reductions in quantitative measures of functional MR, including regurgitant volume and effective regurgitant orifice area, and favorable changes in LV remodeling sustained during 12 months of follow-up. Positive clinical outcomes were reflected in significantly improvement in 6-min walking distances, improvement in functional NYHA class, and quality of life; these effects were sustained or even enhanced during the follow-up period and constantly reported after 24 months. In 17 of the 53 patients, the device could not be permanently implanted, due to difficulties in accessing the coronary sinus, ineffective intraprocedural reduction of MR, or compression of the circumflex artery.

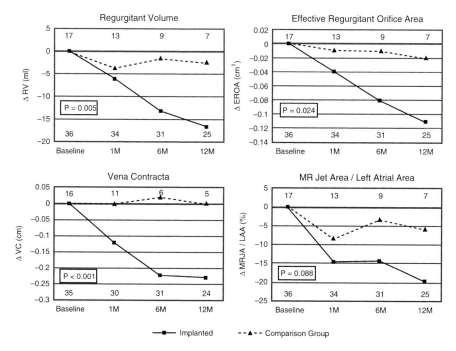

Fig. 15.3 Improvement of parameters determining mitral regurgitation after Carillon implantation during 12 months: Continuous improvement was observed during follow-up of 12 months

The AMADEUS as well as the TITAN study were primarily focused on efficacy of acute reduction of MR grade. Interestingly, although an acute reduction of MR grade was not as good as compared to the MitraClip device, MR reduction was enhanced throughout follow-up time (Fig. 15.3). The authors discussed ongoing pressure on the MV annulus with late-occurring annular and prolonged LV remodeling responsible for this "long-term" effect. However, beneficial effects of the device appear rather modest if compared to other treatment modalities. The Carillon device has received CE mark approval in Europe in 2011.

Other indirect percutaneous mitral annuloplasty devices are no longer in use: The Monarc device (Edwards Lifesciences, Irvine, California) has been studied in a human trial with most patients showing reduction in MR by at least 1 grade. This study has been subsequently stopped due to slow and difficult patient enrollment [21]. The Viacor PTMA system (Viacor, Wilmington, Massachusetts) has been taken off the market due to late, fatal coronary sinus damaging [22].

Direct Annuloplasty

Direct mitral valve annuloplasty is considered the most promising approach for transcatheter mitral valve treatment in patients with secondary MR. It closely reproduces the conventional surgical approach and at this time different technologies are under clinical investigation.

The Mitralign System

The Mitralign system (Mitralign, Inc., Tewksbury, Massachusetts) is a device aiming to achieve partial MV annuloplasty by cinching the annulus at least at two predefined anatomical landmarks on the posterior proportion of the MV annulus. The system is so far inserted retrograde, via an arterial transventricular approach in order to gain access to the mitral annulus. After placing the guide catheter at the ventricular side of the mitral annulus, the MV annulus is penetrated with a wire and radiofrequency. Thereafter, two pairs of anchors (pledgets) made of felt are implanted in the posterior mitral annulus, e.g., next to A1–P1 and A3–P3 using a so-called bident catheter (Fig. 15.4a, b).

Finally, the pledgets are cinched together and locked by a stainless-steel lock at the ventricular side of the implants to reduce the posterior circumference of the mitral annulus (Fig. 15.4c). Preliminary clinical experience with the second-generation device has been reported in 15 high-risk patients with secondary MR. No peri-procedural deaths were observed in this group. At one month, 80 % of the patients had MR ≤2+. Significant quality of life improvements were observed at 6

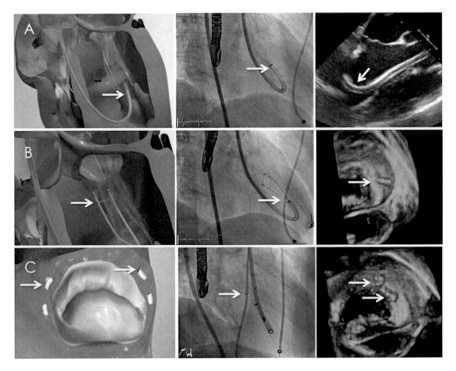

Fig. 15.4 Steps of the Mitralign procedure: (**a**) The guide catheter (*white arrows*) is placed at the ventricular side of the mitral annulus. (**b**) The pledgets are deployed through the "bident" catheter (*white arrows*) using radiofrequency energy. (**c**) The pledgets (*white arrows*) are implanted in the mitral annulus and cinched to achieve a reduction in mitral annular anterior posterior diameter

months. Reduction of the mitral annulus diameters up to 8 mm was observed in this first series of treated patients [23]. A CE approval study has completed patient enrolment, and CE approval is expected in 2015.

The Guided Delivery Systems Accucinch System

The Accucinch system (Guided Delivery Systems, Santa Clara, California) is a direct annuloplasty device that also uses the retrograde transventricular approach. A series of anchors are implanted beneath the MV in the basal LV. A nitinol wire to cinch the basal LV and therefore the mitral annulus connects these anchors (Fig. 15.5). By using this approach, the Accucinch system may cause remodeling of the basal portion of the LV. Feasibility and safety of the Accucinch device have been shown in a small series of 18 patients of whom 28 % had to be converted to surgery, with no reported deaths during 30 days. As reported in an early phase 1 study, this technique leads to a 40 % reduction of regurgitant volumes and effective regurgitant areas, which is accompanied by significant clinical improvement [24]. However, as compared to other interventional devices, this technique has a high invasiveness with a significant conversion rate to surgery; it is technically demanding and several issues must be resolved before introduction for a broad clinical use.

The Valtech CardioBand

The Valtech CardioBand system (Valtech Cardio, Or Yehuda, Israel) is an adjustable, catheter-deliverable, sutureless device. After femoral venous puncture, it is delivered via a transseptal atrial access. The insertion requires a steerable guide and device delivery system that is similar to the MitraClip system. The implant is a Dacron tube that is anchored to the annulus with multiple screw anchors from

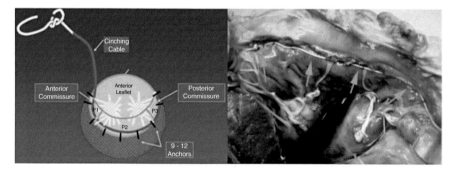

Fig. 15.5 Schematic and in vitro image of the Accucinch device, that is implanted at the ventricular side of the mitral annulus

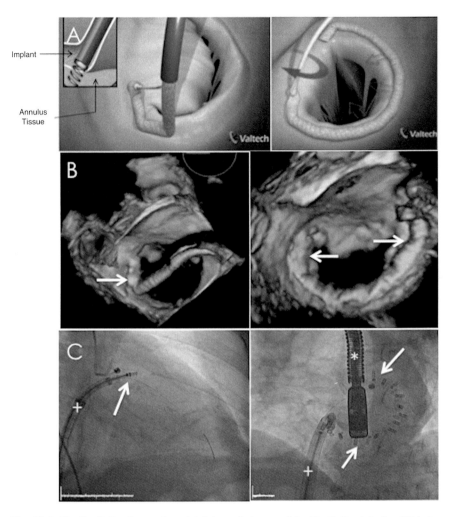

Fig. 15.6 The CardioBand procedure: (**a**) Schematic image of the CardioBand device: With the screw-like anchors, the device is implanted from the anterolateral commissure to the posterome-dial commissure. (**b**) 3D echocardiographic images of the implantation process and the device (*white arrow*) in place. (**c**) Fluoroscopic images of the procedure and the implanted device (*white arrows*; *asterisk* TEE probe; *plus sign* Guide catheter)

commissure to commissure (Fig. 15.6). Thus, the ring is implanted on the atrial side of the mitral annulus. The screw anchors are deployed from the anterolateral commissure to the posteromedial commissure in a counter-clockwise fashion, with the ring extruded from a delivery catheter in small segments. Controlled tension on the band reduces the annular circumference with concomitant reduction of the degree of MR. 3D echocardiography and fluoroscopy guidance is necessary during the interventional process, which makes this procedure well controlled and safe. Once fully anchored, the implant is tensioned to create posterior annuloplasty with septal–lateral dimension reductions of at least 30 % (Fig. 15.6).

Early animal studies demonstrated safety and feasibility in the device, and several patients have had successful percutaneous implants [25]. Although the procedure is technically demanding, this interventional approach is the closest to mimic surgical ring annuloplasty to date with excellent reported acute procedural success and low complication rates of 0 % of device-related major adverse events. MR reduction to ≤2+ was reported to be 91 % after 6 months, with 70 % of patients having mild or none MR at 1 month follow-up. Functional outcome as well improved in 81 % of patients to NYHA class I or II 6 months after CardioBand implantation [25]. First-in-human was performed in 2013 in Milan, Italy, and a European multi-center CE Mark trial with 35 treated patients to date is underway.

Mitral Restriction Ring

Cardiac Implant's Mitral Restriction Ring (Cardiac Implant Solutions LLC, Jacksonville, FL, USA) is another direct annuloplasty device, which is implanted transseptally and is currently under preclinical investigation. It allows the implantation of a complete adjustable mitral ring with an internal cinching wire on the atrial annular side by means of multiple anchor elements, comparable to the Valtech CardioBand device. Of note, the device is designed to enable noninvasive chronic progressive cinching also at follow-up, following the completion of tissue healing. In case of MR recurrence, the complete mitral ring may serve as a retention mechanism for a transcatheter valve-in-ring implantation. Feasibility of this device has been reported so far only in animal models [26].

Other Approaches

Several other devices that address the mitral annulus remain either in preclinical evaluation or involve assisting surgical placement.

The *BOA RF catheter* (QuantumCor Inc., Bothell, WA) uses radiofrequency energy delivered via a transseptal catheter to shrink the tissue of the mitral annulus to somehow mimic surgical ring annuloplasty without implanting a device. In animals, a 20 % reduction in anterior–posterior diameters was achieved with 6-month durability. A first-in-man study during open-heart surgery is planned [27].

MitraSpan Inc. is developing a transapical catheter-based approach utilizing the placement of two sutures, which span and cinch the mitral annulus from the anterior trigones to the posterior annulus, comparable to the Mitralign approach. An outside US feasibility trial is planned [28].

Three other devices, involving hybrid surgical and transcatheter techniques, are under clinical evaluation.

The Adjustable Annuloplasty Ring (St. Jude Medical Inc., St. Paul, MN), the enCor Dynaplasty ring (MiCardia Corp, Irvine, CA), and the CardinalRing

(ValtechCardio Inc., Or Yehuda, Israel) are surgically implanted annuloplasty rings that can be adjusted, after surgery, off-pump under physiological conditions. Both the Adjustable Annuloplasty Ring and the Cardinal Ring allow subsequent reduction with a catheter attachment [29, 30].

The enCor device can be reshaped with radiofrequency energy delivered via removable leads that are connected externally from the left atrium through the incision for connection to a radiofrequency generator. All three devices already have CE Mark, and a U.S. IDE trial involving the enCor device is ongoing. A subcutaneous version that allows for late activation on an outpatient basis as well as a less invasive percutaneous transcatheter version are under development [31]. A catheter-delivered ring is being developed both by MiCardia and Millipede Inc. (Santa Rosa, CA).

MitraClip

As pointed out earlier, the MitraClip procedure is the only transcatheter percutaneous MV device that has been widely used in clinical practice so far [32, 33].

Although the MitraClip device's influence on MR severity is caused by direct MV leaflet edge-to-edge repair, studies showed an acute reduction of the anterior–posterior MV annular diameters after clip implantation in patients with secondary MR. The authors suggested a change in the mitral valve annular diameters due to immediate and persistent tension on the mitral valve annulus via the anterior and posterior mitral valve leaflets. In one study, the amount of acute anterior–posterior diameter reduction was shown to be associated with clinical outcome after 6 months (Fig. 15.7).

These experiences are derived from single center studies, which included only limited patient numbers. However, the results of the cited studies indicate on an "indirect," possibly clinically relevant, impact of interventional-edge-to-edge repair with the MitraClip system on the MV annulus and MV geometry [12, 13].

Conclusion

Several interventional technologies will be available for mitral valve interventions in the near future by using different interventional approaches. Careful patient selection with a patient-tailored treatment strategy will be imperative for optimal interventional results.

When compared to mitral valve replacement, transcatheter mitral valve repair with MV annuloplasty although technically challenging, seems the most promising approach for the treatment of secondary MR; it is more physiological and is associated with superior safety.

In primary MR patients, annuloplasty has to be considered as a complementary approach in combination with leaflet repair.

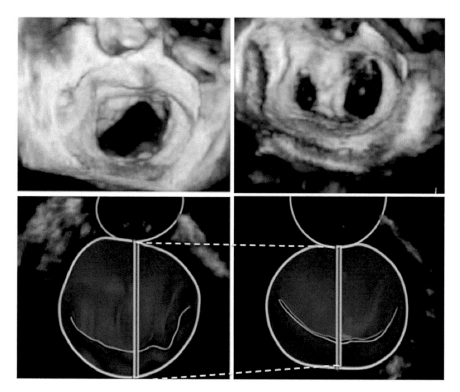

Fig. 15.7 Example of a patient with secondary mitral regurgitation pre (*left*) and post (*right*) MitraClip implantation with reduced anterior posterior diameters after the procedure

Nonetheless, the importance to identify the ideal candidate who could benefit most from different devices or techniques remains the key step for sufficient and durable MR treatment. Patients with predominant annular dilatation and limited valve tethering could be ideal candidates for annuloplasty. Even a combination of different technologies may represent a future option in selected patients.

References

1. Bursi F, Enriquez-Sarano M, Nkomo VT, Jacobsen SJ, Weston SA, Meverden RA, Roger VL. Heart failure and death after myocardial infarction in the community: the emerging role of mitral regurgitation. Circulation. 2005;111:295–301.
2. Trichon BH, Felker GM, Shaw LK, Cabell CH, O'Connor CM. Relation of frequency and severity of mitral regurgitation to survival among patients with left ventricular systolic dysfunction and heart failure. Am J Cardiol. 2003;91:538–43.
3. Vahanian A, Alfieri O, Andreotti F, Antunes MJ, Baron-Esquivias G, Baumgartner H, Borger MA, Carrel TP, Debonis M, Evangelista A, Falk V, Iung B, Lancellotti P, Pierard L, Price S, Schafers HJ, Schuler G, Stepinska J, Swedberg K, Takkenberg J, Von Oppell UO, Windecker S, Zamorano JL, Zembala M. Guidelines in the management of valvular heart disease (version 2012). Eur Heart J. 2012;33:2451–96.

4. Nishimura RA, Otto CM, Bonow RO, Carabello BA, Erwin III JP, Guyton RA, O'Gara PT, Ruiz CE, Skubas NJ, Sorajja P, Sundt III TM, Thomas JD. 2014 AHA/ACC guideline for the management of patients with valvular heart disease. J Am Coll Cardiol. 2014;63:e57–185.
5. Enriquez-Sarano M, Avierinos JF, Messika-Zeitoun D, Detaint D, Capps M, Nkomo V, Scott C, Schaff HV, Tajik AJ. Quantitative determinants of the outcome of asymptomatic mitral regurgitation. N Engl J Med. 2005;352:875–83.
6. Enriquez-Sarano M, Schaff HV, Orszulak TA, Tajik AJ, Bailey KR, Frye RL. Valve repair improves the outcome of surgery for mitral regurgitation. A multivariate analysis. Circulation. 1995;91:1022–8.
7. Gammie JS, O'Brien SM, Griffith BP, Ferguson TB, Peterson ED. Influence of hospital procedural volume on care process and mortality for patients undergoing elective surgery for mitral regurgitation. Circulation. 2007;115:881–7.
8. Mehta RH, Eagle KA, Coombs LP, Peterson ED, Edwards FH, Pagani FD, Deeb GM, Bolling SF, Prager RL, Society of Thoracic Surgeons National Cardiac Registry. Influence of age on outcomes in patients undergoing mitral valve replacement. Ann Thorac Surg. 2002;74:1459–67.
9. Glower DD, Tuttle RH, Shaw LK, Orozco RE, Rankin JS. Patient survival characteristics after routine mitral valve repair for ischemic mitral regurgitation. J Thorac Cardiovasc Surg. 2005;129:860–8.
10. Acker MA, Parides MK, Perrault LP, Moskowitz AJ, Gelijns AC, Voisine P, Smith PK, Hung JW, Blackstone EH, Puskas JD, Argenziano M, Gammie JS, Mack M, Ascheim DD, Bagiella E, Moquete EG, Ferguson TB, Horvath KA, Geller NL, Miller MA, Woo YJ, D'Alessandro DA, Ailawadi G, Dagenais F, Gardner TJ, O'Gara PT, Michler RE, Kron IL, CTSN. Mitral-valve repair versus replacement for severe ischemic mitral regurgitation. N Engl J Med. 2014;370:23–32.
11. Goldstein D, Moskowitz AJ, Gelijns AC, Ailawadi G, Parides MK, Perrault LP, Hung JW, Voisine P, Dagenais F, Gillinov AM, Thourani V, Argenziano M, Gammie JS, Mack M, Demers P, Atluri P, Rose EA, O'Sullivan K, Williams DL, Bagiella E, Michler RE, Weisel RD, Miller MA, Geller NL, Taddei-Peters WC, Smith PK, Moquete E, Overbey JR, Kron IL, O'Gara PT, Acker MA, CTSN. Two year outcomes of surgical treatment of severe ischemic mitral regurgitation. N Engl J Med. 2016;374(4):344–53.
12. Feldman T, Foster E, Glower DD, Glower DG, Kar S, Rinaldi MJ, Fail PS, Smalling RW, Siegel R, Rose GA, Engeron E, Loghin C, Trento A, Skipper ER, Fudge T, Letsou GV, Massaro JM, Mauri L, EVEREST II Herrmann and Maisano Transcatheter Therapy of Mitral Regurgitation 1721 Investigators. Percutaneous repair or surgery for mitral regurgitation. N Engl J Med. 2011;364:1395–406.
13. Feldman T, Wasserman HS, Herrmann HC, Gray W, Block PC, Whitlow P, St Goar F, Rodriguez L, Silvestry F, Schwartz A, Sanborn TA, Condado JA, Foster E. Percutaneous mitral valve repair using the edge-to-edge technique: six-month results of the EVEREST Phase I Clinical Trial. J Am Coll Cardiol. 2005;46:2134–40.
14. Mauri L, Foster E, Glower DD, Apruzzese P, Massaro JM, Herrmann HC, Hermiller J, Gray W, Wang A, Pedersen WR, Bajwa T, Lasala J, Low R, Grayburn P, Feldman T, EVEREST II Investigators. 4-year results of a randomized controlled trial of percutaneous repair versus surgery for mitral regurgitation. J Am Coll Cardiol. 2013;62:317–28.
15. Herrmann HC, Feldman T. Percutaneous mitral valve edge-to-edge repair with the Evalve MitraClip System: rationale and phase 1 results. EuroIntervention. 2006;1(Suppl A):A36–39.
16. Silvestry FE, Rodriguez LL, Herrmann HC, Rohatgi S, Weiss SJ, Stewart WJ, Homma S, Goyal N, Pulerwitz T, Zunamon A, Hamilton A, Merlino J, Martin R, Krabill K, Block PC, Whitlow P, Tuzcu EM, Kapadia S, Gray WA, Reisman M, Wasserman H, Schwartz A, Foster E, Feldman T, Wiegers SE. Echocardiographic guidance and assessment of percutaneous repair for mitral regurgitation with the Evalve MitraClip: lessons learned from EVEREST I. J Am Soc Echocardiogr. 2007;20:1131–40.
17. Wu AH, Aaronson KD, Bolling SF, Pagani FD, Welch K, Koelling TM. Impact of mitral valve annuloplasty on mortality risk in patients with mitral regurgitation and left ventricular systolic dysfunction. J Am Coll Cardiol. 2005;45:381–7.
18. Goodney PP, Stukel TA, Lucas FL, Finlayson EV, Birkmeyer JD. Hospital volume, length of stay, and readmission rates in high-risk surgery. Ann Surg. 2003;238:161–7.

19. Maselli D, Guarracino F, Chiaramonti F, Mangia F, Borelli G, Minzioni G. Percutaneous mitral annuloplasty: an anatomic study of human coronary sinus and its relation with mitral valve annulus and coronary arteries. Circulation. 2006;114:377–80.

20. Schofer J, Siminiak T, Haude M, Herrman JP, Vainer J, Wu JC, Levy WC, Mauri L, Feldman T, Kwong RY, Kaye DM, Duffy SJ, Tübler T, Degen H, Brandt MC, Van Bibber R, Goldberg S, Reuter DG, Hoppe UC. Percutaneous mitral annuloplasty for functional mitral regurgitation: results of the CARILLON Mitral Annuloplasty Device European Union Study. Circulation. 2009;120:326–33.

21. Siminiak T, Wu JC, Haude M, Hoppe UC, Sadowski J, Lipiecki J, Fajadet J, Shah AM, Feldman T, Kaye DM, Goldberg SL, Levy WC, Soloman SD, Reuter DG. Treatment of functional mitral regurgitation by percutaneous annuloplasty: results of the TITAN trial. Eur J Heart Fail. 2012;14:1090–6.

22. Harnek J, Webb JG, Kuck KH, Tschope C, Vahanian A, Buller CE, James SK, Tiefenbachere CP, Stone GW. Transcatheter implantation of the MONARC coronary sinus device for mitral regurgitation. J Am Coll Cardiol Interv. 2011;4:115–22.

23. Sponga S, Bertrand OF, Philippon F, St Pierre A, Dagenais F, Charbonneau E, Bagur R, Sénéchal M. Reversible circumflex coronary artery occlusion during percutaneous transvenous mitral annuloplasty with the Viacor system. J Am Coll Cardiol. 2012;59:288.

24. Mandinov L, Bullesfeld L, Kuck KH, Grube E. Early insight into Mitralign direct annuloplasty for treatment of functional mitral regurgitation. Interv Cardiol Rev. 2011;6:170–2.

25. Feldman T, Young A. Percutaneous approaches to valve repair for mitral regurgitation. J Am Coll Cardiol. 2014;63(20):2057–68.

26. Maisano F, Vanermen H, Seeburger J, Mack M, Falk V, Denti P, Taramasso M, Alfieri O. Direct access transcatheter mitral annuloplasty with a sutureless and adjustable device: preclinical experience. Eur J Cardiothorac Surg. 2012;42:524–9.

27. Herrmann HC, Maisano F. Transcatheter therapy of mitral regurgitation. Circulation. 2014;130(19):1712–22.

28. Langer F, Borger MA, Czesla M, Shannon FL, Sakwa M, Doll N, Cremer JT, Mohr FW, Schäfers HJ. Dynamic annuloplasty for mitral regurgitation. J Thorac Cardiovasc Surg. 2013;145:425–9.

29. Maisano F, Falk V, Borger MA, Vanermen H, Alfieri O, Seeburger J, Jacobs S, Mack M, Mohr FW. Improving mitral valve coaptation with adjustable rings. Eur J Cardiothorac Surg. 2013;44:913–8.

30. Nickenig G, Estevez-Loureiro R, Franzen O, Tamburino C, Vanderheyden M, Lüscher TF, Moat N, Price S, Dall'Ara G, Winter R, Corti R, Grasso C, Snow TM, Jeger R, Blankenberg S, Settergren M, Tiroch K, Balzer J, Petronio AS, Büttner HJ, Ettori F, Sievert H, Fiorino MG, Claeys M, Ussia GP, Baumgartner H, Scandura S, Alamgir F, Keshavarzi F, Colombo A, Maisano F, Ebelt H, Aruta P, Lubos E, Plicht B, Schueler R, Pighi M, Di Mario C. Transcatheter Valve Treatment Sentinel Registry Investigators of the EURObservational Research Programme of the European Society of Cardiology. Percutaneous mitral valve edge-to-edge repair: in-hospital results and 1-year follow-up of 628 patients of the 2011-2012 Pilot European Sentinel Registry. J Am Coll Cardiol. 2014;64(9):875–84.

31. Maisano F, Franzen O, Baldus S, Schäfer U, Hausleiter J, Butter C, Ussia GP, Sievert H, Richardt G, Widder JD, Moccetti T, Schillinger W. Percutaneous mitral valve interventions in the real world: early and 1-year results from the ACCESS-EU, a prospective, multicenter, nonrandomized post-approval study of the MitraClip therapy in Europe. J Am Coll Cardiol. 2013;62:1052–61.

32. Schueler R, Momcilovic D, Weber M, Welz A, Werner N, Mueller C, Ghanem A, Nickenig G, Hammerstingl C. Acute changes of mitral valve geometry during interventional edge-to-edge repair with the MitraClip system are associated with midterm outcomes in patients with functional valve disease: preliminary results from a prospective single-center study. Circ Cardiovasc Interv. 2014;7(3):390–9.

33. Schmidt FP, von Bardeleben RS, Nikolai P, Jabs A, Wunderlich N, Münzel T, Hink U, Warnholtz A. Immediate effect of the MitraClip procedure on mitral ring geometry in primary and secondary mitral regurgitation. Eur Heart J Cardiovasc Imaging. 2013;14(9):851–7.

Chapter 16
Repair of Paravalvular Leaks

Deepak Talreja and Nadim Geloo

Paravalvular leak (PVL) is an important and not uncommon complication of surgically implanted prosthetic valves. Clinically, relevant PVL typically presents as severe hemolysis or congestive heart failure due to significant regurgitation. The incidence of echocardiographically demonstrated regurgitation has been reported to be quite high. Para-mitral regurgitation is encountered more frequently than para-aortic regurgitation representing 80 % of cases [1]. A 5-year echocardiographic follow-up study of aortic prostheses demonstrated an incidence of 47.6 % with the vast majority of these being small and following a benign course [2]. A 2-year follow-up echocardiographic study from the AVERT trial revealed definitive PVL involving 6.8 % of aortic prosthesis and involving 10 % of mitral prosthesis [3]. While the mechanisms of PVL have not been well defined in the literature, clinically relevant PVL occurring early after surgery is likely due to infective endocarditis while late occurring PVL is possibly due to inhibition of fibroblast growth into the valve sewing ring [4] and due to increased mechanical stress on the valve annulus post surgery [5].

Medical treatment of PVL is directed at the sequelae of PVL. Blood cultures should be performed on all patients presenting with PVL and appropriate, prolonged intravenous antibiotics prescribed as appropriate; however, this rarely obviates the need for surgery. Those patients presenting with hemolytic anemia span the spectrum from mild, requiring cautious observation to severe, necessitating frequent red cell transfusions. Those presenting with congestive heart failure are treated with

D. Talreja, MD, FACC (✉)
Department of Cardiology, Sentara Heart Program, Eastern Virginia Medical School,
2353 Haversham Close, Virginia Beach, VA 23454, USA
e-mail: talreja@yahoo.com

N. Geloo, MD
Department of Cardiology, Sentara Rockingham Memorial Hospital,
2010 Health Campus Drive, Harrisonburg, VA 22801, USA

3023 Hamaker Court, Suite 100, Fairfax, VA 22031, USA
e-mail: nadim.geloo@gmail.com

© Springer Science+Business Media New York 2016
G. Ailawadi, I.L. Kron (eds.), *Catheter Based Valve and Aortic Surgery*,
DOI 10.1007/978-1-4939-3432-4_16

diuretics and afterload reduction as tolerated. These treatments do not address the underlying etiology of PVL and are therefore considered palliative [6].

Surgical treatment of PVL has historically been the treatment of choice for patients presenting with clinically relevant PVL associated with severe anemia and/ or congestive heart failure. Surgical options include replacement or repair. Redo valve surgery is associated with adverse mortality with one series reporting a 66 % survival at mean of 2.7 years [7]. Elderly patients undergoing redo valve surgery (mitral or aortic) demonstrated an early death rate of 10.7 % and late death rate of 42 % [8]. Another case series reviewing mitral valve redo surgery in relatively young patients (mean age 36) demonstrated an early mortality of 5.64 % [9]. Moreover, there remains a significant recurrence rate after repeat surgery for PVL with a reported freedom from recurrence of 85 % at 6 months after the first operation, which decreases to 78 % and 65 % after the second and third operation, respectively [10]. Surgical repair of PVL does not fare much better with a 10-year survival of 57.8 % and re-leak-free rate of 67.7 % with no statistically significant difference between leak-site repair and replacement [11]. Unfavorable results from surgery may in part be due to the persistence of the same anatomic and non-anatomic features that predisposed the patient to PVL after the initial operation. This includes the presence of calcified and friable tissue [12], older age, small body size, and degenerative valve disease [13].

Percutaneous closure of PVL has emerged as a feasible and enduring procedure, which offers a less invasive alternative to surgery for appropriately selected patients. Success rates of approximately 90 % have been reported [1, 14, 15] with relatively low morality of 1 % and MACE of 7 % [14]. Long-term outcomes are favorable with 72 % of patients being free of symptoms or repeat intervention (percutaneous or surgical) at 3 years [14]. A significant learning curve has been documented, and success rates and adverse outcomes become more favorable with increasing experience [14]. PVL closure is indicated in patients with moderately severe-to-severe regurgitation, hemolysis (which may occur with less than moderate PVL) with hemoglobin less than 10 g/dL, decreased exercise endurance, and congestive heart failure [1, 6, 14, 16]. Patient selection criteria have not been well defined but include high and intermediate surgical risk patients, those having PVL involving more than 1/3 or less of the valve circumference, absence of dehiscence involving more than ¼ of the valve ring, absence of active endocarditis, and those who have failed surgery for PVL [1, 6, 11]. With the development of purpose-specific devices, percutaneous PVL repair may become the first line of therapy [16, 17].

Para-mitral PVL appears to occur more frequently at the anterolateral and posteromedial sectors of the mitral valve annulus (MVA) [18], which may be due to changes in the MVA post-surgery. After replacement, the MVA becomes rigid, and this imparts a change in the dynamics of valve motion during the cardiac cycle. These altered dynamics may lead to increased mechanical stress in the anterolateral and posteromedial sectors of the MVA possibly explaining the increased incidence of PVL at these sites [5]. Para-mitral defects are often large and oval or crescentic in shape which has important implications for selection of and number of closure devices required in therapy. Those located in the anterolateral sector often follow a superior to inferior, serpiginous course from the left atrium (LA) to the left ventricle (LV). The opening on the LV side may be close to the mechanical prosthesis, and a closure device at this site may affect mechanical leaflet motion [1]. This may impact which closure device is chosen. Para-aortic defects seem to be less complex; they are typically round and smaller than para-mitral defects. Most often, these are located anteriorly [1].

Adequate imaging is critical to the success of the procedure. Pre-procedure imaging is of vital importance in developing a procedural plan; this invariably includes transthoracic echocardiography (TTE) and transesophageal echocardiography (TEE) but may also include CT angiography and MRI. Intraprocedure, various echocardiographic modalities may be employed in conjunction with fluoroscopy to guide access and occluder device delivery. This includes TTE, TEE, and intracardiac echocardiography (ICE) [1, 16, 17, 19, 20]. All the aforementioned echocardiographic techniques become more challenging in these cases due to the universal presence of acoustic shadowing from mechanical valves or struts. The addition of 3D to TEE greatly enhances technological success as it allows excellent definition of the size, shape, and course of the PVL [19–21]. Additionally, 3D TEE allows for a more clear assessment of the orientation of the PVL as it relates to the surrounding structures—this is of particular importance involving para-mitral PVL [19, 22]. For the para-aortic PVL, an ICE catheter placed in the right ventricular outflow tract and directed anteriorly allows for more optimal evaluation of the size and location of the PVL [19]. Fluoroscopy remains a vital imaging tool during PVL closure as this imaging modality is one with which interventionalists have the most experience; biplane fluoroscopy has an important additive role particularly to guide spatial orientation during attempts to engage the PVL with a wire.

A variety of techniques have been described for percutaneous PVL closure. A para-mitral PVL is most often approached using an antegrade technique involving femoral venous access and interatrial septal puncture. A retrograde transfemoral approach may also be employed if the antegrade approach is not feasible (in the case of inability to perform septal puncture). Para-aortic PVLs are almost exclusively approached using the retrograde technique with access primary through the femoral artery. A hybrid approach had also been described and involves a mini left minithoracotomy and direct puncture of the apex of the LV. This allows a retrograde approach for a para-mitral PVL and antegrade approach for a para-aortic defect. While a percutaneous apical puncture can also be performed, the utility of this approach is limited due to the inability to use larger catheters which would significantly increase the risk of bleeding.

The antegrade technique for para-mitral PVL requires transseptal puncture followed by advancement of a deflectable sheath such as an Agilis sheath (St. Jude Medical Inc., St. Paul, Minnesota) across the interatrial septum. Location of septal puncture is of critical importance if the para-mitral PVL is medially located (adjacent to interatrial septum); the puncture site should be sufficiently posterior (≥4 cm from the MVA) to allow enough room for medial deflection of the sheath such that it may hover above the PVL [1]. Additionally, challenging septal anatomy may be encountered which makes septal puncture difficult. Examples include a thick, fibrotic, or calcified septum or a septum that has previously undergone surgical manipulation such as patching. Previous septal punctures or presence of previously placed atrial septal occluder device may also complicate septal puncture. In such circumstances, the addition of radiofrequency (RF) ablation to the septal puncture needle or the use of an NRG RF transseptal needle (Baylis Medical, Montreal, Quebec) may facilitate septal puncture [1]. Once the septum is crossed, a telescoping, coaxial technique is used to cross the PVL; this is accomplished by nesting a 125 cm 5F multipurpose diagnostic catheter inside a 100 cm 6F coronary guide catheter. This assembly is then advanced into the deflectable Agilis sheath; the deflectable sheath is guided above the PVL using echocardiography and fluoroscopy. A 0.035″ exchange-length, stiff Glidewire (Terumo Medical Corp., Somerset, New Jersey) with an angled floppy tip is then advanced across the PVL and into the LV. The wire should subsequently be advanced across the aortic valve and into the descending thoracic aorta to gain adequate wire purchase. An attempt is then made to advance the 5F multipurpose catheter followed by the 6F guide coronary catheter into the left ventricle. Difficulty may be encountered in advancing the guide across small defects and those that demonstrate a serpiginous course through the MVA. To facilitate catheter transit, the wire can be captured in the aorta and externalized using an Amplatz GooseNeck snare (ev3 Encovascular Inc., Plymouth, Minnesota) through a 6F sheath placed in the ipsilateral or contralateral femoral artery. This creates an AV loop or rail and provides excellent support to allow transit of the catheter assembly into the left ventricle. After removal of the 5F diagnostic catheter and wire, the 6F guide is left in position in the LV and used to advance and deploy an appropriately selected closure device. The device remains tethered to the cable until imaging definitively demonstrates resolution of the PVL AND normal function of the prosthetic valve. Special attention should be given to mechanical valves to ensure that the closure device is not adversely affecting normal opening and closing of the mechanical leaflet. This approach works well with small, round defects requiring a single closure device [1, 19, 20]. If the defect is crescentic or oblong, multiple devices may be required. In this case, the technique is modified so that wire access can be maintained across the PVL to allow for multiple device deployments without the need to repeatedly cross the defect; devices can then be deployed either simultaneously or sequentially. The simultaneous technique is performed by passing two Amplatz ExtraStiff (Cook Medical Inc., Bloomington, Indiana) wires with manually preformed atraumatic loops through the 6F guide and into the LV (alternatively, the AV loop is left in place and a single Amplatz ExtraStiff wire is looped into the LV). All catheters are then removed and the bare wires left in place; over each wire, separate catheter assemblies consisting of a 5F multipurpose catheter within a 6F JR4 guide are advanced into the LV (coaxial, telescoping assembly); the multipurpose catheters are then removed leaving both 6F guides in the LV. Using the same technique described above, both occluder devices are deployed simultaneously [1, 19, 20]. Multiple devices may also be deployed using a sequential technique. Once access across the PVL is established and an AV loop created, all catheters are removed and replaced with a 6F Shuttle sheath (Cook Medical) with the tip of the sheath in the left ventricle with the rail left in place. An occluder device is then advanced through the sheath alongside the rail; the device is deployed and the Shuttle sheath removed over the delivery cable. The Shuttle sheath is again placed on the rail and advanced across the PVL; with the rail in place, a second device can now be deployed. This technique works if best utilized with large defects requiring multiple devices for adequate closure.

A retrograde approach for a para-mitral PVL can be attempted from a femoral artery access. A Glidewire is advanced over a coronary diagnostic catheter (JR4, JL4, pigtail) across the aortic valve and into the LV; the wire is then advanced retrograde through the PVL. To create an AV loop, the wire is exteriorized through a transseptal sheath using a GooseNeck snare. Device delivery can then be accomplished across the AV rail [19].

A special circumstance in treating a para-mitral PVL exists if there is an aortic mechanical prosthesis; it may not be desirable to have a stiff wire across the aortic prosthesis impinging leaflet function. A novel approach that involves creating a veno-venous loop may be attempted. This technique involves the placement of a second transseptal sheath. The MV prosthesis is then traversed with a Glidewire antegrade. The Glidewire is subsequently directed retrograde across the PVL from the LV and then snared in the left atrium through the second septal sheath and exteriorized. This creates a rail that can used to deliver the occluder device [20].

A retrograde approach to a para-aortic defect is generally facilitated by using a coaxial catheter assembly (125 cm 5F diagnostic Amplatz Left 1 or multipurpose catheter within a 100 cm 6F coronary guide) and an angled Glidewire. Once the defect is crossed with the Glidewire, difficulty may be encountered in advancing the entire catheter assembly; should this occur, the Glidewire may be exchanged through the 5F diagnostic catheter or a Glide catheter for an 0.035″ Amplatz ExtraStiff (Cook Medical) wire with a manually created, distal atraumatic loop. This should allow for advancement of the 6F guide catheter [1]. If difficulty remains in advancing the guide, an AV loop can be attempted although this would involve septal puncture and exteriorization of the wire using a GooseNeck snare advanced from the left atrial sheath. This is rarely required. Alternatively, percutaneous LV apical access may be considered with insertion of a 4–5F sheath for the sole purpose of wire exteriorization to create a rail. Para-aortic defects are generally small and can be closed with a single device. An Amplatzer Vascular Plug III (AVPIII) (St. Jude Medical Corp., St. Paul, Minnesota) would be an ideal choice as it can be delivered through a 6F coronary guide [17]. If, however, a larger defect is present and a second device is required, an 8F Shuttle Sheath can be advanced over the Amplatz ExtraStiff wire, and a sequential technique can be employed as described previously.

A hybrid technique involving a surgical transapical approach may be considered to deliver an occluder device retrograde for a para-mitral PVL and antegrade to treat a para-aortic PVL. This technique is useful if there are both aortic and mitral mechanical prosthesis present (see Fig. 16.1). Moreover, it serves as an alternate approach if percutaneous techniques have been attempted without success. This technique requires an anterolateral minithoracotomy and exposure of the LV apex followed by placement of a purse string suture and subsequent delivery of a 6F sheath. A Glidewire is then used to traverse the para-mitral or para-aortic

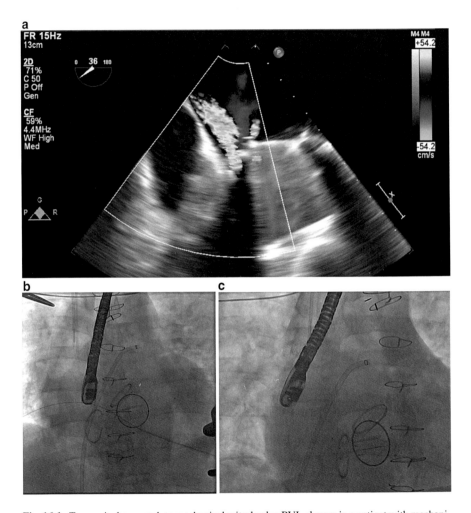

Fig. 16.1 Transapical approach to mechanical mitral valve PVL closure in a patient with mechanical aortic and mitral valves with severe mitral regurgitation through a defect on the septal side of the valve. (**a**) Transesophageal echocardiogram showing an image with color Doppler in long axis demonstrating the paravalvular leak on the septal side of the mechanical mitral valve prosthesis. (**b**) Fluoroscopic image of the mechanical mitral and aortic prosthetic valves and tricuspid valve annuloplasty ring with an Amplatz wire extending through the paravalvular leak from a transapical position extending into the right-sided pulmonary vein. A transeptal sheath is also in place. (**c**) Fluoroscopic image upon completion of the closure of the paravalvular leak with three hugging Amplatzer PDA occluders. Note preserved motion of the bileaflet mechanical mitral valve prosthesis. (**d**) Final Two-dimensional color Doppler transesophageal echocardiogram image showing resolution of the paravalvular keak. (**e**) Final image with three-dimensional echocardiographic reconstruction showing the normally functioning mechanical bileaflet mitral valve and the three hugging Amplatzer PDA occluders

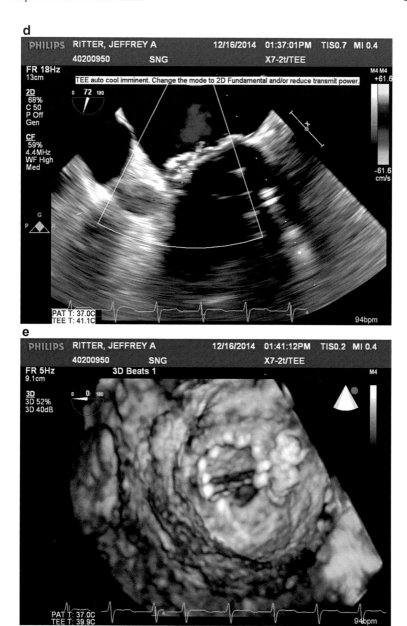

Fig. 16.1 (continued)

PVL. Alternatively, this technique can also be used to support either a retrograde approach to a para-aortic PVL or antegrade approach to a para-mitral PVL as it would allow exteriorization of the wire through the apical sheath and thereby allow formation of a rail over which an occluder device may be delivered [16]. An alternative to surgical apical approach is percutaneous apical access. This approach is somewhat problematic if a larger sheath (≥6F) is required due to the risk of major bleeding [1, 23, 24]. However, as noted above, if a smaller sheath (4–5F) is used for the sole purpose of wire exteriorization, this approach may be considered.

A variety of devices are available for PVL occlusion; however, the initial intent and design of these devices were directed towards other lesions such as atrial septal defects (ASD), patent ductus arteriosus (PDA), and ventricular septal defects (VSD). As such, each device has unique features that must be considered when making a choice. Pre-procedural imaging and planning are of vital importance in this regard. For small defects requiring a single device, an Amplatzer Vascular Plug II (AVPII) (AGA medical Corp. Plymouth, Minnesota) may be effective. This is a multi-segmented device that is weaved of a fine nitinol mesh; this design yields a device that is flexible and low profile and can be delivered through a 6F coronary guide catheter. Additional, its design lacks the large disks that may overhang over the PVL, thus avoiding leaflet impingement [1, 19]. Another specific occluder, the Amplatzer Vascular Plug III (AVPIII), (AGA Medical Corp., Plymouth Minnesota) has an oval shape and relatively small retention rims which may decrease the likelihood of mechanical leaflet impingement [17]. Other options include the Amplatzer Septal Occluder (ASO), Amplatzer Duct Occluder, and Duct Occluder II (all from AGA Medical Corp.). The Duct Occluder has a single retention disk and thus should only be deployed such that the retention rim is on the LV side of a para-mitral defect to reduce the likelihood of embolization which may occur due to the pressure differential between the LV and LA [19] (see Fig. 16.2).

Complications of greatest concern are device embolization and impingement of a mechanical leaflet. Device embolization is a rare but serious complication during the deployment of occluder devices. Several techniques to retrieve these devices have been described. These involve a three-step process; first the device should be oriented, if possible, so that the screw can be more easily approached by a GooseNeck snare. Second, the device should be stabilized distally to create traction and facilitate

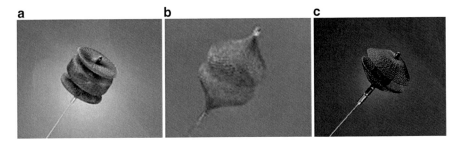

Fig. 16.2 Closure devices commonly used for PVL repair. (**a**) Amplatzer Vascular Plug 2. (**b**) Amplatzer Vascular Plug 4. (**c**) Amplatzer Patent Ductus Arteriosus (PDA) Occluder

lengthening and slenderizing of the device into a large sheath (12F)—this can be accomplished by using a stiff 0.035″ wire [25], bioptome [26–28], second snare, or pigtail [29]. Impingement of a mechanical leaflet is also rare but more common than embolization. The best method to prevent this is to carefully evaluate leaflet function by fluoroscopy as well as echocardiography after device deployment but before cable release. If there is any evidence to suggest mechanical leaflet malfunction, the device should be withdrawn into the delivery sheath and repositioned or a new device should be selected. If the device shifts after cable release, the device must be recaptured using the techniques described above [1]. Hemolysis is a rarely encountered complication and occurs if there is persistent flow through a treated PVL; this is due to high velocity flow through the metal mesh of the occluder device. This seems to occur more often with devices constructed of a larger caliber nitinol mesh (ASO, VSD Occluder, Duct Occluder) and less so with devices constructed with a fine mesh (AVPII, AVPIII, Duct Occluder II) [1, 19].

Paravalvular leak remains an important complication of surgically placed prosthetic valves. Treatment options historically have been limited to redo surgery, which is associated with a relatively high mortality and the need for repeat surgeries. Percutaneous techniques offer a less invasive yet highly successful alternative to surgery. With continuing experience, refinement of technique, and further development of purpose-specific catheters and devices, percutaneous repair of PVL may become the primary approach to treating prosthetic paravalvular leak.

References

1. Rihal CS, Sorajja P, Booker JD, Hagler DJ, Cabalka AK. Principles of percutaneous paravalvular leak closure. JACC Cardiovasc Interv. 2012;5(2):121–30.
2. Rallidis LS, Moyssakis IE, Ikonomidis I, Nihoyannopoulos P. Natural history of early aortic paraprosthetic regurgitation: a five-year follow-up. Am Heart J. 1999;138(2 Pt 1):351–7.
3. Dávila-Román VG, Waggoner AD, Kennard ED, Holubkov R, Jamieson WR, Englberger L, Carrel TP, Schaff HV, Artificial Valve Endocarditis Reduction Trial Echocardiography Study. Prevalence and severity of paravalvular regurgitation in the Artificial Valve Endocarditis Reduction Trial (AVERT) echocardiography study. J Am Coll Cardiol. 2004;44(7):1467–72.
4. Schaff HV, Carrel TP, Jamieson WR, Jones KW, Rufilanchas JJ, Cooley DA, Hetzer R, Stumpe F, Duveau D, Moseley P, van Boven WJ, Grunkemeier GL, Kennard ED, Holubkov R, Artificial Valve Endocarditis Reduction Trial. Paravalvular leak and other events in silzone-coated mechanical heart valves: a report from AVERT. Ann Thorac Surg. 2002;73(3):785–92.
5. Komoda T, Hetzer R, Siniawski H, Oellinger J, Felix R, Uyama C, Maeta H. Effects of prosthetic valve placement on mitral annular dynamics and the left ventricular base. ASAIO J. 2001;47(1):60–5.
6. Pate GE, Al Zubaidi A, Chandavimol M, Thompson CR, Munt BI, Webb JG. Percutaneous closure of prosthetic paravalvular leaks: case series and review. Catheter Cardiovasc Interv. 2006;68(4):528–33.
7. Leontyev S, Borger MA, Davierwala P, Walther T, Lehmann S, Kempfert J, Mohr FW. Redo aortic valve surgery: early and late outcomes. Ann Thorac Surg. 2011;91(4):1120–6.
8. Maganti M, Rao V, Armstrong S, Feindel CM, Scully HE, David TE. Redo valvular surgery in elderly patients. Ann Thorac Surg. 2009;87(2):521–5.
9. Sampath Kumar A, Dhareshwar J, Airan B, Bhan A, Sharma R, Venugopal P. Redo mitral valve surgery-a long-term experience. J Card Surg. 2004;19(4):303–7.

10. Lock J. Catheter closure of paravalvular leaks. In: Fourth international workshop in catheter interventions in congenital heart disease, Frankfurt, Germany; 2001.
11. Choi JW, Hwang HY, Kim KH, Kim KB, Ahn H. Long-term results of surgical correction for mitral paravalvular leak: repair versus re-replacement. J Heart Valve Dis. 2013;22(5):682–7.
12. Erez E, Tam VK, Williams WH, Kanter KR. The Konno aortoventriculoplasty for repeat aortic valve replacement. Eur J Cardiothorac Surg. 2001;19(6):793–6.
13. O'Rourke DJ, Palac RT, Malenka DJ, Marrin CA, Arbuckle BE, Plehn JF. Outcome of mild periprosthetic regurgitation detected by intraoperative transesophageal echocardiography. J Am Coll Cardiol. 2001;38(1):163–6.
14. Sorajja P, Cabalka AK, Hagler DJ, Rihal CS. The learning curve in percutaneous repair of paravalvular prosthetic regurgitation: an analysis of 200 cases. JACC Cardiovasc Interv. 2014;7(5):521–9.
15. Ruiz CE, Jelnin V, Kronzon I, Dudiy Y, Del Valle-Fernandez R, Einhorn BN, Chiam PT, Martinez C, Eiros R, Roubin G, Cohen HA. Clinical outcomes in patients undergoing percutaneous closure of periprosthetic paravalvular leaks. J Am Coll Cardiol. 2011;58(21):2210–7.
16. Taramasso M, Maisano F, Latib A, Denti P, Guidotti A, Sticchi A, Panoulas V, Giustino G, Pozzoli A, Buzzatti N, Cota L, De Bonis M, Montorfano M, Castiglioni A, Blasio A, La Canna G, Colombo A, Alfieri O. Conventional surgery and transcatheter closure via surgical transapical approach for paravalvular leak repair in high-risk patients: results from a single-centre experience. Eur Heart J Cardiovasc Imaging. 2014;5(10):1161–7.
17. Nietlispach F, Johnson M, Moss RR, Wijesinghe N, Gurvitch R, Tay EL, Thompson C, Webb JG. Transcatheter closure of paravalvular defects using a purpose-specific occluder. JACC Cardiovasc Interv. 2010;3(7):759–65.
18. De Cicco G, Russo C, Moreo A, Beghi C, Fucci C, Gerometta P, Lorusso R. Mitral valve periprosthetic leakage: anatomical observations in 135 patients from a multicentre study. Eur J Cardiothorac Surg. 2006;30(6):887–91.
19. Kim MS, Casserly IP, Garcia JA, Klein AJ, Salcedo EE, Carroll JD. Percutaneous transcatheter closure of prosthetic mitral paravalvular leaks: are we there yet? JACC Cardiovasc Interv. 2009;2(2):81–90.
20. García E, Sandoval J, Unzue L, Hernandez-Antolin R, Almería C, Macaya C. Paravalvular leaks: mechanisms, diagnosis and management. EuroIntervention. 2012;8(Suppl Q):Q41–52.
21. Alam M, Serwin JB, Rosman HS, Polanco GA, Sun I, Silverman NA. Transesophageal echocardiographic features of normal and dysfunctioning bioprosthetic valves. Am Heart J. 1991;121(4 Pt 1):1149–55.
22. Marx GR, Su X. Three-dimensional echocardiography in congenital heart disease. Cardiol Clin. 2007;25(2):357–65.
23. Ommen SR, Higano ST, Nishimura RA, Holmes Jr DR. Summary of the Mayo Clinic experience with direct left ventricular puncture. Cathet Cardiovasc Diagn. 1998;44(2):175–8.
24. Jelnin V, Dudiy Y, Einhorn BN, Kronzon I, Cohen HA, Ruiz CE. Clinical experience with percutaneous left ventricular transapical access for interventions in structural heart defects a safe access and secure exit. JACC Cardiovasc Interv. 2011;4(8):868–74. doi:10.1016/j.jcin.2011.05.018.
25. Peuster M, Boekenkamp R, Kaulitz R, Fink C, Hausdorf G. Transcatheter retrieval and repositioning of an Amplatzer device embolized into the left atrium. Catheter Cardiovasc Interv. 2000;51(3):297–300.
26. Levi DS, Moore JW. Embolization and retrieval of the Amplatzer septal occluder. Catheter Cardiovasc Interv. 2004;61(4):543–7.
27. Shirodkar S, Patil S, Pinto R, Dalvi B. Successful retrieval of migrated Amplatzer septal occluder. Ann Pediatr Cardiol. 2010;3(1):83–6.
28. Chan KT, Cheng BC. Retrieval of an embolized amplatzer septal occluder. Catheter Cardiovasc Interv. 2010;75(3):465–8.
29. Goel PK, Kapoor A, Batra A, Khanna R. Transcatheter retrieval of embolized Amplatzer Septal Occluder. Tex Heart Inst J. 2012;39(5):653–6.

Chapter 17
Barriers to Transcatheter Mitral Valve Replacement

Anson Cheung and Kevin Lichtenstein

Overview

For nonsurgical and surgically high risk patients with valvular heart disease, trans-catheter valve repair and replacement has become a rapidly growing option. Initially, aortic valve stenosis was considered for transcatheter treatment because of easy access, simple anatomy, straightforward physiology, and most important with cal-cific stenosis a secure landing spot for transcatheter valve anchorage. However, with transcatheter valve technology improving rapidly, nonsurgical and high-risk surgi-cal patients with mitral regurgitation now have the option to have a transcatheter mitral valve repair.

Some catheter devices are currently available to treat mitral regurgitation, including chordal replacement, indirect (via coronary sinus), direct annuloplasty, and leaflet repair. Only MitraClip (Abbott Laboratories, Abbott Park, Illinois) has long-term results and has enjoyed significant clinical experience. Based on the edge-to-edge suture repair pioneered by Alfierri [1], a catheter delivered clip approximates the mid-portion of the anterior and posterior leaflet to form a double orifice mitral valve. In the pivotal safety trial (Everest I, 2005), the combined primary efficacy endpoint of freedom from death, from surgery for mitral valve dysfunction, and from grade 3+ or 4+ regurgitation was 55 % in the MitraClip group and 73 % in a matched surgical group ($p=.007$) [1]. To

A. Cheung, MD (✉)
Division of Cardiac Surgery, St. Paul's Hospital, 1081 Burroad Street,
Vancouver, BC, Canada V62146
e-mail: acheung@providencehealth.bc.ca

K. Lichtenstein, BM, BS
Division of Cardiac Surgery, University of British Columbia, 1081 Rurrard Street,
Vancouver, BC, Canada V62146
e-mail: kmlichtenstein@gmail.com

© Springer Science+Business Media New York 2016
G. Ailawadi, I.L. Kron (eds.), *Catheter Based Valve and Aortic Surgery*,
DOI 10.1007/978-1-4939-3432-4_17

date, the MitraClip has been implanted in over 25,000 patients for both degenerative leaflet disease (flail, prolapse, etc.) and functional leaflet regurgitation. Nonetheless, the procedure is not without significant limitations both in patient selection and the nature of the mitral regurgitation. The regurgitant jet must be centrally located with a leaflet coaptation length of at least 2 mm and if a mitral leaflet is flail, the flail gap must be less than 10 mm, so there is enough tissue for the clip to grasp on each leaflet. Partial clip detachment identified on echocardiography still remains a problem in 2–10 % of patients and usually requires surgical correction. Care has also to be taken to ensure that baseline mitral valve area is greater than 4 cm^2, because the clip can significantly reduce valve area and lead to mitral stenosis, particularly since nearly 50 % of patients require two clips to reduce the regurgitation to an acceptable level although it is rarely eliminated. The procedure via the femoral vein, transeptal across the left atrium and into the left ventricle, is generally prolonged and it may at times be difficult to capture the leaflets between the arms of the clip. The need for mitral valve replacement was associated with anterior leaflet pathology and that this pathology was a predictor of MV replacement [2]. Only 13.5 % of patients required MV replacement because of injury to the valve sustained during the MitraClip procedure.

Unlike surgical repair of mitral regurgitation which requires specific mitral valve characteristics for a good durable result, mitral valve replacement is universal. However, there are inherent complexities associated with tackling transcatheter mitral valve replacement when compared to the transcatheter aortic valve replacement. First, barriers to transcatheter mitral valve replacement include the complex anatomy of the mitral valve with its leaflets, subvalvular apparatus, the atrial and ventricular components, and the noncircular nature of the mitral annulus. Second, the valve technology, still in its infancy, is slowly adapting to the complex mitral anatomy. Finally, due to its position and function, the mitral valve is exposed to very different physiology compared to the aortic valve. As well, due to its position, accessing the mitral valve is a challenge, and various routes have been attempted with varying degrees of success. These routes include anterograde via the femoral vein with transeptal access and direct atrial approach to the mitral valve and a retrograde transapical approach. With the field of percutaneous mitral valve replacement expanding, industry is rapidly developing new valve technologies to meet this growing field and with this increase in choice, comes varying levels of success. Overall, transcatheter mitral valve replacement is a modality still in its infancy, and there are many challenges to be met in the future that technological improvements will try to address.

Barriers to Minimally Invasive Mitral Valve Replacement

Several barriers to catheter-based mitral valve replacement exist. These can be categorized into anatomical barriers, technological barriers, and longevity barriers.

Anatomically, there are many more barriers to transcatheter mitral valve replacement than there were for the aortic valve. The mitral valve is in close proximity to the aortic valve with the anterior mitral leaflet, a curtain suspended from the right and left trigone part of the left ventricular outflow tract (LVOT) and immediately confluent with the aortic valve.

Obstruction of the LVOT is one such barrier since any implantable valve with a rigid structure could potentially, based on its deployment, result in significant left ventricular outflow obstruction with related morbidity and mortality [3]. Even if the transcatheter valve itself were no more obstructive than a surgically implanted valve, the redundant retained large anterior leaflet held constantly open might interfere with ventricular outflow. Besides outflow tract compromise, damage or distortion of the native aortic valve may occur.

Another anatomical difficulty lies in the fact that the left circumflex coronary artery is closely associated with the posterolateral mitral annulus and an rigid, self-expanding valve, deployed within the annulus, may compress or occlude the left circumflex coronary artery [3]. This has been a major problem for the clinical adoption of indirect annuloplasty via the coronary sinus. In the same regard, the valve should not be so rigid or require a degree of expansion that may obstruct the coronary sinus which is anatomically closely related to the posteromedial mitral annulus [3]. In terms of cardiac anatomy, the ideal transcatheter mitral valve should not disturb or damage the myocardium or papillary muscles, spare the chordal structures while restoring physiologic anterograde flow, eliminate retrograde regurgitation, without causing aortic valve incompetence, or obstructing left ventricular outflow [3]. In essence, in the absence of dense circumferential mitral annular calcification, transcatheter mitral valve replacement suffers from lack of an easy, safe, and secure landing zone.

Finally, all transcatheter valves are prone to postimplantation perivalvular and transvalvular leaks secondary to poor valve placement expansion or distortion [4].

In terms of technological barriers, the current challenges for any transcatheter mitral valve are formidable. For a transcatheter mitral valve replacement to be successful, the valves themselves have to have certain characteristics that contribute to their success. If one were to imagine the ideal transcatheter valve, it would be one that first and foremost addresses the above anatomical concerns and obtains and holds a stable position in the mitral position without compromising the aortic valve, LVOT, and with minimal risk of migration or embolization [3]. The valve structure must also be pliable enough not to be disturbed or fail from fatigue by the continuous dynamic movements of the mitral valve apparatus nor damage these biologic structures [3]. The mitral valve is exposed to high pressure gradients, and the ideal transcatheter mitral valve would remain competent and not be displaced by the high pressures that are generated across it during ventricular systole [3]. As alluded to above, if one compares the mitral valve to the aortic valve, one major difference when it comes to transcatheter implantation is that in the aortic position, the calcified aortic root provides an excellent landing zone for a stented valve, whereas the mitral valve has no such rigid structure to facilitate landing a stent-based bioprosthesis [5]. Thus, any stent-based bioprothetic valve must have appropriate anchoring mechanisms to prevent migration of the valve either into the atrial chamber or ventricular chamber and remain competent.

Longevity or durability of any implanted bioprosthetic valve, exposed to chronic ongoing biologic and mechanical stresses, can only be accurately determined in retrospect. However, the materials from which the mitral valves are constructed must be able to tolerate the pressures generated by the systolic function of the left ventricle. Furthermore, the valve materials should ideally be biologically inert and resistant to degradation of the leaflet material to avert regurgitation or stenosis at the mitral position, both poorly tolerated [3]. It is known that despite all efforts, surgically implanted bioprosthetic mitral valves have a durability free from structural valve failure inferior to bioprosthesis in the aortic position. At present, candidates for transcatheter mitral valve replacement have limited life expectancy, but as this proves to be a viable modality, the long-term durability of the valve will become increasingly more important.

Access Points

Transvenous–Transseptal Approach

An obvious point of access to the mitral valve would be via a femoral vein puncture up into the right atrium and across the atrial septum at the foramen ovale into the left atrium and the mitral valve. The right femoral vein would be the site of choice since it is a straighter route to the right atrium, and the right femoral-iliac vein does not have to pass under the aorto-iliac artery which has been known to impede long venous catheters introduced via the left femoral. Care must be taken to cross as always crossing the foramen ovale not to inadvertently puncture the closely applied proximal aorta. Once in the left atrium, a steerable catheter should allow easy navigation through the mitral valve. An advantage of femoral venous access is the low venous pressure that can be easily controlled with hand pressure to maintain hemostasis when the introducing sheath is withdrawn. Femoral vein cannulation can result in an arterio-venous shunt if initial access to the femoral vein unknowingly occurred through the femoral artery.

Transapical Access: Why Is It the Best Approach Right Now?

Access for transcatheter valves is limited by the deployment catheter size which are large in the early stages of development and limit arterial and to a lessor degree venous introduction. The present transcatheter mitral valves being evaluated come with reported sheath sizes varying from 42F to 18F, with only 42F and 32F (10.6 to 14 mm diameter) sheaths used to date clinically. Catheter size, however, does not compromise the transapical approach to ventricular valves and for many reasons is a favored approach.

The transapical approach to the mitral valve is direct and the shorter distance providing accurate control and positioning of the device. The downside is dealing with the left ventricular apex which can be problematic in elderly frail patient.

The field of percutaneous mitral valve replacement is still in its relative infancy, and therefore different approaches and studies comparing them have yet to be undertaken.

Surgeons have become familiar with the transapical approach through their experience with TAVI. In a recent study, it was found when the transapical TAVI approach was compared to the transfemoral approach, there was no difference in 30-day mortality between the two approaches [6]. The same study found no difference in the rate of myocardial infarction, postoperative bleeding, stroke, requirement for pacemaker implantation, and moderate aortic insufficiency between the transfemoral and the transapical approaches [6]. Finally, survival probability over the long term was no different between the two approaches [6]. The transapical approach with greater control and accuracy in achieving small corrections in position was initially adopted for all left-sided valve-in-valve procedures [4]. Successful deployment of a transcatheter valve-in-valve or even valve-in-ring in the mitral position via the apex of the left ventricle has been excellent with a 30-day and 1-year mortality of 12 and 25 %, respectively, and important improvement in symptoms after the procedure as reported by Dvir [7]. Given the limited safe and secure landing zone available for a transcatheter mitral valve replacement makes the transapical approach ideal.

Transcatheter mitral valve replacement is a relatively new area compared to transcatheter aortic valve replacement; however, given the mitral valve position within the heart makes femoral access that much more challenging since femoral venous access has to be followed by potentially complicated antegrade atrial septal puncture to access the mitral valve. The transapical approach seems to lend itself more easily to transcatheter mitral replacement as compared to the transfemoral venous approach, simply due to proximity and anatomy.

Tiara

The Tiara bioprosthesis is a D-shaped transcatheter device (Neovasc Inc, Richmond, Canada) [8]. The valve is constructed from cross-linked bovine pericardial tissue leaflets that are held within a self-expanding nitinol alloy frame, and the valve is implanted using the transapical approach [3, 9]. Shaped to match the saddle-shaped native mitral valve annulus, the Tiara is designed to minimize left ventricular outflow tract obstruction [3, 9]. A covered skirt design of the atrial portion of the Tiara prevents paravalvular leakage [9].

Tiara implantation is performed via the transapical approach under fluoroscopic and echocardiographic guidance. The valve is deployed from a 32F delivery catheter. Once seated in the appropriate position, a retractable sheath keeps the Tiara valve in place until fully expanded [3]. The two anterior ventricular anchoring structures capture the fibrous trigones on each side of the anterior mitral leaflet, and a posterior tab

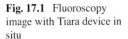
Fig. 17.1 Fluoroscopy image with Tiara device in situ

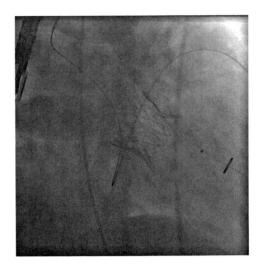

anchors behind the posterior mitral leaflet onto the posterior shelf [9]. During deployment, the leaflets and chordae are engaged from the ventricular side further securing the valve and minimizing paravalvular leak. One of the major benefits of the Tiara valve is that the valve is able to be repositioned and recaptured during all stages of deployment other than the final release phase [3].

The D-shape of the Tiara valve itself mimics the natural mitral orifice with the aim for full reduction of the risk of left circumflex impingement as well as left ventricular outflow obstruction.

In preclinical trials, a short-term porcine and long-term ovine models were used. In both models, the Tiara showed excellent valve alignment and function with no coronary artery obstruction, left ventricular outflow obstruction, or transvalvular gradients. Human cadaver models showed that implantation of the Tiara achieved proper anatomical alignment and valve seating in both the atrial and ventricular portions of the valve [3].

The first two human implantations of the 35 mm Tiara prosthesis were performed in early 2014. In both cases, the transapical approach was used under a general anesthetic. In both patients, the Tiara deployment was uneventful, and both patients were hemodynamically stable throughout the procedure with no need for cardiopulmonary bypass (Fig. 17.1). Post-procedure echocardiogram at 48 h, 1 month, and 2 months showed excellent valvular function with no sign of left ventricular outflow obstruction, paravalular leak, and minimal transvalvular pressure gradients [10] (Fig. 17.2).

Currently, the Tiara-1 feasibility trial is being conducted in Canada, Western Europe, and United States to assess the safety and efficacy of the Tiara device. First patient was enrolled in Begium, and enrollment is expected to be complete by the end of 2015.

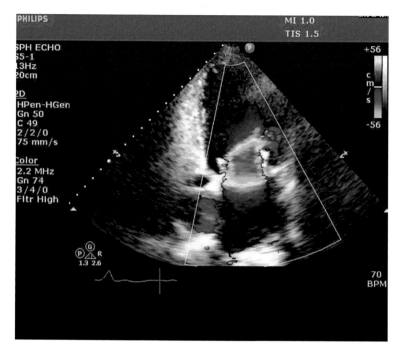

Fig. 17.2 Transthoracic echocardiography 9-month post-Tiara implant demonstrating good valvular function with no evidence of paravalvular leak

CardiAQ

The CardiAQ valve, produced by CardiAQ Valve Technologies Inc., is a bovine pericardial self-expanding prosthesis on a nitinol frame. It anchors itself to native anatomy on self-expansion via two sets of anchor barbs and does not apply radial force to the mitral annulus [8, 9]. The two anchor barbs grasp the mitral leaflets from the left atrial and left ventricular side [9]. The valve structure is foreshortened to apply a clamping action to aid in valve anchoring once deployed; the valve resides supraannularly with the majority of the valve structure in the left atrium. In terms of access, the CardiAQ valve can be implanted anterograde through transeptal access of the left atrium with the initial point of access being the femoral vein. Alternatively, the CardiAQ valve can also be implanted transapically. First in human implant was carried out in 2012 using the transeptal approach with cardiopulmonary bypass support [8]. An addition transapical system has been developed, and successful implant has been announced in Denmark in May, 2014. Subsequently, other success implantations were carried out via the apex, though no data has been published at this point. A multicenter feasibility trial is expected in 2015.

Fortis

The Fortis device (Edwards Lifesciences, Irvine, USA) is a cloth covered, self-expanding nitinol stent with three bovine pericardial leaflets [3, 8]. It consists of a valve body, paddles to hold unto the existing mitral leaflets, and an atrial skirt. A 29 mm size is presently available for clinical use and is cylindrical in cross section. The atrial flange at the inflow portion of the valve body is made of nitinol struts with two more flexible struts aligned with the A2 segment of the anterior leaflet to prevent aortic valve distortion. It is deployed via the transapical approach [8] by a delivery system 42F in diameter (Fig. 17.3). Bapat et al. reported use of the FORTIS device in five patients deemed high risk for surgery. Their results in the first 5 patients found 3 of the 5 patients survived beyond 30 days after device implantation [9, 11].

Tendyne

The Tendyne trileaflet valve is produced by Tendyne Medical Inc. [9]. Inserted via the transapical approach, this porcine, stent-based, self-expanding valve was trialed in the porcine animal model initially [12]. Of the 8 test animals, 7 died of either failure of valve fixation, perivalvular leakage, or poor positioning with their prototype [12]. Subsequently, the latest version consists of an atrial fixation system, a nitinol self-expanding stent-based ventricular body, and a ventricular fixation system composed of tethering strings that are attached to the left ventricular apex. No PVL was noted in the subsequent animal implants [13]. Due to its design, the Tendyne valve allows precise deployment with adjustable intraannular positioning and the valve itself fully retrievable [12, 13].

The first Tendyne valve implantations were performed in 2013 at the French Hospital in Ascuncion, Paraguay [9]. Using the transapical method, two patients were treated with one patient having complete elimination of grade IV mitral regurgitation and the other having a reduction in mitral regurgitation from grade IV to grade I [9].

Fig. 17.3 Final deployment of the Fortis transcatheter mitral valve. Courtesy of Dr. Jian Ye, St. Paul's Hospital, Vancouver, Canada

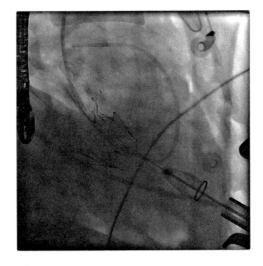

Three successful chronic first-in-human cases were performed by Moat at the Royal Brompton Hospital in the United Kingdom. A multicenter Tendyne TMVI feasibility trial is being conducted, and enrollment has commenced in Australia (Fig. 17.4).

Device		Route of Delivery	Sheath Size	Current Status
CardiAQ	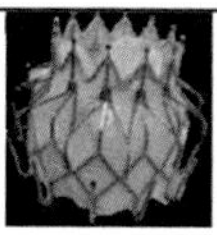	TF/TA	32F	First in Man
Tendyne	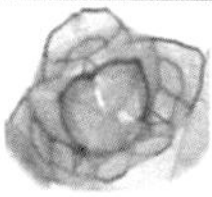	TA	30F	Feasibility Trial
Neovasc Tiara	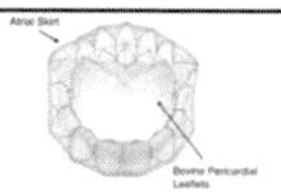	TA	32F	Feasibility Trial
Edwards Fortis	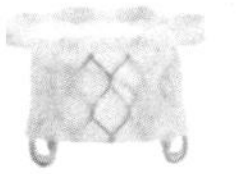	TA	42F	Feasibility Trial
Medtronic	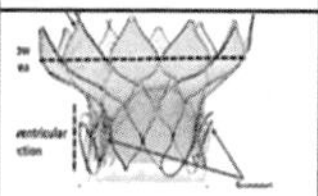	Trans-atrial	N/A	Preclinical
Cardiovalve	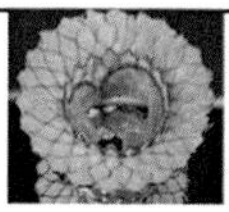	TF	26F	Preclinical
HighLife	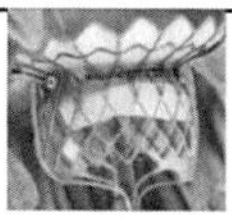	Trans-atrial	N/A	Preclinical
Endovalve	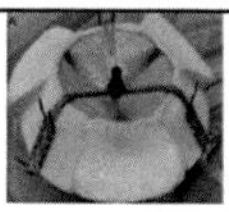	TA	N/A	Preclinical
Gorman	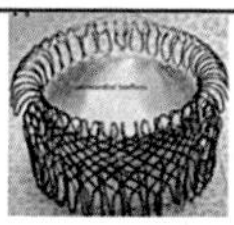	Trans-atrial	30F	Preclinical
MitrAssist	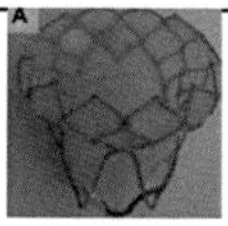	TAo	18F	Preclinical

Fig. 17.4 Tendyne TMVI device in situ. Courtesy of Dr. Paul Jansz

Conclusions

Transcatheter mitral valve replacement is a new burgeoning technology. Early apparent success in human implants proves feasibility. Most of the early clinical cases were performed on extreme risk patients and likely a major contributor for the less than favorable outcomes. However, with better patient selection and further refinement in implant techniques and technology, clinical outcomes will improve. It will no doubt undergo innumerable improvements over the years to come in an attempt to improve life for our patients.

References

1. Feldman T, Young A. Percutaneous approach to valve repair for mitral regurgitation. J Am Coll Cardiol. 2014;63:2057–68.
2. Glower D, Ailawadi G, Argenziano M, Mack M, Trento A, Wang A, et al. EVEREST II randomized clinical trial: predictors of mitral valve replacement in de novo surgery or after the MitraClip procedure. J Thorac Cardiovasc Surg. 2012;143(4 Suppl):S60–3.
3. Banai S, Verheye S, Cheung A, Schwartz M, Marko A, Lane R, et al. Transpical mitral implantation of the Tiara bioprothesis: pre-clinical results. JACC Cardiovasc Interv. 2014;7(2): 154–62.
4. Cheung A, Webb JG, Wong DR, Ye J, Masson JB, Carere RG, et al. Transapical transcatheter mitral valve-in-valve implantation in a human. Ann Thorac Surg. 2009;87(3):e18–20.
5. Anyanwu AC, Adams DH. Transcatheter mitral valve replacement: the next revolution? J Am Coll Cardiol. 2014;64(17):1820–4.
6. Schymik G, Würth A, Bramlage P, Herbinger T, Heimeshoff M, Pilz L, et al. Long-term results of transapical versus transfemoral TAVI in a real world population of 1000 patients with severe symptomatic aortic stenosis. Circ Cardiovasc Interv. 2014;8(1)
7. Dvir D. Update from the global valve-in-valve registry, TCT Meeting, Miami 2012.
8. Herrmann HC, Maisano F. Transcatheter therapy of mitral regurgitation. Circulation. 2014;130(19):1712–22.
9. De Backer O, Piazza N, Banai S, Lutter G, Maisano F, Herrmann HC, et al. Percutaneous transcatheter mitral valve replacement: an overview of devices in preclinical and early clinical evaluation. Circ Cardiovasc Interv. 2014;7(3):400–9.
10. Cheung A, Webb J, Verheye S, Moss R, Boone R, Leipsic J, et al. Short-term results of transapical transcatheter mitral valve implantation for mitral regurgitation. J Am Coll Cardiol. 2014;64(17):1814–9.
11. Bapat V, Buellesfeld L, Peterson MD, Hancock J, Reineke D, Buller C, et al. Transcatheter mitral valve implantation (TMVI) using the Edwards FORTIS device. EuroIntervention. 2014;10(Suppl U):U120–8.
12. Lutter G, Lozonschi L, Ebner A, et al. First-in-human off-pump transcatheter mitral valve replacement. J Am Coll Cardiol Interv. 2014;7(9):1077–8.
13. Lutter G, Pokorny S, Frank D, Cremer J, Lozonschi L. Transapical mitral valve implantation: the Lutter valve. Heart Lung Vessel. 2013;5(4):201–6.

Chapter 18
Mitral Valve

M. Andrew Morse, Rick Meece, and Evelio Rodriguez

Introduction

There are over 210,000 mitral valve operations performed in the United States every year with over 50 % of these patients undergoing mitral valve replacement. Despite shorter durability compared to mechanical valves, bioprosthetic valve usage has continued to rise. This is related to advancements in surgical valve technology, patient preference, and avoidance of long-term anticoagulation [1]. Bioprosthetic structural valve degeneration (SVD) can overtime lead to valvular regurgitation, stenosis, or mixed pathology. It occurs via a variety of mechanisms including leaflet perforation, leaflet tears, commissural tears, cuspal detachment, and restricted leaflet motion. Leaflet dysfunction is most commonly related to collagen degeneration and dystrophic calcification within the bioprosthetic tissue. The true incidence of bioprosthetic valve failure is likely underreported in the published literature and varies greatly between studies. In general, younger patients (less than 65 years of age) have much higher rates of SVD compared to their older counterparts and reoperation more frequently. A number of publications have done subgroup analysis to determine the effect of age at time of surgical mitral valve replacement on the rate of SVD. Table 18.1 shows the differences of published rates of SVD based on age at time of valve implantation. Although older patients have lower rates of SVD compared to their younger counterparts, it still occurs at relatively high frequency. These high rates of SVD in combination with good long-term survival after initial mitral valve surgery has led to increasing numbers of patients requiring reoperations.

The published mitral valve reoperation rates in surgical series vary greatly and can range from 19.7 to 84 % on long-term follow-up [2–9]. There are confounders and selection bias in how patients are chosen to undergo redo mitral valve surgery.

M.A. Morse, MD • R. Meece, ACS, RDCS, RCIS, FASE • E. Rodriguez, MD (✉)
Department of Cardiology, St. Thomas Hospital, 4220 Harding Pike,
Nashville, TN 37205, USA
e-mail: m.andrew.morse@gmail.com; Evelio.Rodriguez@sth.org

© Springer Science+Business Media New York 2016   237
G. Ailawadi, I.L. Kron (eds.), *Catheter Based Valve and Aortic Surgery*,
DOI 10.1007/978-1-4939-3432-4_18

Table 18.1 Summary of published rates of structural valve deterioration depending on age of patients at time of surgery [2–5]

Author	# of MVR patients	Follow-up duration (years)	Younger patient cohort (years)	% of SVD	Older patient cohort (years)	% of SVD
Borger et al.	559	20	<65	73	>65	41
Hammermeister et al.	93	15	<65	44	>65	20
Bourguignon et al.	404	20	<65	80.9	>65	38.5
Jamieson et al.	1135	18	51–60	85.3	>70	31

In contemporary practice, the overall rate of bioprosthetic mitral valve reoperation is felt to be lower due to improvements in valve design including anti-calcification leaflet treatments. In a recent study published by Kaneko et al. of patients less than 65 years of age undergoing mitral valve replacement, 24.7 % required reoperation at 15 years [7]. In general, each reoperation brings increased surgical morbidity and mortality. Mitral valve reoperations are not uncommon practice with the median time from the original surgery ranging from 8 to 11.8 years [6, 10, 11]. In a recent publication by Bourguignon et al. of 404 bioprosthetic mitral valve replacement patients, the expected durability of the valve in patients less than 60 years of age was 11.4 years [4]. In addition, redo mitral valve operations are increasingly prevalent in US practice and currently account for over 10 % of all mitral valve surgeries performed each year [1]. In a large surgical series reported by Fukunaga et al., redo mitral valve replacement for structural valve deterioration accounted for 37.5 % of all redo cardiac valve surgeries [12]. It is clear that mitral bioprosthetic failure is becoming more prevalent and will need alternative therapeutic options for high risk patients.

This chapter will review transcatheter mitral valve-in-valve (MiVIV) implantation within an existing failed mitral bioprosthesis or mitral annuloplaty ring and demonstrate it as a viable therapeutic option for this challenging patient population.

Risk of Reoperation

Redo valvular operations can be associated with high morbidity and mortality rates, especially in the elderly. Perioperative mortality rates in lower risk isolated mitral valve reoperations can be as low as 4.7 % to 6.3 % in experienced centers [11, 13]. These published reports have in general focused on lower risk redo surgical patients. In contrast, patients with additional medical comorbidities, multiple prior cardiac surgeries, higher NYHA classes, the need for urgent/emergent surgery, and older age have substantially higher surgical mortality rates [12, 13]. The elderly (age >75 years) are especially vulnerable population with redo valvular surgical mortality rates reported to be 13.8 % to 32 % [12, 14–16]. The majority of these patients would be categorized as high (STS Score ≥ 8 %) or prohibitive surgical risk and would likely not have a therapeutic option. These mortality rates are similar to the thresholds chosen by the current Centers for Medicare & Medicaid Services (CMS) guidelines that most clinicians choose transcatheter aortic valve replacement (TAVR) instead of traditional aortic valve replacement (AVR).

Access, Procedure Planning, and Technical Considerations

A variety of procedural approaches have been utilized including transapical, transeptal (via femoral vein or jugular vein), and direct left atrial. Presurgical imaging including 3D transesophageal echocardiography and cardiac CT are critical for understanding the valvular pathology, adjacent anatomical structures, and for procedural planning (Fig. 18.1). Transapical is the most common access route and accounted for over 80 % of the cases in the Global Valve-in-Valve Registry [17]. Transapical (retrograde) approach has the advantages of providing direct access to the mitral valve, coaxiallity enabling valve alignment, and stability during deployment. However, transapical procedures are more invasive and can have serious

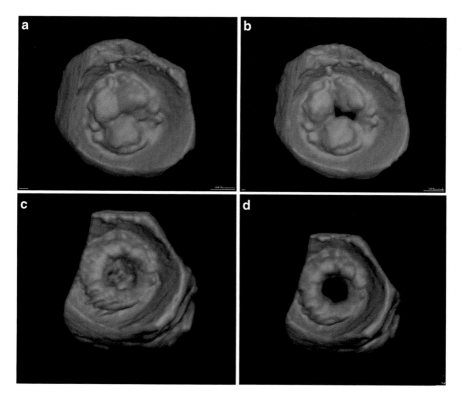

Fig. 18.1 Systolic and diastolic 3D transesophageal echocardiography images of a degenerated (stenotic) 29 mm Epic Biocor bioprosthetic mitral valve pre- and post-transcatheter mitral valve-in-valve (26 mm Edwards Sapien Valve). Panel (**a**)=Preop Systolic, Panel (**b**)=Preop Diastolic, Panel (**c**)=Postop Systolic, Panel (**d**)=Postop Diastolic

complications due to the access site. The transeptal (antegrade) approach is less invasive and can be potentially done under local anesthesia. The challenges with this type of approach are that it is technically challenging, positioning/coaxiallity can be difficult, and there is a residual septal defect after the procedure. Some centers have advocated creating an arterial–venous loop by externalizing the transeptal wire through the femoral artery or the left ventricular apex. A percutaneous approach to accessing the left ventricular apex can be used to snare and externalize the wire. This technique can help with delivery system stability and coaxiallity; however, it can also increase the rate of serious complications (i.e., hemothorax and coronary laceration). Whether crossing the mitral prosthesis in an antegrade or retrograde fashion, care should be taken to avoid entanglement in any retained subvalvular apparatus or papillary muscles. In addition, a balloon valvuloplasty is generally not required unless there is difficulty crossing a severely stenotic valve with the delivery system. Balloon valvuloplasty may be detrimental given the friable nature of the degenerated bioprosthetic valve and the risk of particle embolization. Rapid right ventricular pacing is recommended to reduce cardiac motion and to allow precise placement of the transcatheter valve. Implanting teams can consider temporary circulatory support during implantation for patients with significant ventricular dysfunction.

One of the key elements to a successful MiVIV procedure is meticulous pre-procedure planning. This includes, but is not limited to, understanding the design of the previously placed bioprosthetic valve and the anatomical challenges within each patient. A detailed prior surgical report is also critical to understanding the anatomic issues faced during the original surgery and to correctly identify the surgical prosthesis used. Surgical bioprosthetic valves, as compared to surgical rings, achieve near circularity making them ideal for this intervention with transcatheter heart valves. Surgical valves can either be stented or stentless; however, stentless valves are rarely, if ever, used in the mitral position. Some of the valve frames, but not all, contain radiopaque makers that aid in coaxiality and positioning during the procedures (Fig. 18.2). The valve leaflets are usually constructed of either porcine valve or bovine pericardial tissue. Valve manufacturers label surgical valves based on the valve's inner or outer diameters. The true inner diameter, which takes into account the valve stent frame and leaflets, is the critical measurement needed for appropriate sizing. Depending on the manufacturer, leaflet configuration, and material, this can vary greatly. Through his innovative work, Bapat et al. developed a comprehensive database of surgical valves that is crucial to procedure planning [18, 19]. From the compilation of this data, a Valve-in-Valve Application was constructed that gives physician an in-depth understanding of valve positioning and correct sizing (http://www.ubqo.com/viv). In order to avoid unacceptably, high post-procedure transmitral gradients, biprosthetic surgical valves with small inner diameters should be avoided. To date, there are only three transcatheter valves that have been used for MiVIV procedures which include the Edwards Sapien/Sapien XT (Edwards Lifesciences, Irvine, CA), Medtronic Melody (Minneapolis, Medtronic. MN), and the Inovare transcatheter (Braile Biomedica, São José do Rio Preto/SP Brazil) valves. In the vast majority of these cases, an Edwards Sapien or Sapien XT valve has been implanted. There are also small case series using the Medtronic Melody

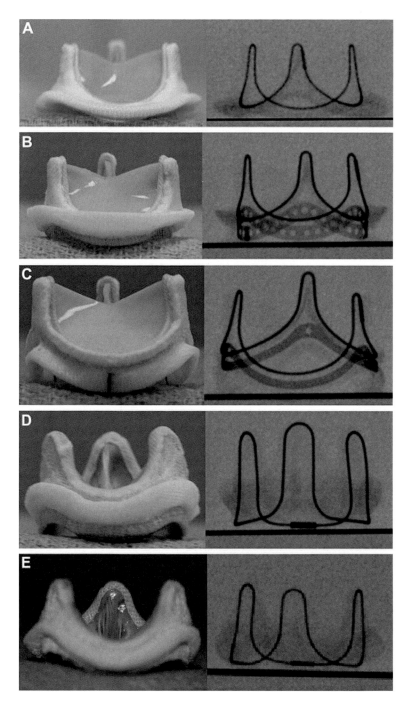

Fig. 18.2 Radiographic images of stented surgical bioprosthetic valves. (**a**) Perimount 2700. (**b**) Perimount. (**c**) Magna. (**d**) CE porcine. (**e**) CE S.A.V. (**f**) Mosaic. (**g**) Hancock II. (**h**) Epic. (**i**) Epic Supra. (**j**) Trifecta. (**k**) Mitroflow. (**l**) Soprano. (**m**) Aspire. Taken from Bapat et al. [19]

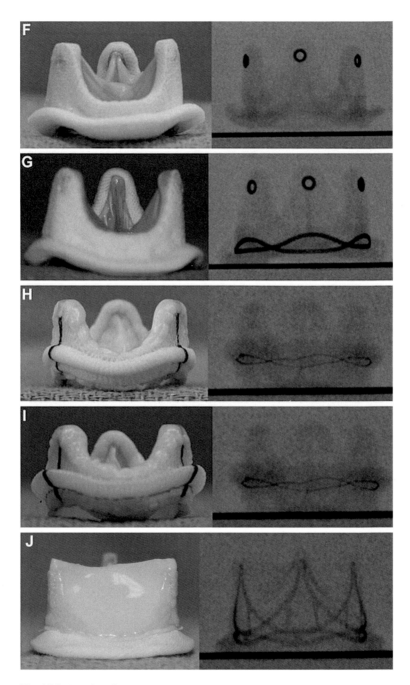

Fig. 18.2 (continued)

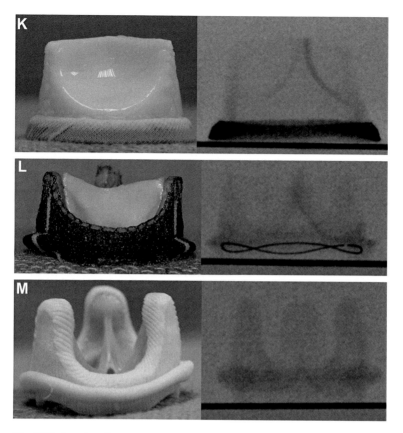

Fig. 18.2 (continued)

and the Inovare Valve [20–22] (Braile Biomedica). It is generally recommended to oversize the transcatheter heart valve by at least 10 % compared to true inner diameter of the surgical prosthesis to obtain secure anchoring. The accurate positioning is obtained by understanding the location of sewing ring of the bioprosthetic that will form with "neo-annulus" [23]. Ideally achieving a slight "hour glass" or "flower pot" shape at the level of sewing ring is preferable to securely anchor the valve and avoid migration (Fig. 18.3). However, significant distortion of the transcatheter valve stent frame from over inflation can lead to leaflet malcoaptation and central regurgitation.

We strongly recommend that the implanting team practices deploying the appropriate size trascatheter prosthesis within the mitral prosthesis prior to the actual patient case. In this way, they will familiarize themselves with the valve-in-valve interaction and proper depth of implantation. The importance of proper pre-procedure planning cannot be overemphasized. It is also very important to determine bail out strategies in the event of a complication. This should have been clearly discussed with the patient prior to the procedure.

Fig. 18.3 Fluoroscopic images of an Edwards Sapien Valve deployed within a degenerated Epic Biocor mitral prosthesis

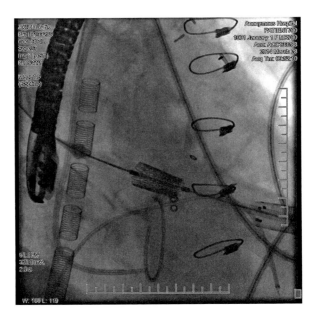

Post-procedure Management/Follow-up

There is currently no clear consensus of the anticoagulation strategy following a transcatheter MiVIV procedure. In the 2014 AHA/ACC Guideline for the Management of Patients with Valvular Heart Disease, aspirin (75–100 mg) is recommended after receiving a bioprosthetic mitral valve. In addition, it is reasonable to consider vitamin K antagonist therapy for 3 months as well (Class IIa, Level of Evidence C). If the patient is not a candidate for a vitamin K antagonist, consideration should be given for a dual antiplatelet strategy. The AHA/ACC guidelines give an IIb indication for Clopidogrel following TAVR for 6 months in addition to lifelong aspirin (75–100 mg). Whether this can be extrapolated to transcatheter MiVIV procedures is unclear [24].

A baseline echocardiogram prior to hospital discharge following any transcatheter valve-in-valve is recommended to provide baseline transvalvular gradients and any degree of bioprosthetic or perivalvular regurgitation. In addition, repeat studies can be performed at 1 month and 1 year after implantation. Every year thereafter patients should have an echocardiogram or if there is any change in clinical status.

Clinical Outcomes

There is a clear paucity of data surrounding this therapy. In a recent meta-analysis of transcatheter valve-in-valve (TVIV) implantation by Raval et al., there were a total of 66 published cases of mitral TVIV procedures. This included the largest single center cohort by Cheung et al. with 23 patients considered at high surgical risk with an average calculated STS score of 12.2 ± 6.9 %. The median follow-up was 357 days. The patients had favorable hemodynamics results with an average mean gradient of 6.9 ± 2.2 mmHg at 30 days and 7.7 ± 2.6 mmHg at 1 year. No patients had moderate or severe mitral regurgitation following the procedure. There were remarkably no mortalities at 30 days. Finally, at a median follow-up of 753 days, the survival rate was 90.4 % [25, 26].

The Valve-In-Valve International Registry reported on 190 patients undergoing a MiViV procedure ($n = 157$) or mitral valve-in-ring procedure ($n = 33$). The average STS Score was elevated at 14.8 ± 12.6 %, and the average age was 74.5 ± 12.4 years. The all-cause death at 30 days was 8.9 % which was substantially lower than the predicted operative mortality. The post-procedure valve performance was excellent with the average mean gradient of 6.2 ± 2.7 mmHg and very little mitral regurgitation (95.8 % with none or mild). The majority of the patients (85.8 %) had improved to NYHA Class I/II symptoms at 30 days. At 1 year, there was a 22.3 % mortality rate reported [17].

Mitral Valve in Ring

Mitral valve repair has become the surgical treatment of choice in patients with mitral regurgitation and suitable anatomy. The ACC/AHA Valvular Guidelines recommend surgical repair over replacement for primary mitral regurgitation [24] (Class I; LOE B). Surgical mitral valve repair continues to rise in the United States and accounts for over two-thirds of isolated mitral valve regurgitation surgeries [1]. The durability of mitral valve repair has been demonstrated to be quite robust. This was demonstrated in two large cohorts reported by Seeburger et al. and David et al. In a surgical series of 1339 mitral valve repair patients, the freedom from reoperation at 5 years was 96.3 % [27]. David et al. series of 840 mitral valve repairs demonstrated a low reoperation probability, at 20 years, of 5.9 %. However, the freedom from moderate-to-severe recurrent mitral regurgitation was only 69.2 % [28]. Other reports, including the surgical series by Flameng et al. reported higher rates of recurrent mitral regurgitation following mitral repair. At 7 years, the freedom from severe (>2/4) mitral regurgitation was 71.1 %. In addition, the yearly rate of recurrence of significant mitral regurgitation was found to be 3.7 % [29].

Annuloplasty rings are used in the vast majority of mitral valve repairs. Rings are defined whether they are complete or incomplete and by their structural rigidity (i.e., rigid, semi-rigid, and flexible). In addition, mitral annuloplasty rings can come in variety of shapes including D-shaped, D-shaped planar, saddle shaped, C-shaped, and bands. Due to this often noncircular shape, placing a transcatheter valve in a prior surgical ring can present an additional anatomical challenge. Rigid complete and incomplete rings have the largest potential for poor results with valve-in-ring therapy. Due to the non-conformable nature of rigid complete bands, this tends to distort the normally circular shape of the trancatheter valve. This can lead to central valvular regurgitation due to stent frame deformation and leaflet malcoaptation. In addition, there can be residual gaps between the annuloplasty ring and the trancatheter valve, which can lead to significant paravalvular regurgitation. The first published case of mitral valve-in-ring procedure was reported by de Weger et al. in 2010. This case report demonstrated the feasibility of this therapy in a high-risk surgical candidate [30]. The largest published cohort of mitral valve-in-ring patients by Descoutures et al. included 17 total high-risk (average STS score = 13 ± 9 %) surgical patients. The route of access was equally split between transeptal ($n = 8$) and transapical ($n = 9$). The procedural success rate was 88 %, and the 30-day survival was 82 %. At a mean follow-up of 13 ± 5 months, the survival rate was 71 %. The hemodynamic outcomes were acceptable with a mean mitral valve gradient of 7 ± 3 mmHg, and the majority of patients had none to mild residual mitral regurgitation [31]. Although technically and anatomically challenging, this therapy may offer an alternative to an extreme risk mitral valve reoperation in highly selected patients.

Conclusions

It is clear that mitral valve bioprosthesis failure is becoming increasingly prevalent and may pose a significant problem for our patients. In addition, based on the high morbidity and mortality associated with redo mitral valve operations in a large proportion of patients, other less invasive options should be explored. Currently, there are also nested registries within the PARTNER and US Core-Valve Pivotal Trials for transcatheter aortic valve-in-valve procedures in order to obtain FDA approval. However, there is no such study for failed mitral prosthesis despite the similarly high mortality and morbidity rates for redo-mitral valve surgery. Transcatheter valve-in-valve for a failed mitral bioprosthesis is a technique that has offered encouraging initial published results and has recently received CE Mark in Europe. This procedure may offer a safer alternative to redo cardiac surgery and avoid the need for cardiopulmonary bypass and cardioplegic arrest. In experienced centers, MiVIV therapy has emerged as a potentially safe and feasible option for high-risk patients with failed mitral bioprosthesis.

Transcatheter valve in ring procedures for failed mitral valve repairs may also become a feasible option for high-risk patients requiring mitral valve reoperations.

References

1. Gammie JS, Sheng S, Griffith BP, et al. Trends in mitral valve surgery in the United States: results from the Society of Thoracic Surgeons Adult Cardiac Surgery Database. Ann Thorac Surg. 2009;87(5):1431–7.
2. Borger MA, Ivanov J, Armstrong S, Christie-hrybinsky D, Feindel CM, David TE. Twenty-year results of the Hancock II bioprosthesis. J Heart Valve Dis. 2006;15(1):49–55.

3. Hammermeister K, Sethi GK, Henderson WG, Grover FL, Oprian C, Rahimtoola SH. Outcomes 15 years after valve replacement with a mechanical versus a bioprosthetic valve: final report of the Veterans Affairs randomized trial. J Am Coll Cardiol. 2000;36(4):1152–8.
4. Bourguignon T, Bouquiaux-stablo AL, Loardi C, et al. Very late outcomes for mitral valve replacement with the Carpentier-Edwards pericardial bioprosthesis: 25-year follow-up of 450 implantations. J Thorac Cardiovasc Surg. 2014;148(5):2004–2011.e1.
5. Jamieson WR, Von Lipinski O, Miyagishima RT, et al. Performance of bioprostheses and mechanical prostheses assessed by composites of valve-related complications to 15 years after mitral valve replacement. J Thorac Cardiovasc Surg. 2005;129(6):1301–8.
6. Ruel M, Chan V, Bédard P, et al. Very long-term survival implications of heart valve replacement with tissue versus mechanical prostheses in adults <60 years of age. Circulation. 2007;116(11 Suppl):I294–300.
7. Kaneko T, Aranki S, Javed Q, et al. Mechanical versus bioprosthetic mitral valve replacement in patients <65 years old. J Thorac Cardiovasc Surg. 2014;147(1):117–26.
8. Jamieson WR, Gudas VM, Burr LH, et al. Mitral valve disease: if the mitral valve is not reparable/failed repair, is bioprosthesis suitable for replacement? Eur J Cardiothorac Surg. 2009;35(1):104–10.
9. Mykén PS. Seventeen-year experience with the St. Jude medical biocor porcine bioprosthesis. J Heart Valve Dis. 2005;14(4):486–92.
10. Chan V, Malas T, Lapierre H, et al. Reoperation of left heart valve bioprostheses according to age at implantation. Circulation. 2011;124(11 Suppl):S75–80.
11. Potter DD, Sundt TM, Zehr KJ, et al. Risk of repeat mitral valve replacement for failed mitral valve prostheses. Ann Thorac Surg. 2004;78(1):67–72.
12. Fukunaga N, Okada Y, Konishi Y, et al. Clinical outcomes of redo valvular operations: a 20-year experience. Ann Thorac Surg. 2012;94(6):2011–6.
13. Jamieson WR, Burr LH, Miyagishima RT, et al. Reoperation for bioprosthetic mitral structural failure: risk assessment. Circulation. 2003;108 Suppl 1:II98–102.
14. Balsam LB, Grossi EA, Greenhouse DG, et al. Reoperative valve surgery in the elderly: predictors of risk and long-term survival. Ann Thorac Surg. 2010;90(4):1195–200.
15. Kirsch M, Nakashima K, Kubota S, Houël R, Hillion ML, Loisance D. The risk of reoperative heart valve procedures in Octogenarian patients. J Heart Valve Dis. 2004;13(6):991–6.
16. Jones JM, O'kane H, Gladstone DJ, et al. Repeat heart valve surgery: risk factors for operative mortality. J Thorac Cardiovasc Surg. 2001;122(5):913–8.
17. Dvir, D. (2014, September 14th). Perspectives from Valve-in-Valve Experiences. TCT 2014, Washington DC.
18. Bapat VN, Attia RQ, Condemi F, et al. Fluoroscopic guide to an ideal implant position for Sapien XT and CoreValve during a valve-in-valve procedure. JACC Cardiovasc Interv. 2013;6(11):1186–94.
19. Bapat VN, Attia R, Thomas M. Effect of valve design on the stent internal diameter of a bioprosthetic valve: a concept of true internal diameter and its implications for the valve-in-valve procedure. JACC Cardiovasc Interv. 2014;7(2):115–27.
20. Cullen MW, Cabalka AK, Alli OO, et al. Transvenous, antegrade Melody valve-in-valve implantation for bioprosthetic mitral and tricuspid valve dysfunction: a case series in children and adults. JACC Cardiovasc Interv. 2013;6(6):598–605.
21. Gaia DF, Breda JR, Ferreira CB, De Souza JA, Buffolo E, Palma JH. Double transapical aortic and mitral valve-in-valve implant: an alternative for high risk and multiple reoperative patients. Int J Cardiol. 2013;164(3):e32–4.
22. Gaia DF, Palma JH. De souza JA, et al. Transapical mitral valve-in-valve implant: an alternative for high risk and multiple reoperative rheumatic patients. Int J Cardiol. 2012;154(1):e6–7.
23. Bapat V, Adams B, Attia R, Noorani A, Thomas M. Neo-annulus: A reference plane in a surgical heart valve to facilitate a valve-in-valve procedure. Catheter Cardiovasc Interv. 2014.
24. Nishimura RA, Otto CM, Bonow RO, et al. 2014 AHA/ACC guideline for the management of patients with valvular heart disease: a report of the American College of Cardiology/American

Heart Association Task Force on Practice Guidelines. J Thorac Cardiovasc Surg. 2014;148(1):e1–132.

25. Cheung A, Webb JG, Barbanti M, et al. 5-year experience with transcatheter transapical mitral valve-in-valve implantation for bioprosthetic valve dysfunction. J Am Coll Cardiol. 2013;61(17):1759–66.

26. Raval J, Nagaraja V, Eslick GD, Denniss AR. Transcatheter valve-in-valve implantation: a systematic review of literature. Heart Lung Circ. 2014;23(11):1020–8.

27. Seeburger J, Borger MA, Falk V, et al. Minimal invasive mitral valve repair for mitral regurgitation: results of 1339 consecutive patients. Eur J Cardiothorac Surg. 2008;34(4):760–5.

28. David TE, Armstrong S, Mccrindle BW, Manlhiot C. Late outcomes of mitral valve repair for mitral regurgitation due to degenerative disease. Circulation. 2013;127(14):1485–92.

29. Flameng W, Herijgers P, Bogaerts K. Recurrence of mitral valve regurgitation after mitral valve repair in degenerative valve disease. Circulation. 2003;107(12):1609–13.

30. De Weger A, Ewe SH, Delgado V, Bax JJ. First-in-man implantation of a trans-catheter aortic valve in a mitral annuloplasty ring: novel treatment modality for failed mitral valve repair. Eur J Cardiothorac Surg. 2011;39(6):1054–6.

31. Descoutures F, Himbert D, Maisano F, et al. Transcatheter valve-in-ring implantation after failure of surgical mitral repair. Eur J Cardiothorac Surg. 2013;44(1):e8–15.

Chapter 19
Percutaneous Treatment of Adverse Left Ventricular Remodeling

Firas Zahr and Phillip A. Horwitz

Introduction

Heart failure remains a major public health problem. Almost 5,000,000 patients in the United States are affected, and 30–40 % of patients die from heart failure within 1 year after receiving the diagnosis [1].

Despite the application of best available medical therapy, the percentage of patients suffering from signs and symptoms of heart failure remains high. This supports the concept that heart failure progresses independently of neurohormonal activation due to abnormal and excessive increase in left ventricular volume. This theory, the biomechanical model of heart failure, was first proposed by Mann and Bristow [2]. The concept of biomechanical model of heart failure introduces the need for strategies aimed at reducing left ventricular volumes and restoring heart geometry.

Surgical ventricular restoration has been introduced to restore left ventricular shape, size, and function in patient with ischemic dilated cardiomyopathy and heart failure. The technique, initially introduced by Dor and Jatene [3, 4], has been refined over the last 10 years. More recently, percutaneous approaches to restore ventricular geometry have been developed.

Left Ventricular Remodeling

Myocardial infarction, particularly large, transmural infarcts, results in a number of structural changes involving both the infarcted and non-infarcted zones [5]. This process begins shortly after the infarction, and progresses over time causing

F. Zahr, MD • P.A. Horwitz, MD (✉)
Department of Internal Medicine, University of Iowa Carver College of Medicine,
200 Hawkins Dr, Iowa City, IA 52242, USA
e-mail: firas-zahr@uiowa.edu; phillip-horwitz@uiowa.edu

© Springer Science+Business Media New York 2016   249
G. Ailawadi, I.L. Kron (eds.), *Catheter Based Valve and Aortic Surgery*,
DOI 10.1007/978-1-4939-3432-4_19

abnormal thinning and dilatation of the necrotic zones. This process, while is initially considered as a compensatory mechanism to maintain stroke volume, is accompanied by secondary volume overload in the uninfarcted regions. Wall stress is increased leading to eccentric hypertrophy of noninfarcted regions. This results in conditions that promote further dilatation and global ventricular dysfunction. Structural and geometrical ventricular changes proceed along with increased myocyte stress, neurohormonal activation, collagen synthesis, fibrosis, and remodeling of the extracellular matrix resulting in further deterioration of cardiac function [6]. Patients with adverse remodeling and increased ventricular volumes after myocardial infarction are at increased risk for adverse cardiac events including symptomatic heart failure and cardiac death. While pharmacologic interventions such as inhibition of the renin–angiotensin system and beta blockade help reduce remodeling and improve clinical outcomes, the effect is only moderate [7]. Heart failure and increased mortality continue to be seen in this patient population highlighting the need for new therapies to reduce adverse remodeling after myocardial infarction.

Surgical Procedures for Adverse Left Ventricular Remodeling

Surgical methods to prevent adverse ventricular remodeling after myocardial infarction (surgical ventricular restoration (SVR)) have evolved over the years. A linear suture closure technique for excision of left ventricular aneurysm was described by Cooley in 1958 [8], and circular external suture was by reported by Jatene in 1984 [4]. In 1985, Vincent Dor MD, introduced the endoventricular circular patch plasty (Dor Procedure), where a circular patch was used to reconstruct the left ventricle by opening the ventricle in the center of the affected area, performing a thromboembolectomy when indicated, then excluding the dyskinetic or akinetic left ventricular free wall with an endoventricular circular suture passed through the fibrous tissue above the infarct transitional zone. A Dacron patch was secured at the junction of the endocardial muscle and scar tissue, thereby excluding the noncontractile portion of the left ventricle (LV) and septum. The excluded scar was folded over the patch to assure hemostasis [3].

Surgical Ventricular Remodeling: Cardiac Function and Survival

The first consistent results were reported by Dor and coauthors. They showed that the procedure improved left ventricular function, NYHA functional class, and survival by reducing ventricular volumes and increasing the ejection fraction. These results were observed not only in the patients with classic dyskinetic aneurysms but also with dilated ischemic cardiomyopathy and severe LV dysfunction [9].

A few years later in the first international registry, the RESTORE group (Reconstructive Endoventricular Surgery, returning Torsion Original Radius Elliptical shape to the left ventricle) confirmed the safety and efficacy of this technique in 1198 patients between 1998 and 2003. This study reported improvement in the ejection fraction from 29.6 ± 11 % preoperatively to 39.5 ± 12.3 % post-procedure ($p < 0.001$). An improvement in left ventricular end-systolic volume index from 80.4 ± 51.4 mL/m^2 preoperatively to 56.6 ± 34.3 mL/m^2 postoperatively was observed. 30-day mortality after the procedure was 5.3 % with this value being higher in patients whom mitral valve repair was performed (8.7 %). The overall 5-year survival was 68.6 %, and 78 % of patients were not readmitted to the hospital for congestive heart failure [10]. Excellent results have been reported from SVR procedures at the Cleveland Clinic as well, with that series showing 30-day mortality of 1 %, and survival at 1, 3, and 5 years was 92 %, 90 %, and 80 % respectively [11]. While this registry and case series data appeared encouraging for the technical feasibility, safety, and initial efficacy of surgery for ventricular restoration, they all suffered from the limitations of their non-randomized study design.

The Surgical Treatment for Ischemic Heart Failure (STICH) trial was an international multicenter randomized trial to determine whether surgical ventricular reconstruction performed at the time of coronary bypass surgery (CABG) would decrease the rate of death or hospitalization in patients with ischemic cardiomyopathy (LV ejection fraction <35 %) with anterior myocardial akinesia amenable to SVR [12]. 1000 patients from 2002 to 2006 were randomized between coronary bypass surgery plus ventricular reconstruction versus bypass surgery alone. Ventricular reconstruction successfully reduced end-systolic LV volume index by 19 % as compared with 6 % in CABG alone ($p < 0.001$). However, this reduction in ventricular volume did not translate into improvements in clinical endpoints of survival, exercise capacity, and repeat hospitalizations.

A number of patient selection issues and hemodynamic effects of LV volume reduction have been proposed to explain these contradictory results. It is possible that current heart failure therapies are themselves effective at limiting adverse remodeling leaving little room for the benefit of surgical interventions. It is also possible that the highly invasive nature of surgical ventricular reconstruction in the sickest heart failure patients may limit the benefits of the procedure in those likely to benefit the most. This leads to the hope for less invasive approaches of mitigating adverse left ventricular remodeling to demonstrate clinical improvement in this patient population.

New Therapies for Adverse Remodeling

A number of novel therapies to prevent or improve adverse ventricular remodeling are under current study. Animal and human studies of various cellular-based therapies have been performed and are currently underway. Interventions with fetal cardiomyocytes, allogeneic, and autologous stem cell treatments are in various stages of study—this large topic is outside the scope of the current text [13, 14]. Additionally, components of the extracellular matrix have been identified as potential targets for affecting postinfarction adverse remodeling. For example, matrix metalloprotease inhibition, in some animal models, has shown some promise in altering adverse healing after infarction [15]. Possibly, cellular or pharmacologic therapies directly targeted at preventing adverse remodeling will prove to be effective.

Another novel approach to the management of adverse remodeling postinfarction might be percutaneous therapies to reduce ventricular volumes and mimic surgical ventricular restoration procedures. Patients undergoing percutaneous therapies may enjoy the benefits of improvements in ventricular geometry but avoid the complications and morbidity associated with more invasive techniques. The first such device is the PARACHUTE ventricular partitioning device (VPD) (Cardiokinetix Inc., Menlo Park, CA).

Percutaneous Left Ventricular Partitioning Device

The PARACHUTE (Cardiokinetix, Inc., Menlo Park, CA) is a novel percutaneous device that partitions the dysfunctional portion of the left ventricle from the functioning portion in patient with chronic heart failure with prior anterior wall myocardial infarction (MI). The device is a partitioning membrane deployed within the aneurysmal left ventricle. This novel device partitions an enlarged scarred ventricle into a dynamic and a static chamber. The static chamber is the portion of the left ventricle volume that is distal to the device and is taken out of the circulation. Stress placed on the partitioned myocardium and the forces previously transmitted to the apical segment are decreased both in systole and diastole, lessening the forces responsible for left ventricular dilatation. In addition to this regional unloading, the reduction in size of the dynamic chamber results in decreased myocardial stress in the normal myocardium via Laplace law, providing global unloading of the ventricle. The device, in effect, is designed to mimic surgical ventricular remodeling procedures by excluding rather than excising the noncontractile ventricular apex.

The PARACHUTE VPD device is composed of a self-expanding nitinol frame, an expanded polytetrafluoroethylene occlusive membrane, and a distal foot. The nitinol frame is shaped like an umbrella with 16 struts each ending with a 2-mm anchor (Fig. 19.1). Upon expansion of the VPD by the delivery catheter balloon, these anchors engage the tissue, stabilize the device, and prevent dislodgment and migration after the device is detached from the delivery catheter [16]. After the device is expanded, the occlusive membrane provides a barrier to seal off the static chamber on the distal side of the device. The VPD is designed to be inserted percutaneous via femoral arterial access. The device is advanced retrograde across the aortic valve and positioned in the ventricular apex under fluoroscopic and echocardiographic guidance. Once positioned, the device is unsheathed and expanded (Fig. 19.2). After full deployment, it is released and the delivery catheter removed.

Fig. 19.1 Right anterior oblique angiographic image of the ventricular partitioning device being deployed

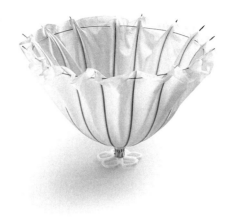

Fig. 19.2 The PARACHUTE Ventricular Partitioning Device Implant. Photo courtesy CardioKinetex, Menlo Park, CA

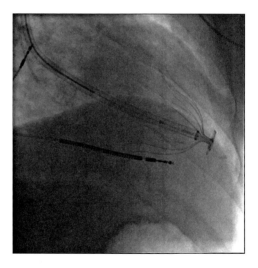

Ventricular Partitioning Device Clinical Outcomes/Clinical Trials

The feasibility and preliminary safety and efficacy of percutaneous LV partitioning in patients with heart failure with a prior anterior wall MI was published by Mazzaferri et al. [17]. The study enrolled 39 patients in the United States and Europe with anteroapical akinesis due to previous myocardial infarction, New York Heart Association (NYHA) class II–IV heart failure, and an ejection fraction of ≤40 %.

The device was implanted in 34 patients (94 %). At 6-month follow-up, overall success rate was 74 %, defined as successful deployment of the VPD without a major adverse cardiac event. Improvements in end-diastolic volume index (127.2 ± 4.2 vs. 110.4 ± 4.6 (ml/m^2); $p < 0.001$) and end-systolic volume index (93.6 ± 4.1 vs. 79.5 ± 3.6 (ml/m^2); $p < 0.001$) were seen after VPD insertion. Additionally, statistically significant improvements in NYHA class and quality of life assessments were seen. Ejection fraction and stroke volume were unchanged after VPD implantation.

This study demonstrated the potential for a percutaneous device to successfully reduce ventricular volumes in patients with adverse ventricular remodeling after acute infarction up to 3 years [18]. Of course, limited conclusions regarding clinical benefit to VPD insertion can be drawn from this small, uncontrolled, initial registry.

A number of additional non-randomized studies of this percutaneous VPD are in various stages of enrollment or follow-up in Europe, China, and the United States. Additional clinical data on procedural success, major adverse cardiac events, and hemodynamic and imaging measures will be available in the near future from some of these sources.

The Pivotal Trial to Establish the Efficacy and Long-term Safety of the Parachute Implant System (PARACHUTE IV) trial is a randomized (VPD vs. optimal medical therapy), multicenter trial designed to evaluate the PARACHUTE implant [19]. This study will enroll approximately 560 patients with ischemic cardiomyopathy (ejection fraction ≤ 35 %) due to anterior infarction and NYHA Class III–IV heart failure despite optimal medical therapy in up to 80 centers in the USA. The event driven primary endpoint includes all-cause mortality and rehospitalization for worsening heart failure. Other key endpoints include hemodynamic measures by echocardiography and imaging measures by computed tomography. This currently enrolling randomized trial is hoped to provide the most robust information on the safety and efficacy of VPD insertion in this patient population.

Conclusion

Adverse ventricular remodeling following myocardial infarction has been associated with increased mortality and progressive heart failure in patients with ischemic cardiomyopathy. Surgical procedures to improve ventricular geometry, such as the Dor procedure, have been shown to successfully improve ventricular volumes, but this has not translated into improved clinical outcomes in the limited clinical trial data to date. A single percutaneous device for the treatment of adverse ventricular remodeling, the PARACHUTE device, is currently under investigation in postinfarction cardiomyopathy. This, and future such devices, may allow for minimally invasive methods for reducing ventricular volumes without the morbidity associated with open surgical procedures in an advanced heart failure population. The currently enrolling PARACHUTE IV randomized trial should shed light on the potential for ventricular partitioning devices to improve outcomes in patients with adverse remodeling.

References

1. McMurray JJ, Pfeffer MA. Heart failure. Lancet. 2005;365(9474):1877–89.
2. Mann DL, Bristow MR. Mechanisms and models in heart failure: the biomechanical model and beyond. Circulation. 2005;111(21):2837–49.
3. Dor V, Saab M, Coste P, Kornaszewska M, Montiglio F. Left ventricular aneurysm: a new surgical approach. Thorac Cardiovasc Surg. 1989;37(1):11–9.
4. Jatene AD. Left-ventricular aneurysmectomy – resection or reconstruction. J Thorac Cardiov Sur. 1985;89(3):321–31.
5. Pfeffer MA, Braunwald E. Ventricular remodeling after myocardial infarction. Experimental observations and clinical implications. Circulation. 1990;81(4):1161–72.
6. Braunwald E. Biomarkers in heart failure. N Engl J Med. 2008;358(20):2148–59.
7. Pfeffer MA, Braunwald E, Moye LA, Basta L, Brown EJ, Cuddy TE, et al. Effect of captopril on mortality and morbidity in patients with left-ventricular dysfunction after myocardial-infarction – results of the survival and ventricular enlargement trial. New Engl J Med. 1992;327(10):669–77.
8. Cooley DA, Collins HA, Morris GC, Chapman DW. Ventricular aneurysm after myocardial infarction – surgical excision with use of temporary cardiopulmonary bypass. JAMA. 1958;167(5):557–60.
9. Dor V, Sabatier M, Di Donato M, Montiglio F, Toso A, Maioli M. Efficacy of endoventricular patch plasty in large postinfarction akinetic scar and severe left ventricular dysfunction: comparison with a series of large dyskinetic scars. J Thorac Cardiovasc Surg. 1998;116(1):50–9.
10. Athanasuleas CL, Buckberg GD, Stanley AW, Siler W, Dor V, DiDonato M, et al. Surgical ventricular restoration: the RESTORE Group experience. Heart Fail Rev. 2004;9(4):287–97.
11. O'Neill JO, Starling RC, McCarthy PM, Albert NM, Lytle BW, Navia J, et al. The impact of left ventricular reconstruction on survival in patients with ischemic cardiomyopathy. Eur J Cardio-Thorac. 2006;30(5):753–9.
12. Velazquez EJ, Lee KL, Deja MA, Jain A, Sopko G, Marchenko A, et al. Coronary-Artery Bypass Surgery in Patients with Left Ventricular Dysfunction. New Engl J Med. 2011;364(17):1607–16.
13. Hare JM, Traverse JH, Henry TD, Dib N, Strumpf RK, Schulman SP, et al. A randomized, double-blind, placebo-controlled, dose-escalation study of intravenous adult human mesenchymal stem cells (prochymal) after acute myocardial infarction. J Am Coll Cardiol. 2009;54(24):2277–86.
14. Abdel-Latif A, Bolli R, Tleyjeh IM, Montori VM, Perin EC, Hornung CA, et al. Adult bone marrow-derived cells for cardiac repair: a systematic review and meta-analysis. Arch Intern Med. 2007;167(10):989–97.
15. Iyer RP, de Castro Bras LE, Jin YF, Lindsey ML. Translating Koch's postulates to identify matrix metalloproteinase roles in postmyocardial infarction remodeling: cardiac metalloproteinase actions (CarMA) postulates. Circ Res. 2014;114(5):860–71.
16. Sharkey H, Nikolic S, Khairkhahan A, Dae M. Left ventricular apex occluder. Description of a Ventricular Partitioning Device. EuroIntervention. 2006;2(1):125–7.
17. Mazzaferri Jr EL, Gradinac S, Sagic D, Otasevic P, Hasan AK, Goff TL, et al. Percutaneous left ventricular partitioning in patients with chronic heart failure and a prior anterior myocardial infarction: results of the PercutAneous Ventricular RestorAtion in Chronic Heart failUre PaTiEnts Trial. Am Heart J. 2012;163(5):812–20.e1.
18. Costa MA, Mazzaferri Jr EL, Sievert H, Abraham WT. Percutaneous ventricular restoration using the parachute device in patients with ischemic heart failure: three-year outcomes of the PARACHUTE first-in-human study. Circ Heart Fail. 2014;7(5):752–8.
19. Costa MA, Pencina M, Nikolic S, Engels T, Templin B, Abraham WT. The PARACHUTE IV trial design and rationale: percutaneous ventricular restoration using the parachute device in patients with ischemic heart failure and dilated left ventricles. Am Heart J. 2013;165(4):531–6.

Chapter 20
Anatomic Considerations for the Pulmonary Valve

Matthew L. Stone and James J. Gangemi

Introduction

The pulmonary valve is a semilunar valve with anterior, left, and right leaflets, no trans-valvular pressure gradient, and a valve orifice area in the normal adult of 2.0 cm^2/m^2 of body surface area [1]. The spectrum of pulmonary valve disease ranges from physiologic pulmonic flow murmurs to significant stenoses that results in changes to the structure and function of the native valve. Neonatal stenosis is a distinct entity characterized by thickened valve leaflets. This condition may resolve with time and result in a functionally normal pulmonic valve; however, infants may also progress from mild pulmonary stenosis to severe disease with time [2, 3]. While various discriminatory standards have been used in diagnosis, pulmonary stenosis is defined as a systolic gradient at cardiac catheterization of 25 mmHg or a flow velocity over 120 cm/s by echocardiography [4, 5]. Central to preoperative planning and determination of candidacy for pulmonary valve replacement or the Ross procedure is an understanding of congenital and adult heart disease pathophysiology and the effect of each on the valve architecture, function, and annulus diameter. This understanding has been revolutionized by the advancement of two- and three-dimensional real-time imaging techniques, most notably color and continuous-wave Doppler, computed tomography (CT), and dynamic magnetic resonance imaging (MRI) [6, 7]. While long-term prospective study remains limited, applied knowledge of pulmonary valve development and morphologic change provides insight into appropriate thresholds for symptomatic treatment and subsequent surveillance to prevent irreversible changes within the right heart.

The anatomic pulmonary valve is characterized by thin leaflets with a relatively small content of elastic tissue. While this composition has important implications for native pulmonary valve disease, it is also critical to understanding long-term effects of elevated

M.L. Stone, MD • J.J. Gangemi, MD (✉)
Department of Surgery, University of Virginia Medical Center, 1215 Lee Street,
Charlottesville, VA 22908, USA
e-mail: mstone@virginia.edu; jjg5d@virginia.edu

© Springer Science+Business Media New York 2016
G. Ailawadi, I.L. Kron (eds.), *Catheter Based Valve and Aortic Surgery*,
DOI 10.1007/978-1-4939-3432-4_20

left ventricular outflow tract pressures on the native pulmonary valve following the Ross procedure and after arterial switch operations for transposition of the great arteries. Additional congenital heart conditions that involve pulmonary valve mechanics and systemic hemodynamics include the well-established palliative surgical approaches to hypoplastic left heart syndrome with Damus–Kaye–Stansel procedure reconstruction [8]. Isolated pulmonary valve stenosis remains a relatively common congenital heart defect that constitutes 7 % of congenital heart disease with an estimated median incidence of 532 per million live births [9]. While stenosis is most commonly an isolated lesion, it also shares association with d-transposition of the great arteries, double-outlet right ventricle, single ventricle pathology, congenitally corrected transposition of the great arteries, and concomitant valvular aortic stenosis [10]. Of patients with right ventricular outflow obstruction, 80–90 % have valvular obstruction with the remainder being sub-valvular or supra-valvular [1, 11]. Subvalvular stenosis is a rare entity and accounts for less than 10 % of pulmonary stenosis and is most commonly associated with a ventricular septal defect and may necessitate repair at the time of ventricular septal defect repair [10]. Valvular stenosis most commonly results from commissural fusion; however, it may result from valve dysplasia in up to 15 % of patients and is characterized by thickened, immobile leaflets that are composed of myxomatous tissue and often annular hypoplasia with non-fused commissures [1, 9]. Syndromes that involve stenosis of the pulmonary valve include Holt–Oram syndrome, Noonan syndrome, and Leopard syndrome [12, 13]. Rare acquired etiologies for pulmonary stenosis include carcinoid syndrome, rheumatic heart disease, and extrinsic compression [1].

Tetralogy of Fallot (TOF) affects 5 out of every 10,000 babies and remains the most common cyanotic heart defect [14]. TOF is defined by the presence of a ventricular septal defect, pulmonary stenosis, right ventricular hypertrophy, and an overriding aorta. As outcomes for children with TOF have significantly improved over the past decade, an adult population with late pulmonary valve regurgitation is emerging. The most common presentation for TOF patients with late pulmonary failure is a progressive decrease in functional capacity that may more severely lead to decreased right ventricular flow and dysrhythmia. Therefore, strategies directed at either pulmonary valve replacement or balloon dilatation are needed to preserve right ventricular function and augment pulmonary blood flow. Following initial valve replacement, approximately 20–30 % of patients will need another valve replacement within 10 years. Thus, an understanding of right ventricular pressures and valve characteristics is guided by imaging and patient functional capacity to determine the appropriate timing for re-intervention [14].

Embryologic Development

The human semilunar valves develop as a part of the endocardial cushion material at the distal aspect of the cardiac tube and emerge by cellular proliferation and the margins of the conus arteriosus [15]. Right and left cushions develop at each corresponding margin and fuse with one another to only be further subdivided into two parts, one going to each orifice. Entry of anterior and posterior cushions results in three cushions for each valve, resulting in the three native cusps [16].

Surface blood flow results in flat endothelial cell development on the ventricular aspect of the valve and cuboidal endothelium on the arterial side of the valve, correlating with respective high and low shear forces across the valve. Separate yet coordinated ejection streams lead to the distinct separation of aortic and pulmonic tricuspid semilunar valve geometries from the common truncus arteriosus [15]. Later stages of valve development are characterized by increases in elastic and collagenous fiber content secondary to fluctuating and static tensions [15]. These inherent changes within development are critical to understanding pulmonary valve reconstruction techniques and to an understanding for long-term implications following translation of the pulmonary valve to the neoaortic position.

Pulmonary Valve Structure and Function

Stenosis of the pulmonary valve most commonly results in leaflet thickening that renders the valve flexible and competent yet limited in function due to commissural fusion. Valve structure may be domed with no commissures or exhibit fused commissures with monocuspid, bicuspid (10–20 %), tricuspid, or quadricuspid valve leaflet morphology [17, 18]. Calcification is rare and occurs most commonly after the age of 40 years [10, 19]. As described, valve dysplasia resulting in obstruction secondary to thickened and immobile valve cusps is less common and shares association with Noonan syndrome most commonly. This minority of patients with myxomatous valvular change has annular obstruction secondary to thickened and relatively immobile valve cusps with absent or trivial commissural fusion [10, 18]. In the study of percutaneous balloon valvotomy, thickening of valve leaflets decreased from 93 % to 4 % with improved leaflet mobility in all patients and a freedom from re-intervention of 84 % at 8 years, supporting a degree of reversibility in undesired valve characteristics with an improved transvalvular gradient and overall native valve geometry [20].

Post-stenotic dilatation of the right ventricular outflow tract has been hypothesized to result in a decrease in the severity of pulmonary stenosis through annular dilatation. This phenomenon had a demonstrated 58 % decrease in the severity of pulmonary stenosis with standard echocardiographic follow-up and in contrast to congenital aortic stenosis resulted in no rapid increase in pulmonary stenosis throughout early childhood [2]. Post-stenotic dilatation may be massive and extend into the left main pulmonary artery and is postulated to occur secondary to disruption of elastic tissues from the turbulent flow through the stenotic valve [10, 21, 22]. It has also been observed that neonates with critical pulmonary stenosis do not exhibit post-stenotic dilation likely secondary to the low flow and pressure within the main pulmonary artery. This subgroup of patients also exhibits hypoplasia of the tricuspid valve with concomitant decrease in right ventricular volume [10]. An understanding of these morphologic changes accompanying pulmonary stenosis is imperative to guide operative reconstruction and post-repair surveillance.

Pathophysiology

Narrowing of the pulmonary valve orifice results in varying degrees of strain on the right ventricle that in the most severe stages may result in right ventricular diastolic dysfunction secondary to ventricular hypertrophy and resultant increased right-sided heart pressures that lead to congestive failure. Variability exists in the estimation of pulmonary stenosis with classification systems being contingent upon the imaging modality utilized in diagnosis. Pulmonary stenosis severity is principally determined by the transpulmonary pressure gradient as required image planes are generally not available to assess pulmonic valve area. Echocardiographic assessment is notably limited with sequential areas of subvalvular or infundibular stenosis, with infundibular obstruction being characterized by a late peaking systolic jet [23]. While no specific Doppler gradient is agreed upon as an indication for intervention, the American College of Cardiology/American Heart Association stratifies pulmonary stenosis as mild, moderate, or severe [24] (Table 20.1).

Right ventricular pressures and pulmonary valvular gradients are commonly incongruent when measuring by Doppler echocardiography and heart catheterization, with the mean pressure gradient most accurately correlating with peak-to-peak systolic pressure gradients as measured by catheterization [25]. Prior study has demonstrated that outpatient mean gradient is most predictive of peak-to-peak gradient and should be used for the determination of candidacy for intervention, as maximal gradients lead to systematic overstatement of the degree of stenosis [25].

While recognizing limitations in the ability for echocardiography to detect pulmonary valve disease and outflow tract stenosis, CT and MRI have introduced adjunct modalities for both detailed cross-sectional and dynamic imaging of the pulmonary valve (Fig. 20.1). Specifically, cardiac MRI has often replaced cardiac catheterization as the preferred imaging modality for the pulmonary valve while optimizing follow-up and preoperative treatment protocols. In prospective study, MRI reproducibly demonstrated marked hemodynamic improvement of RV function after pulmonary valve replacement in adult patients late after the correction of tetralogy of Fallot, validating this imaging modality in both structural and functional assessment [26]. In addition to MRI, electrocardiogram (ECG)-gated multidetector-computed tomography provides the capacity to detect functional changes in the pulmonary valve with a demonstrated potential for identification of valve thrombus and potential avoidance of operative re-intervention after pulmonary valve replacement [27]. CT is also

Table 20.1 Classification of pulmonary stenosis

	Mild	Moderate	Severe
Peak velocity (m/s)	<3	3–4	>4
Peak gradient (mmHg)	<36	36–64	>64

Adapted from Baumgartner et al. [23]

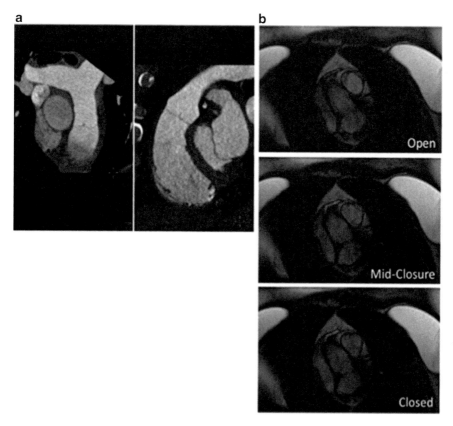

Fig. 20.1 Dynamic imaging modalities of the pulmonary valve. (**a**) Selected CT angiography images depicting a normal pulmonary valve and right ventricular outflow tract. (**b**) MRI phase imaging demonstrating a normal pulmonary valve in the open, mid-closure, and closed positions. Images courtesy of David Mauro, MD, Clinical Instructor of Radiology, University of Virginia Health System

adopted as an approach to defining potential safe sites for cannulation should cardiopulmonary bypass be needed and for re-operative approaches to sternal reentry that may necessitate early cardiopulmonary bypass access (see Fig. 20.1).

Important to understanding the pathophysiology of pulmonary valve stenosis is the distinction from pulmonary artery hypertension, as pulmonary valve stenosis alone results in significantly less right ventricular dilation, improved ventricular performance, and reduced myocardial stress biomarkers when compared to patients with isolated pulmonary hypertension [28]. Differential effects on right ventricular function are also inherent to operative repair, as strain measurements in patients with tetralogy of Fallot and RVOT patch augmentation are significantly lower than that of patients with valvular pulmonary stenosis after balloon valvuloplasty, indicating that RV strain is a regional phenomenon [29]. Additionally, native pulmonary valve stenosis must be distinguished from functional pulmonary stenosis that is characterized by an increased pressure gradient across a normal valve secondary to a massive increase in pulmonary blood flow secondary to a large left-to-right arterial shunt [10, 30].

Right ventricular volume is most commonly normal in patients with pulmonary stenosis; however, in utero severe stenosis may result in an increased right-to-left atrial shunt and decreased right-sided heart volumes that predispose infants to maldevelopment of right-sided heart structures [10]. Correction of the valvular obstruction increases right-heart blood flow and restores right ventricular volume and morphology. Approximately, 75 % of infants with mild stenosis have a patent foramen ovale or an atrial septal defect that results in left-to-right shunt early in life that may progress to a right-to-left shunt through a patent foramen ovale or atrial septal defect as right ventricular distensibility decreases and end diastolic pressure increases [10, 31]. Infundibular hypertrophy most commonly occurs after 10 years of life and distends with increased right-sided heart pressures. Important to this finding is a predisposition to subvalvular stenosis following correction of valvular stenosis which most commonly resolves slowly, yet may lead to acute right heart failure following correction [32]. Older patients may exhibit a degree of right ventricular myocardial fibrosis of subendocardial ischemic etiology secondary to right heart pressures exceeding aortic pressures and resulting in decreased coronary perfusion. Similarly, infants with critical stenosis and right ventricular hypoplasia may exhibit subendocardial fibroelastosis. Moderate or severe pulmonary valve regurgitation following balloon valvuloplasty during a mean follow-up period of 12 years has been demonstrated to be present in 57 % of children with correlation to smaller body surface area, younger age at initial intervention, and non-syndromic etiology, yet is well-tolerated as demonstrated by a 10-year freedom from re-intervention of 83 % [33]. Importantly, prior study has demonstrated a capacity for the pulmonary valve to grow concordant with the annulus and age (PV z-score: -1.3 vs. -0.7 at follow-up) [33].

Surgical Approaches and Outcomes

Outcomes for children and adults with pulmonary stenosis remain excellent, with a 25-year survival of 96 %. Additionally, a minority of patients with gradients less than 25 mmHg experience an increase in gradient and a resultant indication for intervention, which is estimated to approach only 4 % [1]. Patients with more severe degrees of stenosis, however, have high intervention rates with only 40 % remaining free of intervention at 10 years following diagnosis [34]. Infants born with critical pulmonary stenosis or membranous pulmonary atresia with intact ventricular septum are primarily treated by balloon dilation. While this treatment serves as an effective treatment and a bridge to more definitive repair, right ventricular dysfunction is estimated to occur in up to 35 % and is most commonly seen in infants with larger right ventricles [35].

In addition to pulmonary stenosis, advancement of operative repair techniques for tetralogy of Fallot has resulted in significant improvements in survival into adulthood and has introduced late-term implications inherent to each technical approach. Infundibular sparing strategies have demonstrated potential for avoidance of early reoperation and seek to decrease the progressive right ventricular failure introduced by transventricular repair [36]. While the infundibular sparing technique has been demonstrated to have lower end diastolic volumes than the classic repair, it commonly results in significant pulmonary regurgitation following repair [36]. In addition to infundibular sparing approaches, there is also demonstrated promise in pulmonary valve preservation at the initial repair with the performance of balloon dilation. This approach has resulted in improved mid-term right ventricular function in selected patients with annular preservation when compared to patients undergoing cusp reconstruction [37].

Conclusion

Pulmonary valve-directed therapies are guided by an understanding of underlying valve mechanics, leaflet composition, and potential changes in each as a result of the underlying pathophysiology. Multidisciplinary planning supports an informed approach to each repair. Further long-term longitudinal study is needed to provide more effective standards for intervention and treatment advancement.

References

1. Mehta V, Sengupta PP, Khandheria BK. Hemodynamic evaluation of pulmonary valve disease. Part II: adult perspectives. In: Hijazi ZM, Ruiz CE, Bonhoeffer P, Feldman T, editors. Transcatheter valve repair. United Kingdom: Taylor & Francis Group; 2006. p. 51.
2. Gielen H, Daniels O, van Lier H. Natural history of congenital pulmonary valvar stenosis: an echo and Doppler cardiographic study. Cardiol Young. 1999;9(2):129–35.
3. Mody MR. The natural history of uncomplicated valvular pulmonic stenosis. Am Heart J. 1975;90(3):317–21.
4. Bound JP, Logan WF. Incidence of congenital heart disease in Blackpool 1957-1971. Br Heart J. 1977;39(4):445–50.
5. Ooshima A, Fukushige J, Ueda K. Incidence of structural cardiac disorders in neonates: an evaluation by color Doppler echocardiography and the results of a 1-year follow-up. Cardiology. 1995;86(5):402–6.
6. Tajik AJ, Seward JB, Hagler DJ, Mair DD, Lie JT. Two-dimensional real-time ultrasonic imaging of the heart and great vessels. Technique, image orientation, structure identification, and validation. Mayo Clin Proc. 1978;53(5):271–303.
7. Hatle L, Angelsen B. Doppler ultrasound in cardiology: physical principles and clinical applications. 2nd ed. Philadelphia: Lea and Febiger; 1985.
8. Jenkins KJ, Hanley FL, Colan SD, Mayer Jr JE, Castaneda AR, Wernovsky G. Function of the anatomic pulmonary valve in the systemic circulation. Circulation. 1991;84(5 Suppl):Iii173–9.
9. Hoffman JI, Kaplan S. The incidence of congenital heart disease. J Am Coll Cardiol. 2002;39(12):1890–900.

10. Hoffman JIE, editor. The natural and unnatural history of congenital heart disease. San Francisco, CA: Blackwell; 2009.
11. Fyler D. Pulmonary stenosis. In: Fyler DC, editor. Nadas pediatric cardiology. Philadephia, PA: Hanley and Belfus; 1992. p. 459–70.
12. Armstrong EJ, Bischoff J. Heart valve development: endothelial cell signaling and differentiation. Circ Res. 2004;95(5):459–70.
13. Hatemi AC, Gursoy M, Tongut A, Bicakhan B, Guzeltas A, Cetin G, et al. Pulmonary stenosis as a predisposing factor for infective endocarditis in a patient with Noonan syndrome. Tex Heart Inst J. 2010;37(1):99–101.
14. Naser A, Adult congenital heart association. [cited 2015 April 30]. Available from http://www.achaheart.org/resources/for-patients/health-information/tetralogy-of-fallot.aspx
15. Maron BJ, Hutchins GM. The development of the semilunar valves in the human heart. Am J Pathol. 1974;74(2):331–44.
16. Singh I. In: Singh I, editor. Human embryology. 10th ed. New Delhi, India: Jaypee Brothers Medical Publishers; 2014.
17. Altrichter PM, Olson LJ, Edwards WD, Puga FJ, Danielson GK. Surgical pathology of the pulmonary valve: a study of 116 cases spanning 15 years. Mayo Clin Proc. 1989;64(11): 1352–60.
18. Gikonyo BM, Lucas RV, Edwards JE. Anatomic features of congenital pulmonary valvar stenosis. Pediatr Cardiol. 1987;8(2):109–16.
19. Hoffman JI. The natural history of congenital isolated pulmonic and aortic stenosis. Annu Rev Med. 1969;20:15–28.
20. Tabatabaei H, Boutin C, Nykanen DG, Freedom RM, Benson LN. Morphologic and hemodynamic consequences after percutaneous balloon valvotomy for neonatal pulmonary stenosis: medium-term follow-up. J Am Coll Cardiol. 1996;27(2):473–8.
21. Roach MR. Reversibility of poststenotic dilatation in the femoral arteries of dogs. Circ Res. 1970;27(6):985–93.
22. Guntheroth WG. Causes and effects of poststenotic dilation of the pulmonary trunk. Am J Cardiol. 2002;89(6):774–6.
23. Baumgartner H, Hung J, Bermejo J, Chambers JB, Evangelista A, Griffin BP, et al. Echocardiographic assessment of valve stenosis: EAE/ASE recommendations for clinical practice. Eur J Echocardiogr. 2009;10(1):1–25.
24. Bonow RO, Carabello BA, Chatterjee K, de Leon Jr AC, Faxon DP, Freed MD, et al. ACC/AHA 2006 guidelines for the management of patients with valvular heart disease: a report of the American College of Cardiology/American Heart Association Task Force on Practice Guidelines (writing Committee to Revise the 1998 guidelines for the management of patients with valvular heart disease) developed in collaboration with the Society of Cardiovascular Anesthesiologists endorsed by the Society for Cardiovascular Angiography and Interventions and the Society of Thoracic Surgeons. J Am Coll Cardiol 2006;48(3):e1–148.
25. Silvilairat S, Cabalka AK, Cetta F, Hagler DJ, O'Leary PW. Echocardiographic assessment of isolated pulmonary valve stenosis: which outpatient Doppler gradient has the most clinical validity? J Am Soc Echocardiogr. 2005;18(11):1137–42.
26. Vliegen HW, van Straten A, de Roos A, Roest AA, Schoof PH, Zwinderman AH, et al. Magnetic resonance imaging to assess the hemodynamic effects of pulmonary valve replacement in adults late after repair of tetralogy of fallot. Circulation. 2002;106(13):1703–7.
27. Kakizaki S, Tazawa S, Kure S, Saiki Y. Visualization of thrombosis on a prosthetic pulmonary valve using electrocardiogram-gated multidetector computed tomography. Thorac Cardiovasc Surg Rep. 2014;3(1):6–8.
28. Jurcut R, Giusca S, Ticulescu R, Popa E, Amzulescu MS, Ghiorghiu I, et al. Different patterns of adaptation of the right ventricle to pressure overload: a comparison between pulmonary hypertension and pulmonary stenosis. J Am Soc Echocardiogr. 2011;24(10):1109–17.

29. Anwar S, Harris MA, Whitehead KK, Keller MS, Fogel MA, Mercer-Rosa LM. Right ventricular outflow tract strain is reduced in tetralogy of fallot compared to valvar pulmonary stenosis patients; regional RV function defined by strain cardiac magnetic resonance imaging. Circulation. 2013;128:A18777. http://circ.ahajournals.org/cgi/content/meeting_abstract/128/22_MeetingAbstracts/A18777.
30. Johnson AM. Functional infundibular stenosis: its differentiation from structural stenosis and its importance in atrial septal defect. Guys Hosp Rep. 1959;108:373–87.
31. Roberts WC, Shemin RJ, Kent KM. Frequency and direction of interatrial shunting in valvular pulmonic stenosis with intact ventricular septum and without left ventricular inflow or outflow obstruction. An analysis of 127 patients treated by valvulotomy. Am Heart J. 1980;99(2):142–8.
32. Ben-Shachar G, Cohen MH, Sivakoff MC, Portman MA, Riemenschneider TA, Van Heeckeren DW. Development of infundibular obstruction after percutaneous pulmonary balloon valvuloplasty. J Am Coll Cardiol. 1985;5(3):754–6.
33. Garty Y, Veldtman G, Lee K, Benson L. Late outcomes after pulmonary valve balloon dilatation in neonates, infants and children. J Invasive Cardiol. 2005;17(6):318–22.
34. Hayes CJ, Gersony WM, Driscoll DJ, Keane JF, Kidd L, O'Fallon WM, et al. Second natural history study of congenital heart defects. Results of treatment of patients with pulmonary valvar stenosis. Circulation. 1993;87(2 Suppl):I28–37.
35. Ronai C, Rathod RH, Marshall AC, Oduor R, Gauvreau K, Colan SD, et al. Left ventricular dysfunction following neonatal pulmonary valve balloon dilation for pulmonary atresia or critical pulmonary stenosis. Pediatr Cardiol. 2015;36(6):1186–93.
36. McKenzie ED, Maskatia SA, Mery C. Surgical management of tetralogy of fallot: in defense of the infundibulum. Semin Thorac Cardiovasc Surg. 2013;25(3):206–12.
37. Vida VL, Guariento A, Castaldi B, Sambugaro M, Padalino MA, Milanesi O, et al. Evolving strategies for preserving the pulmonary valve during early repair of tetralogy of Fallot: midterm results. J Thorac Cardiovasc Surg. 2014;147(2):687–94. discussion 94–6.

Chapter 21
Pulmonary Insufficiency: Melody Valve

Transcatheter Therapy for the Dysfunctional Right Ventricular Outflow Tract

Michael L. O'Byrne and Matthew J. Gillespie

Introduction

To date, research and development for transcatheter valve replacement devices in patients with congenital heart disease has focused on dysfunction of the right ventricular outflow tract (RVOT), and it is in this population that safety and efficacy of transcatheter pulmonary valve replacement (TCPVR) has been clearly demonstrated. Reconstruction of the RVOT with homograft conduits is performed in patients with stenotic or atretic RVOT (e.g., tetralogy of Fallot or truncus arteriosus) and in patients with left ventricular outflow obstruction in whom the pulmonary valve is used as a neo-aortic valve (e.g., the Ross operation). RVOT augmentation can also be performed by patch augmentation (e.g., transannular patch in tetralogy of Fallot). In either case, progressive RVOT obstruction and/or insufficiency can develop. Neither obstruction nor insufficiency typically causes dramatic symptoms for years, but both proximal functional limitation (ascertainable on cardiopulmonary exercise testing) [1, 2] and insidious, progressive detriment to the RV, including systolic dysfunction and increased risk of arrhythmia and sudden death [1–3], have been demonstrated. This has been best demonstrated in long-term follow-up studies of patients following operative correction of tetralogy of Fallot, which have demonstrated accelerating risk of dysrhythmia and mortality in the second decade following repair [3–5]. The risk of arrhythmia and all-cause mortality are correlated with more extensive transannular RVOT patches [3]. Replacement of the pulmonary valve effectively addresses pulmonary regurgitation, potentially mitigating RV dysfunction and risk of adverse outcome. The presuppositions (1) that all prosthetic valves have finite life spans and (2) that the technical complexity and associated morbidity of reoperations increase

M.L. O'Byrne, MD, MSCE (✉) • M.J. Gillespie, MD
Division of Cardiology, Department of Pediatrics, The Children's Hospital of Philadelphia,
Perelman School of Medicine, University of Pennsylvania,
34th Street and Civic Center Boulevard, Philadelphia, PA 19104, USA
e-mail: mlobyrne@childrensnational.org; GILLESPIE@mail.chop.edu

© Springer Science+Business Media New York 2016   267
G. Ailawadi, I.L. Kron (eds.), *Catheter Based Valve and Aortic Surgery*,
DOI 10.1007/978-1-4939-3432-4_21

with repetition have resulted in consensus to delay operative reintervention as long as possible [1, 6–9]. The influence of these presuppositions is reflected in a number of observational studies that attempt to identify threshold values from imaging data that identify the point beyond which the RV is not recoverable [1–3, 6, 10–13]. TCPVR provides a less invasive alternative therapy with potential reductions in morbidity and mortality. Moreover, serial reinterventions with TCPVR have similar or reduced complexity and morbidity, while in operative valve replacement, repeat open-heart procedures become increasingly complex and hazardous. This challenges the prevailing calculations of risk and benefit of pulmonary valve replacement. However, at this time, there remains no consensus on timing of pulmonary valve replacement (PVR), and there is tremendous heterogeneity in practice for patients with congenital heart disease [14–16].

Brief History of TCPVR in CHD

TCPVR was first reported in 2000 by Bonhoeffer and colleagues in a lamb [17], quickly followed by a report of a successful procedure in a human patient with a dysfunctional RV to pulmonary artery (PA) conduit [1, 6, 18]. The Melody transpulmonary valve (TPV) (Medtronic Inc., Minneapolis, MN) is the only available device designed specifically for TCPVR (Fig. 21.1). A prospective nonrandomized study of the Melody TPV was completed in 2010 [2, 3, 11, 19], and in January 2010, the Melody TPV was approved for use in the United States under a Humanitarian Device Exemption (HDE) (http://www.accessdata.fda.gov/cdrh_docs/pdf8/H080002a.pdf). The SAPIEN transcatheter heart valve (Edwards Lifesciences LLC, Irvine, CA), first developed as a

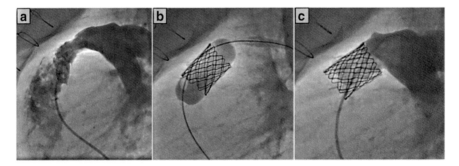

Fig. 21.1 Melody transcatheter pulmonary valve (TPV) implantation. (**a**) Lateral projection of a power injection angiogram through an antegrade pigtail catheter whose side holes are distal to the valve in a calcified homograft right ventricle to pulmonary artery conduit. There is significant narrowing of the homograft conduit and significant regurgitation of contrast. (**b**) Digital acquisition image of Melody TPV with balloon inflated in the same patient's homograft conduit. (**c**) Repeat power injection angiogram through antegrade pigtail catheter following deployment of the Melody TPV. Even with the pigtail bridging the transcatheter valve, there is no regurgitation of contrast across the valve

device for transcatheter aortic valve replacement, has since been used for transcatheter valve replacement in the pulmonary position but is currently only available in the United States as part of an investigational device exemption (IDE) trial.

Current Indications for TCPVR in CHD

The current indications for Melody TPV deployment under HDE are a circumferential RVOT conduit and either greater than moderate regurgitation or stenosis with peak-to-peak gradient ≥35 mmHg. The IDE stated that the narrowest portion of the conduit should be at least 16 mm in diameter at the time of TPV deployment. No upper limit to conduit size was included in the HDE, but the outer diameter of the deployed valve is 1.4 mm larger than the available delivery systems (18, 20, and 22 mm) limiting the use of the Melody TPV in larger conduits and in non-conduit dilated RVOTs. Successful deployment of the Melody TPV on 24 mm balloons or post-dilating with a 24mm balloon with no more than minimal insufficiency of the transcatheter valve has been reported [20]. The initial IDE established a lower weight limit of 30 kg [7–9, 19], but the valve has been subsequently implanted in smaller patients. A recent series reported the outcomes of TCPVR in 23 subjects under 30 kg with successful valve implantation in subjects as small as 13.8 kg [21]. Currently there are no explicit age or size limits.

The SAPIEN transcatheter heart valve is a balloon-expandable stent-mounted valve designed for implantation in the aortic position in adults with acquired calcific aortic stenosis. The range of diameters available includes 23, 26, and in some countries 29 mm, which make it potentially suitable for larger diameter conduits and native outflow tracts than the Melody TPV.

Technical Challenges

There are several technical challenges to TCPVR. The systems used to deliver the current transcatheter valves are large in diameter (22 French for the Melody TPV). Reports of major vascular complications have been infrequent, with 8 events in 618 cases (1.1 % with 95 % CI: 0.5–2.3 %) [22–29], but this may represent an issue for both smaller patients and those who undergo serial transcatheter interventions. Though typically femoral venous access has been used, the right internal jugular vein and subclavian vein have also been used [28] even in relatively small patients [21].

Second, a subset of individuals have one or more coronary arteries that are at risk of compression by a stent-mounted transcatheter valve. Compression of a coronary artery or arteries by conduit or RVOT stent is a catastrophic complication and has been reported in many large series [23, 26, 28, 30–32]. Two multi-institution series assessing the risk for coronary compression in transcatheter RVOT stent procedures have been published recently [30, 31] in which 5–6 % of referred subjects demonstrated coronary compression on test angioplasty of the RVOT. In both series, abnormal coronary artery anatomy was associated with a higher risk of coronary artery compression though in the smaller series this did not reach statistical significance. Pre-procedure cross-sectional imaging (either through CT or MRI) of the coronaries and conduit is useful, but measurement of the distance between conduit and coronary is insufficient. The displacement of the conduit during stent angioplasty is unpredictable. In the only series assessing this, pre-procedure imaging only identified 50 % of the patients at risk [31]. Static angiographic imaging of the coronary arteries (either through root angiography or selective coronary angiography) is insufficient for similar reasons. A method of reversibly testing whether the coronaries are at risk of compression is simultaneous coronary angiography and balloon angioplasty of the RVOT with a balloon of the same diameter and size as the planned transcatheter pulmonary valve delivery system [33] (Fig. 21.2). If there are concerns regarding the risk of conduit rupture, serial angiography and conduit angioplasty can be performed with increasing balloon diameters. No consensus exists regarding the specific method of angiography, with advocates existing for selective coronary angiography, root angiography, and even rotational angiography. However, it should be noted that there are reports of coronary compression that was initially missed because the proximal coronary was stented open by a selective coronary catheter [31].

Another relatively frequent major procedural adverse event is rupture of the RVOT conduit (Fig. 21.3). This is not unique to transcatheter pulmonary valve replacement and was initially reported in an earlier era during stent or balloon angioplasty of stenotic conduits [34]. Conduit rupture, some fraction of which have required open surgical intervention, is consistently reported in multiple large series [19, 22, 23, 26, 28, 32]. One recent multicenter series identified homograft conduits (vs. other materials) and more severe calcification as risk factors for

Fig. 21.2 Compression of a coronary artery during test inflation with simultaneous angiography. A selective hand injection angiogram through a Judkins left coronary artery catheter was performed while a 22 mm diameter balloon was inflated in a homograft RV to PA conduit. This left axial oblique projection demonstrates compression of the left anterior descending coronary artery (*yellow arrow*), due to displacement of accrued calcium, which can be seen between the inflated balloon and compressed coronary

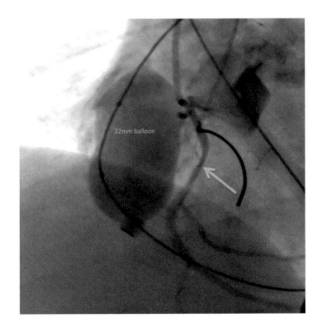

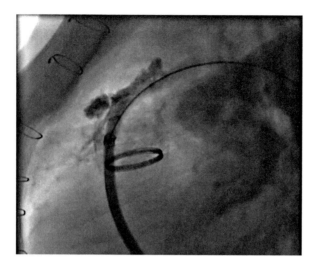

Fig. 21.3 Rupture of a right ventricle to pulmonary artery conduit. A hand injection of through an antegrade long sheath was performed following balloon angioplasty of a ringed Gore-Tex conduit. On the lateral projection of the angiogram, contrast can be seen layering on the greater curvature of the conduit along its irregular border. Contrast was contained and did not dissipate suggesting that the tear was contained within scar tissue

rupture, while balloon size and pressure were not significant risk factors [35]. Judicious pre-procedural planning and organization (including, where possible, immediate access to appropriately sized covered stents and sufficient vascular access, appropriately large sheaths, and wire position with which to deploy them) for possible conduit rupture is recommended. A potential nightmare scenario, which has yet to be described in the literature combines both of these concerns, where serial balloon angioplasty with coronary angiography is attempted and results in a conduit rupture with a balloon that is smaller than the planned trans-catheter valve system. This poses the risk of attempting to deploy the system without knowing if there is significant risk of coronary compression or discontinuing the procedure.

Short- and Medium-Term Outcomes

Case series of TVR with Melody TPV in RV to PA conduits from the United States and Europe have demonstrated >90 % technical success, procedural mortality <1 %, and infrequent adverse events in appropriately selected patients [10, 12, 13, 19, 22, 23, 27–29, 36, 37], with uniform reductions in RV systolic pressure, RVOT stenosis, and RVOT regurgitation [17, 22, 23, 28, 29, 38, 39], along with subsequent improvement in RV end-diastolic volume [39–41], diastolic function [42], and strain [42] after TCPVR. Short-term outcomes following TCPVR with SAPIEN transcatheter valve are similar to the Melody TPV [1–3, 6, 10–13, 43–45].

The effect of TCPVR with Melody TPV on exercise capacity (measured by maximal oxygen consumption) has been equivocal in studies, whether subjects with RVOT stenosis, regurgitation, or a combination of both were pooled [23, 38, 40, 46, 47] or divided into subgroups with predominant stenosis or predominant regurgitation [38–40, 47]. No trials have directly compared SVR to TCPVR for clinical or functional outcomes. A parallel case series of a single center's experience with TCPVR and SVR reported similar short-term results in both groups [48], demonstrating that, with some caveats, TCPVR has comparable safety and efficacy to operative valve replacement. Durability of the Melody TPV has been good in published case series, but few series have median follow-up greater than a year [22, 26, 29, 49]. Progressive stenosis is the more commonly cited cause of reintervention. In early series, this was most commonly due to stent fracture [19, 50], but implantation of a bare metal stent prior to TCPVR with the Melody transcatheter valve has reduced that risk [1, 6, 22, 23, 27, 50, 51]. Currently, freedom from reintervention is 92–95 % at 1 year and 86–87% at 2 years [1–3, 6, 11, 26, 51], with most reintervention able to be accomplished via catheter-based procedure. Pre-stenting is part of the standard deployment of the SAPIEN transcatheter valve, but to date no studies have specifically addressed the risk of progressive stenosis or stent fracture in this population.

Endocarditis has been identified as a potential adverse event [1, 6–9, 52–54], but it is not yet clear how the risk compares to that in surgical prosthetic valves. The only study to date that has compared the incidence of endocarditis following surgical and transcatheter pulmonary valve replacement demonstrated increased risk in the transcatheter group but was not able to account for confounding factors, and caution should be exercised in inferring from this data until larger multicenter studies can be performed [55].

Challenge of the Dilated Right Ventricular Outflow Tract

Returning to TCPVR for RVOT dysfunction, only a fraction of affected patients have an RV to PA conduit or bioprosthetic valve that is appropriately sized for TCPVR with current technology. There are reports the off-label use of both Melody and SAPIEN valves deployed in native outflow tracts [10, 12, 13, 19, 22–24, 27–29, 36, 37, 56–58], but even with pre-stenting, these are limited to RVOT that are the appropriate size to anchor the device, usually ≤24 mm. The dilated RVOT typical of transannular patch used in tetralogy of Fallot is simply too large in most cases for current devices, though there are case reports of TCPVR in larger diameter RVOT [17, 20, 22, 23, 28, 29, 38, 39]. In addition, it is often more compliant than a similar diameter conduit. We recommend testing the compliance of the RVOT by inflating a low pressure balloon with an appropriately large diameter to determine whether the RVOT will exert enough pressure hold stent-mounted valve. Deployment of

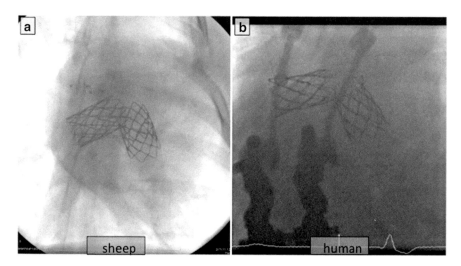

Fig. 21.4 Deployment of melody transcatheter pulmonary valve (TPV) in bilateral branch pulmonary arteries. Digital acquisition images after deployment of melody TPV in both branch pulmonary arteries of a sheep [59] (**a**) and human patient [25] (**b**). In the human patient, the right ventricular outflow tract was too large to accommodate a Melody TPV and was judged to be too medically frail for an operative pulmonary valve replacement

transcatheter valves in the branch pulmonary arteries is one solution, which has been reported in an animal model [39–41, 59] and subsequently in human patients [25, 42, 60] (Fig. 21.4). Deploying a nested series of stents from a branch PA back into the MPA to provide a stable position for TCPVR has also been used [42, 57, 58]. Thirdly, the Medtronic Native Outflow Tract device, a self-expanding transcatheter device, has been enrolling subjects at limited centers for an IDE trial since April 2013 [23, 38, 40, 46, 47, 61] (clinicaltrials.gov identifier: NCT01762124). Another approach aims to reduce the diameter of the RVOT with a transcatheter device, leaving a smaller diameter internal channel in which to deploy a transcatheter valve; these devices are currently in preclinical trials [38–40, 47, 62–65]. Despite these novel approaches, studies with CMR have demonstrated that postsurgical anatomy is highly variable [48, 66] and will likely represent a persistent technical and technological challenge.

Expanding Indications for TCPVR in the Pulmonary Position

Pulmonary valve TCPVR in patients with pulmonary hypertension [17, 47, 67] demonstrates the capacity of current valves to function under higher pressures. The off-label use of Melody valve for failed bioprosthetic valves in the pulmonary position has also been reported with good safety, efficacy, and short-term durability [1, 6, 18, 49,

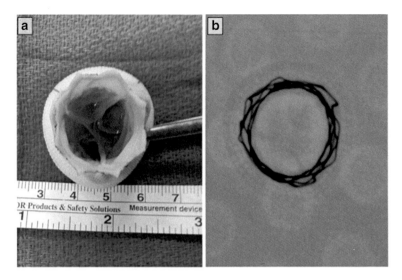

Fig. 21.5 Ex vivo implantation of a melody transcatheter pulmonary valve (TPV) in a biopros-thetic valve. Melody TPV deployed in a Carpentier-Edwards aortic porcine bioprosthesis in an en face view in a digital photograph (**a**) and under fluoroscopy (**b**). The fluoroscopic image demon-strates the good apposition of the covered stent, in which the TPV is sewn, and the bioprosthesis

68]. This is a logical extension of the current TCPVR approach and allows for valve deployment in orthotopic position seated in the failed surgical hardware, providing a stable, uniform substrate for seating the transcatheter valve (Figs. 21.5 and 21.6). The valve-in-valve TCPVR concept has been further expanded to include deployment in both tricuspid [2, 3, 11, 19, 69–75] and mitral [7–9, 19, 70, 76] positions.

Adapting Surgical Practice in the Face of TCPVR

TCPVR is less invasive than operative pulmonary valve replacement. This probably results in reduced mortality and almost certainly is accompanied by reduced mor-bidity, hospital stay, and recovery time. These differences are likely magnified in patients undergoing repeat procedures over time. How the development of TCPVR technologies should affect surgical and medical practice is a difficult question, but what is clear is that (1) chronic valvular dysfunction contributes to decrements in function and increased morbidity and mortality and (2) a minimally invasive approach alters the balance of risk and benefit (in at least some patients). This will exert pressure to intervene earlier on dysfunctional valves. While TCPVR technol-ogy evolves to address a broader range of indications and anatomic substrates, there may be an intermediate stage, during which adjustments in surgical technique for

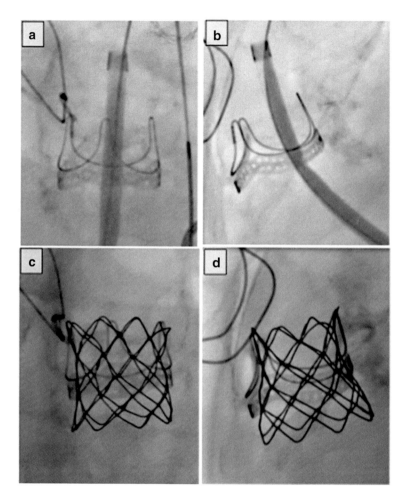

Fig. 21.6 Deployment of Melody transcatheter pulmonary valve (TPV) in a bioprosthetic valve. Digital acquisition images of Melody TPV in two different Carpentier-Edwards porcine bioprosthetic valves in situ are shown. Pre-image (**a** and **b**) and post-image (**c** and **d**) are shown. The TPV in both cases conforms to the waist created by the annulus of the bioprosthesis

procedures that have high or even certain risk of reintervention to facilitate future TCPVR may have real benefits. The goal for any such strategy would be to continue to provide competent valve function with the minimum risk and morbidity. At the same time, an added goal would be to consider a longer time horizon in considering postoperative outcome and try to minimize the number of operative procedures over the course of the patient's lifetime. This could be accomplished by providing an anatomic substrate for TCPVR during the initial operation.

The following strategies are possible initial steps in this process. The first would be to consider the possibility of TCPVR when selecting the size of bioprosthetic valves for SVR. We would advocate (within reason) maximizing the size of bioprosthetic valves to facilitate future (and multiple) valve-in-valve TCPVR, effectively delaying another surgical procedure. Valve replacement with larger diameter valves in younger patients has been shown to be associated with shorter time to reintervention [77–79]. However, reducing the number of open-heart procedures (even if replaced by multiple TCPVR procedures) could potentially reduce total mortality, morbidity, and economic cost, and if a slightly larger bioprosthetic valve allows for TCPVR, there may be a net benefit even if the original operative valve lasts a shorter time. Finally, for RVOT augmentation in tetralogy of Fallot, use of techniques that limit the size of RVOT (e.g., monocusp technique or partial annuloplasty) might increase the probability that TCPVR could be attempted as the patient's second procedure. Again, the chance to avoid a second open-heart operation may prove beneficial in spite of increased risk of residual RVOT obstruction. The common theme among these strategies is that they balance some potential risk of early reintervention or "imperfect hemodynamics" in the short term to facilitate future transcatheter intervention and also reduce long-term morbidity, mortality, and cost by replacing open-heart operation(s) with transcatheter procedure(s). All of these innovations would require cooperation between interventional cardiologists and surgeons, and we acknowledge that demonstrating the benefit of this type of approach is a challenge. It requires analysis that considers a broader range of ramifications (including cost and quality of life) of clinical decisions to a more distant time horizon than is the current standard. Both of these factors represent an obstacle to testing these ideas in a conventional clinical trial and alternative strategies such as clinical decision analysis may be necessary to determine whether these strategies provide benefit.

Disclosures

Dr. Gillespie is a consultant to Medtronic Inc., the manufacturer of the Melody valve.
Dr. O'Byrne has no conflicts to disclose.

Funding Sources

Dr. O'Byrne is supported by a grant from the National Institutes of Health (T32HL007915-15) and the ENTELLIGENCE Young Investigator Grant. Dr. Gillespie receives funding from the American Heart Association and National Institutes of Health.

References

1. Wessel HU, Paul MH. Exercise studies in tetralogy of Fallot: a review. Pediatr Cardiol. 1999;20(1):39–47. discussion 48.
2. Gatzoulis MA, Till JA, Somerville J, Redington AN. Congestive heart diseases: mechanoelectrical interaction in tetralogy of Fallot: QRS prolongation relates to right ventricular size and predicts malignant arrhythmias and sudden death. Circulation. 1995;92(2):231–7.
3. Gatzoulis MA, Balaji S, Webber SA, Siu SC, Hokanson JS, Poile C, et al. Risk factors for arrhythmia and sudden cardiac death late after repair of tetralogy of Fallot: a multicentre study. Lancet. 2000;356(9234):975–81.

4. Deanfield JE, McKenna WJ, Presbitero P, England D, Graham GR, Hallidie-Smith K. Ventricular arrhythmia in unrepaired and repaired tetralogy of Fallot. Relation to age, timing of repair, and haemodynamic status. Br Heart J. 1984;52(1):77–81.
5. Nollert G, Fischlein T, Bouterwek S, Böhmer C, Klinner W, Reichart B. Long-term survival in patients with repair of tetralogy of Fallot: 36-year follow-up of 490 survivors of the first year after surgical repair. J Am Coll Cardiol. 1997;30(5):1374–83.
6. Mulla N, Simpson P, Sullivan NM, Paridon SM. Determinants of aerobic capacity during exercise following complete repair of tetralogy of Fallot with a transannular patch. Pediatr Cardiol. 1997;18(5):350–6.
7. Geva T. Indications and timing of pulmonary valve replacement after tetralogy of Fallot repair. Semin Thorac Cardiovasc Surg Pediatr Card Surg Annu. 2006;9(1):11–22.
8. Mertens L. Timing of pulmonary valve replacement in post-operative tetralogy of Fallot patients in asymptomatic patients: Based on RV volumes only? Prog Pediatr Cardiol. 2012;34:35–7.
9. Tweddell JS, Simpson P, Li S-H, Dunham-Ingle J, Bartz PJ, Earing MG, et al. Timing and technique of pulmonary valve replacement in the patient with tetralogy of fallot. Semin Thorac Cardiovasc Surg Pediatr Card Surg Annu. 2012;15(1):27–33.
10. Oosterhof T, van Straten A, Vliegen HW, Meijboom FJ, van Dijk APJ, Spijkerboer AM, et al. Preoperative thresholds for pulmonary valve replacement in patients with corrected tetralogy of Fallot using cardiovascular magnetic resonance. Circulation. 2007;116(5):545–51.
11. Frigiola A, Redington AN, Cullen S, Vogel M. Pulmonary regurgitation is an important determinant of right ventricular contractile dysfunction in patients with surgically repaired tetralogy of Fallot. Circulation. 2004;110(11 Suppl 1):II153–7. doi:10.1161/01.CIR.0000138397.60956.c2.
12. Therrien J, Provost Y, Merchant N, Williams W, Colman J, Webb G. Optimal timing for pulmonary valve replacement in adults after tetralogy of Fallot repair. Am J Cardiol. 2005;95(6):779–82.
13. Therrien J, Siu SC, McLaughlin PR, Liu PP, Williams WG, Webb GD. Pulmonary valve replacement in adults late after repair of tetralogy of Fallot: are we operating too late? J Am Coll Cardiol. 2000;36(5):1670–5.
14. Cheung EW-Y, Wong WH-S, Cheung Y-F. Meta-analysis of pulmonary valve replacement after operative repair of tetralogy of fallot. Am J Cardiol. 2010;106(4):552–7.
15. Ferraz Cavalcanti PE, Sá MPBO, Santos CA, Esmeraldo IM, de Escobar RR, de Menezes AM, et al. Pulmonary valve replacement after operative repair of tetralogy of fallot: meta-analysis and meta-regression of 3,118 patients from 48 studies. J Am Coll Cardiol. 2013;62(23):2227–43.
16. O'Byrne ML, Glatz AC, Mercer-Rosa L, Gillespie MJ, Dori Y, Goldmuntz E, Kawut S, Rome JJ. Trends in pulmonary valve replacement in children and adults with tetralogy of Fallot. Am J Cardiol. 2014;115(1):118–24.
17. Bonhoeffer P, Boudjemline Y, Saliba Z, Hausse AO, Aggoun Y, Bonnet D, et al. Transcatheter implantation of a bovine valve in pulmonary position a lamb study. Circulation. 2000;102(7):813–6.
18. Bonhoeffer P, Boudjemline Y, Saliba Z, Merckx J, Aggoun Y, Bonnet D, et al. Percutaneous replacement of pulmonary valve in a right-ventricle to pulmonary-artery prosthetic conduit with valve dysfunction. Lancet. 2000;356(9239):1403–5.
19. Zahn EM, Hellenbrand WE, Lock JE, McElhinney DB. Implantation of the melody transcatheter pulmonary valve in patients with a dysfunctional right ventricular outflow tract conduit early results from the US Clinical trial. J Am Coll Cardiol. 2009;54(18):1722–9.
20. Cheatham SL, Holzer RJ, Chisolm JL, Cheatham JP. The Medtronic Melody® transcatheter pulmonary valve implanted at 24-mm diameter--it works. Catheter Cardiovasc Interv. 2013;82(5):816–23.
21. Berman DP, McElhinney DB, Vincent JA, Hellenbrand WE, Zahn EM. Feasibility and short-term outcomes of percutaneous transcatheter pulmonary valve replacement in small (<30 kg) children with dysfunctional right ventricular outflow tract conduits. Circ Cardiovasc Interv. 2014;7(2):142–8.
22. Butera G, Milanesi O, Spadoni I, Piazza L, Donti A, Ricci C, et al. Melody transcatheter pulmonary valve implantation. Results from the registry of the Italian society of pediatric cardiology. Catheter Cardiovasc Interv. 2013;81(2):310–6.

23. Eicken A, Ewert P, Hager A, Peters B, Fratz S, Kuehne T, et al. Percutaneous pulmonary valve implantation: two-centre experience with more than 100 patients. Eur Heart J. 2011;32(10): 1260–5.

24. Boshoff DE, Cools BLM, Heying R, Troost E, Kefer J, Budts W, et al. Off-label use of percutaneous pulmonary valved stents in the right ventricular outflow tract: time to rewrite the label? Catheter Cardiovasc Interv. 2013;81(6):987–95.

25. Gillespie MJ, Dori Y, Harris MA, Sathanandam S, Glatz AC, Rome JJ. Bilateral branch pulmonary artery melody valve implantation for treatment of complex right ventricular outflow tract dysfunction in a high-risk patient. Circ Cardiovasc Interv. 2011;4(4):e21–3.

26. Lurz P, Coats L, Khambadkone S, Nordmeyer J, Boudjemline Y, Schievano S, et al. Percutaneous pulmonary valve implantation: impact of evolving technology and learning curve on clinical outcome. Circulation. 2008;117(15):1964–72.

27. Martins JDF, Ewert P, Sousa L, Freitas I, Trigo C, Jalles N, et al. Percutaneous pulmonary valve implantation: initial experience. Rev Port Cardiol. 2010;29(12):1839–46.

28. McElhinney DB, Hellenbrand WE, Zahn EM, Jones TK, Cheatham JP, Lock JE, et al. Short- and medium-term outcomes after transcatheter pulmonary valve placement in the expanded multicenter US melody valve trial. Circulation. 2010;122(5):507–16.

29. Vezmar M, Chaturvedi R, Lee K-J, Almeida C, Manlhiot C, McCrindle BW, et al. Percutaneous pulmonary valve implantation in the young 2-year follow-up. JACC Cardiovasc Interv. 2010;3(4):439–48.

30. Morray BH, McElhinney DB, Cheatham JP, Zahn EM, Berman DP, Sullivan PM, et al. Risk of coronary artery compression among patients referred for transcatheter pulmonary valve implantation: a multicenter experience. Circ Cardiovasc Interv. 2013;6(5):535–42.

31. Fraisse A, Assaidi A, Mauri L, Malekzadeh-Milani S, Thambo J-B, Bonnet D, et al. Coronary artery compression during intention to treat right ventricle outflow with percutaneous pulmonary valve implantation: incidence, diagnosis, and outcome. Catheter Cardiovasc Interv. 2014;83(7):E260–8.

32. Kostolny M, Tsang V, Nordmeyer J, van Doorn C, Frigiola A, Khambadkone S, et al. Rescue surgery following percutaneous pulmonary valve implantation. Eur J Cardiothorac Surg. 2008;33(4):607–12.

33. Sridharan S, Coats L, Khambadkone S, Taylor AM, Bonhoeffer P. Images in cardiovascular medicine. Transcatheter right ventricular outflow tract intervention: the risk to the coronary circulation. Circulation. 2006;113(25):e934–5.

34. Peng LF, McElhinney DB, Nugent AW, Powell AJ, Marshall AC, Bacha EA, et al. Endovascular stenting of obstructed right ventricle-to-pulmonary artery conduits: a 15-year experience. Circulation. 2006;113(22):2598–605.

35. Boudjemline Y, Malekzadeh-Milani S, Patel M, Thambo J, Bonnet D, Iserin L, Fraisse A. Predictors and outcomes of right ventricular outflow tract conduit rupture during percutaneous pulmonary valve implantation: a multicentre study. EuroIntervention. 2014. doi:10.4244/EIJY14M09_06.

36. Demkow M, Biernacka EK, Śpiewak M, Kowalski M, Siudalska H, Wolski P, et al. Percutaneous pulmonary valve implantation preceded by routine prestenting with a bare metal stent. Cathet Cardiovasc Interv. 2011;77(3):381–9.

37. Khambadkone S, Coats L, Taylor A, Boudjemline Y, Derrick G, Tsang V, et al. Percutaneous pulmonary valve implantation in humans: results in 59 consecutive patients. Circulation. 2005;112(8):1189–97.

38. Coats L, Khambadkone S, Derrick G, Sridharan S, Schievano S, Mist B, et al. Physiological and clinical consequences of relief of right ventricular outflow tract obstruction late after repair of congenital heart defects. Circulation. 2006;113(17):2037–44.

39. Coats L, Khambadkone S, Derrick G, Hughes M, Jones R, Mist B, et al. Physiological consequences of percutaneous pulmonary valve implantation: the different behaviour of volume- and pressure-overloaded ventricles. Eur Heart J. 2007;28(15):1886–93.

40. Lurz P, Nordmeyer J, Giardini A, Khambadkone S, Muthurangu V, Schievano S, et al. Early versus late functional outcome after successful percutaneous pulmonary valve implantation:

are the acute effects of altered right ventricular loading all we can expect? J Am Coll Cardiol. 2011;57(6):724–31.

41. Romeih S, Kroft LJ, Bokenkamp R, Schalij MJ, Grotenhuis H, Hazekamp MG, et al. Delayed improvement of right ventricular diastolic function and regression of right ventricular mass after percutaneous pulmonary valve implantation in patients with congenital heart disease. Am Heart J. 2009;158(1):40–6.

42. Moiduddin N, Asoh K, Slorach C, Benson LN, Friedberg MK. Effect of transcatheter pulmonary valve implantation on short-term right ventricular function as determined by two-dimensional speckle tracking strain and strain rate imaging. Am J Cardiol. 2009;104(6):862–7.

43. Ewert P, Horlick E, Berger F. First implantation of the CE-marked transcatheter Sapien pulmonic valve in Europe. Clin Res Cardiol. 2011;100(1):85–7.

44. Boone RH, Webb JG, Horlick E, Benson L, Cao Q-L, Nadeem N, et al. Transcatheter pulmonary valve implantation using the edwards SAPIEN™ transcatheter heart valve. Cathet Cardiovasc Interv. 2010;75(2):286–94.

45. Kenny D, Hijazi ZM, Kar S, Rhodes J, Mullen M, Makkar R, et al. Percutaneous implantation of the Edwards SAPIEN transcatheter heart valve for conduit failure in the pulmonary position: early phase 1 results from an international multicenter clinical trial. J Am Coll Cardiol. 2011;58(21):2248–56.

46. Batra AS, McElhinney DB, Wang W, Zakheim R, Garofano RP, Daniels C, et al. Cardiopulmonary exercise function among patients undergoing transcatheter pulmonary valve implantation in the US Melody valve investigational trial. Am Heart J. 2012;163(2):280–7.

47. Lurz P, Nordmeyer J, Coats L, Taylor AM, Bonhoeffer P, Schulze-Neick I. Immediate clinical and haemodynamic benefits of restoration of pulmonary valvar competence in patients with pulmonary hypertension. Heart. 2009;95(8):646–50.

48. Frigiola A, Tsang V, Nordmeyer J, Lurz P, van Doorn C, Taylor AM, et al. Current approaches to pulmonary regurgitation. Eur J Cardiothorac Surg. 2008;34(3):576–81.

49. Gillespie MJ, Rome JJ, Levi DS, Williams RJ, Rhodes JF, Cheatham JP, et al. Melody valve implant within failed bioprosthetic valves in the pulmonary position a multicenter experience. Circ Cardiovasc Interv. 2012;5(6):862–70.

50. Nordmeyer J, Lurz P, Khambadkone S, Schievano S, Jones A, McElhinney DB, et al. Presenting with a bare metal stent before percutaneous pulmonary valve implantation: acute and 1-year outcomes. Heart. 2011;97(2):118–23.

51. McElhinney DB, Cheatham JP, Jones TK, Lock JE, Vincent JA, Zahn EM, et al. Stent fracture, valve dysfunction, and right ventricular outflow tract reintervention after transcatheter pulmonary valve implantation: patient-related and procedural risk factors in the US Melody Valve Trial. Circ Cardiovasc Interv. 2011;4(6):602–14.

52. McElhinney DB, Benson LN, Eicken A, Kreutzer J, Padera RF, Zahn EM. Infective endocarditis after transcatheter pulmonary valve replacement using the melody valve combined results of 3 prospective north american and european studies. Circ Cardiovasc Interv. 2013;6(3):292–300.

53. Bhat DP, Forbes TJ, Aggarwal S. A case of life-threatening staphylococcus aureus endocarditis involving percutaneous transcatheter prosthetic pulmonary valve. Congenit Heart Dis. 2013; 8(6):E161–4.

54. Patel M, Iserin L, Bonnet D, Boudjemline Y. Atypical malignant late infective endocarditis of Melody valve. J Thorac Cardiovasc Surg. 2012;143(4):e32–5.

55. Malekzadeh-Milani S, Ladouceur M, Iserin L, Bonnet D, Boudjemline Y. Incidence outcomes of right-sided endocarditis in patients with congenital heart disease after surgical or transcatheter pulmonary valve implantation. J Thorac Cardiovasc Surg. 2014;148(5):2253–9.

56. Momenah TS, El Oakley R, Najashi Al K, Khoshhal S, Qethamy Al H, Bonhoeffer P. Extended application of percutaneous pulmonary valve implantation. J Am Coll Cardiol. 2009;53(20): 1859–63.

57. Boudjemline Y, Legendre A, Ladouceur M, Boughenou M-F, Patel M, Bonnet D, et al. Branch pulmonary artery jailing with a bare metal stent to anchor a transcatheter pulmonary valve in patients with patched large right ventricular outflow tract. Circ Cardiovasc Interv. 2012;5(2):e22–5.

58. Boudjemline Y, Brugada G, Van-Aerschot I, Patel M, Basquin A, Bonnet C, et al. Outcomes and safety of transcatheter pulmonary valve replacement in patients with large patched right ventricular outflow tracts. Arch Cardiovasc Dis. 2012;105(8-9):404–13.

59. Robb JD, Harris MA, Minakawa M, Rodriguez E, Koomalsingh KJ, Shuto T, et al. Melody valve implantation into the branch pulmonary arteries for treatment of pulmonary insufficiency in an ovine model of right ventricular outflow tract dysfunction following tetralogy of Fallot repair. Circ Cardiovasc Interv. 2011;4(1):80–7.

60. Maschietto N, Milanesi O. A concert in the heart. Bilateral melody valve implantation in the branch pulmonary arteries. J Invasive Cardiol. 2013;25(4):E69–71.

61. Schievano S, Taylor AM, Capelli C, Coats L, Walker F, Lurz P, et al. First-in-man implantation of a novel percutaneous valve: a new approach to medical device development. EuroIntervention. 2010;5:745–50.

62. Amahzoune B, Szymansky C, Fabiani J-N, Zegdi R. A new endovascular size reducer for large pulmonary outflow tract. Eur J Cardiothorac Surg. 2010;37(3):730–2.

63. Mollet A, Basquin A, Stos B, Boudjemline Y. Off-pump replacement of the pulmonary valve in large right ventricular outflow tracts: a transcatheter approach using an intravascular infundibulum reducer. Pediatr Res. 2007;62(4):428–33.

64. Basquin A, Pineau E, Galmiche L, Bonnet D, Sidi D, Boudjemline Y. Transcatheter valve insertion in a model of enlarged right ventricular outflow tracts. J Thorac Cardiovasc Surg. 2010;139(1):198–208.

65. Boudjemline Y, Agnoletti G, Bonnet D, Sidi D, Bonhoeffer P. Percutaneous pulmonary valve replacement in a large right ventricular outflow tract: an experimental study. J Am Coll Cardiol. 2004;43(6):1082–7.

66. Schievano S, Coats L, Migliavacca F, Norman W, Frigiola A, Deanfield J, et al. Variations in right ventricular outflow tract morphology following repair of congenital heart disease: implications for percutaneous pulmonary valve implantation. J Cardiovasc Magn Reson. 2007;9(4):687–95.

67. Hasan BS, McElhinney DB, Brown DW, Cheatham JP, Vincent JA, Hellenbrand WE, et al. Short-term performance of the transcatheter melody valve in high-pressure hemodynamic environments in the pulmonary and systemic circulations. Circ Cardiovasc Interv. 2011;4(6):615–20.

68. Asoh K, Walsh M, Hickey E, Nagiub M, Chaturvedi R, Lee K-J, et al. Percutaneous pulmonary valve implantation within bioprosthetic valves. Eur Heart J. 2010;31(11):1404–9.

69. Bentham J, Qureshi S, Eicken A, Gibbs J, Ballard G, Thomson J. Early percutaneous valve failure within bioprosthetic tricuspid tissue valve replacements. Catheter Cardiovasc Interv. 2013;82(3):428–35.

70. Cullen MW, Cabalka AK, Alli OO, Pislaru SV, Sorajja P, Nkomo VT, et al. Transvenous, antegrade melody valve-in-valve implantation for bioprosthetic mitral and tricuspid valve dysfunction: a case series in children and adults. J Am Coll Cardiol Cardiovasc Interv. 2013;6(6):598–605.

71. Kenny D, Hijazi ZM, Walsh KP. Transcatheter tricuspid valve replacement with the Edwards SAPIEN valve. Catheter Cardiovasc Interv. 2011;78(2):267–70.

72. Petit CJ, Justino H, Ing FF. Melody valve implantation in the pulmonary and tricuspid position. Catheter Cardiovasc Interv. 2013;82(7):E944–6.

73. Riede FT, Dähnert I. Implantation of a Melody valve in tricuspid position. Catheter Cardiovasc Interv. 2012;80(3):474–6.

74. Roberts PA, Boudjemline Y, Cheatham JP, Eicken A, Ewert P, McElhinney DB, et al. Percutaneous tricuspid valve replacement in congenital and acquired heart disease. J Am Coll Cardiol. 2011;58(2):117–22.

75. Eicken A, Fratz S, Hager A, Vogt M, Balling G, Hess J. Transcutaneous melody valve implantation in "tricuspid position" after a Fontan Björk (RA-RV homograft) operation results in biventricular circulation. Int J Cardiol. 2010;142(3):e45–7.

76. Michelena HI, Alli O, Cabalka AK, Rihal CS. Successful percutaneous transvenous antegrade mitral valve-in-valve implantation. Cathet Cardiovasc Interv. 2012;81(5):E219–24.

77. Chen PC, Sager MS, Zurakowski D, Pigula FA, Baird CW, Mayer JE, Del Nido PJ, Emani SM. Younger age and valve oversizing are predictors of structural valve deterioration after

pulmonary valve replacement in patients with tetralogy of Fallot. J Thorac Cardiovasc Surg. 2012;143(2):352–60.

78. Batlivala SP, Emani S, Mayer JE, McElhinney DB. Pulmonary Valve Replacement Function in Adolescents: A Comparison of Bioprosthetic Valves and Homograft Conduits. Annals of Thoracic Surgery. 2012;93(6):2007–16.

79. Tweddell JS, Pelech AN, Frommely PC, Mussatto KA, Wyman JD, Fedderly RT, Berger S, Frommelt MA, Lewis DA, Friedberg DZ, Thomas JP, Sachdeva R, Litwin SB. Factors affecting longevity of homograft valves used in right ventricular outflow tract reconstruction for congenital heart disease. Circulation. 2000;102:Iii130–5. doi:10.1161/01.CIR.102.suppl_3.III-130.

Chapter 22
Transventricular Approaches to Pulmonary Valve Replacement

Joseph W. Turek and Abhay A. Divekar

Background

It is estimated that between one and two million people in the United States carry a diagnosis of congenital heart disease (CHD) [1]. Decades of advances in medical, interventional, and surgical cardiac care have resulted in an increasing proportion of these patients surviving to adulthood (95 % of those with noncritical CHD and 69 % of those with critical CHD) [2]. Pulmonary valve insufficiency, with or without stenosis, typified by repaired tetralogy of Fallot, remains the most common indication for cardiac reintervention. At the same time, multiple studies have convincingly shown the deleterious effects of chronic volume load from pulmonary insufficiency on right and left ventricular function and adverse clinical outcomes [3–5]. More recent studies continue to define the optimal timing and indications for pulmonary valve replacement [6, 7]. With over 100,000 Americans currently surviving with repaired tetralogy of Fallot and ever-lowering thresholds for pulmonary valve replacement, interventions on the right ventricular outflow tract will continue to drive the practice of reoperative congenital cardiac care well into the future.

Without question, the gold standard for pulmonary valve replacement remains the open surgical approach. Operative replacement of the pulmonary valve can be done with low morbidity and mortality, despite the vast majority of these cases occurring in the reoperative setting [8, 9]. Additionally, an open operation enables

J.W. Turek, MD, PhD (✉)
Division of Pediatric Cardiac Surgery, University of Iowa Children's Hospital,
200 Hawkins Dr, Iowa City, IA 52242, USA
e-mail: joseph-turek@uiowa.edu

A.A. Divekar, MBBS, MD
Division of Pediatric Cardiology, University of Iowa Children's Hospital,
200 Hawkins Dr, Iowa City, IA 52242, USA
e-mail: abhay-divekar@uiowa.edu

© Springer Science+Business Media New York 2016
G. Ailawadi, I.L. Kron (eds.), *Catheter Based Valve and Aortic Surgery*,
DOI 10.1007/978-1-4939-3432-4_22

adequate upsizing of the valve to match patient size by allowing for patch augmentation of the right ventricular outflow tract. Concomitant proximal branch pulmonary artery stenosis repair and correction of residual intracardiac defects can be simultaneously performed. Furthermore, the ability to choose the site of valve placement at the discretion of the surgeon allows one to attain an unobstructed right ventricular outflow and avoid compression of the coronaries, one of the limitations of transcatheter intervention. Nonetheless, surgical replacement does require cardiopulmonary bypass, risks of sternal reentry, and, in cases with small intracardiac shunts, the need for fibrillatory or cardioplegic cardiac arrest. Hospitalization, recovery time, and return to work are also more protracted for operative pulmonary valve replacement. These factors, in addition to the constant hazard of bioprosthetic valve deterioration over time, lack growth potential, and the need for multiple procedures during the patient's lifetime weighs in heavily on the timing for initial and subsequent referral for pulmonary valve replacement.

Transcatheter techniques for relief of right ventricular outflow tract obstruction with balloon angioplasty and/or balloon-expandable bare-metal stent implantation are well described. In 2000, a landmark event, namely, transcatheter implantation of a bovine jugular valve mounted on a stent for a failed surgically implanted right ventricle to pulmonary artery conduit, changed the landscape of transcatheter intervention and pulmonary valve replacement [10]. Since then, the field has grown rapidly with the Melody® transcatheter pulmonary valve first introduced in the American market in July 2007 with humanitarian use device designation and attained humanitarian device exemption approval in January 2010. In February of 2015, the Melody® valve received pre-market approval from the US Food and Drug Administration based on strong evidence from three clinical studies demonstrating the valve's effectiveness in delaying open-heart reoperation [11–13]. Now, however, the most important milestone that needs to be achieved is the ability to translate minimally invasive pulmonary valve replacement to all patients with an incompetent pulmonary valve when indicated. This includes not only patients with a surgically implanted valve or right ventricle to pulmonary artery conduit but also those who have a native right ventricular outflow tract with an incompetent pulmonary valve.

As with any new technology with growing experience, a number of challenges have come to attention. Some of the major limitations to current transcatheter pulmonary valve replacement are limited patient and vessel size, large native outflow tracts, lack of suitable venous access, hemodynamic instability secondary to stiff wires and the delivery system, and tortuosity of the venous pathway from the access site to the right ventricular outflow tract precluding manipulation of the delivery system. Further, when the procedure is complicated by device malpositioning and cannot be retrieved by transcatheter techniques, alternate strategies are necessary. Finally, newer prototypes, especially for the large outflow tracts, will require even larger delivery systems. Most animal models used to develop these new prototypes show significant hemodynamic instability using standard transcatheter techniques in addition to the limitations mentioned above.

The natural evolution of improving surgical and transcatheter techniques is for surgical approaches to become more minimally invasive and transcatheter approaches to become bolder and more complex. Yet both interventional and surgical approaches have inherent limitations. The ability to combine these two skills with a team approach helps to minimize the limitations of each approach and maximize the patient benefit and has been described as the hybrid approach. As accurately described by del Nido et al., the hybrid procedure and a minimally invasive procedure are not the same [14]. A hybrid procedure is a true collaborative effort with extensive use of fluoroscopy, echocardiographic imaging, and working on a beating heart. The success of such collaborative efforts has already been demonstrated in other procedures such as closure of muscular ventricular septal defects, the hybrid Norwood procedure, and transcatheter aortic valve replacement.

This chapter will review the indications for a hybrid approach to pulmonary valve replacement and detail the surgical and interventional considerations, including preplanning, equipment, technique, and potential pitfalls.

Indications

The indications for pulmonary valve replacement by any method (surgical, transcatheter, or hybrid) are similar to traditional criteria as put forth by Geva et al. [7]. The common indications for considering a hybrid approach for pulmonary valve replacement include:

1. Patient or vascular size not suitable to accommodate the large delivery system. Typically patients <30 kg should prompt consideration for alternate approaches; although this is decided on a case by case basis, as some younger patients can accommodate the delivery system [15].
2. Tortuosity of the venous pathway that is negotiated by the delivery system. This is typically discovered during the actual procedure, although there are increasing attempts to define this patient population during the diagnostic portion of the procedure by measurements such as the angle between the tricuspid and pulmonary annulus [16].
3. Lack of venous access due to chronic occlusion of vessels.
4. Hemodynamic instability related to manipulation of stiff wires and/or larger delivery systems that preclude positioning of the valve for deployment. Again, this is determined during attempted transcatheter intervention.
5. Bailout option during an unsuccessful transcatheter attempt, such as when the valve is deployed in an undesirable position and cannot be percutaneously retrieved [17, 18].
6. Need for creation of a landing zone in a larger native or surgically reconstructed right ventricular outflow tract [19].
7. Patient who is deemed to be a high-risk surgical candidate due to comorbidities such as decompensated heart failure, dense adhesions, chest wall, or musculoskeletal deformities.
8. Need for novel delivery technique such as the flower-blossom technique—the valve is mounted on two balloons and then deployed over two guidewires placed in the right and the left pulmonary arteries [20].

With increasing experience, these indications are subject to changes and additions. In this context, there are a large number of prototypes being developed for large-sized balloon or self-expanding pulmonary valves, especially for the native outflow tract. As these devices are being developed, the delivery systems, at least initially, will tend to be quite large. Both for animal studies as well as initial human studies, there will be a growing need for the hybrid approach. Several authors have already commented on the fact that animals tend to poorly tolerate stiff interventional wires and a large delivery system across the tricuspid and pulmonary valve [21]. The perventricular hybrid approach has shown to be quite useful in this situation. Similarly, novel prototypes such as the injectable pulmonary valve have already been shown to successfully utilize the hybrid approach [22, 23].

Approach

Surgical

The operative component of transventricular pulmonary valve replacement requires a heightened level of concern regarding sternal reentry. After all, outside of the patient that is believed to be too sick to tolerate an open operation, a prohibitively high-risk sternal reentry remains the most likely indication for opting for an alternate approach to pulmonary valve replacement. As such, preoperative imaging using a limited chest computed tomography (CT) scan or magnetic resonance imaging (MRI) study, as used in many congenital reoperative cases to look at the proximity of the right ventricle to the posterior sternal plate, is recommended. These studies also provide valuable insight into anatomical considerations for device deployment through the right ventricular free wall. Specifically, the alignment of the right ventricular free wall with the right-sided outflow tract can be ascertained. Furthermore, the presence of coronary arteries crossing the right ventricle may alter the right ventricular entry site. Lower extremity duplex imaging is preferred if there exists any suspicion of groin vessel occlusion, in case emergent bypass is needed during reentry. In patients greater than 40 years of age, or those with significant risk factors for coronary artery disease, coronary angiography is indicated to rule out the need for concomitant bypass grafting.

The interdisciplinary participation of cardiac surgeons and interventional cardiologists in these procedures necessitates a full array of equipment and resources from each discipline. Consequently, these procedures are best performed in the hybrid operating room setting. While cardiopulmonary bypass is not a standard component of the perventricular approach, it may be indicated in an emergent situation. In these cases, arrangements should be made for cardiopulmonary bypass backup. It remains of utmost importance to preoperatively determine suitability for cardiopulmonary bypass as many of these patients carry prohibitive risks for such invasive maneuvers. Wishes of the family and patient must be well-delineated prior to embarking on an interventional plan.

Typically, the right ventricular free wall is accessed through a subxiphoid incision (Fig. 22.1). This can usually be managed quite well even in the multi-reoperative

Fig. 22.1 Subxiphoid access in the reoperative setting for transventricular pulmonary valve replacement

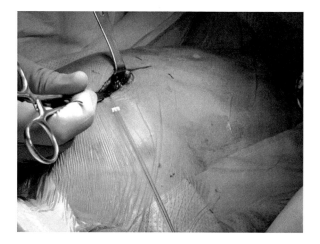

environment. In fact, most cardiac surgeons performing reoperative cases through a full sternotomy initially perform an extensive dissection in the subxiphoid region prior to proceeding superiorly under the sternum. The plane between the acute margin of the heart and the diaphragmatic pericardium is often devoid of significant adhesions and allows an access point wherein damage to the heart is minimized. Dissection is then continued under the right hemi-sternum to expose the right ventricular free wall. In some cases, a full median sternotomy may be required to appropriately access the right ventricle. Dense adhesions or anatomic variants where the right ventricular outflow tract does not align with the right ventricular free wall (i.e., dextrocardia) may necessitate full mobilization of the heart to optimize sheath alignment. The precise site for right ventricular access can be localized by palpation with simultaneous triangulation using echocardiography.

Bleeding around the sheath constitutes the most common pitfall from the surgical approach. To minimize this complication, a double-pledgeted purse-string suture can be used. Importantly, the purse-string diameter should be large, as manipulation of the cannula will widen the ventriculotomy throughout the procedure. Additionally, the anticipated access site on the right ventricle may need to be altered by crossing coronary branches that are not always evident despite preoperative imaging. Finally, a severe pectus excavatum or chest wall deformity may preclude the subxiphoid approach.

Interventional

The hybrid procedure does not allow one to sidestep the standard planning for interventional procedures (Fig. 22.2). This includes detailed evaluation of the anatomy, the most recent echocardiogram, advanced imaging studies (CT or MRI), and surgical notes. Different from the usual practice, the preplanning ritual needs to include the surgical team, the cardiac anesthesiologist, as well as the imaging cardiologist. If the hybrid procedure suite is not the usual cardiac catheterization laboratory,

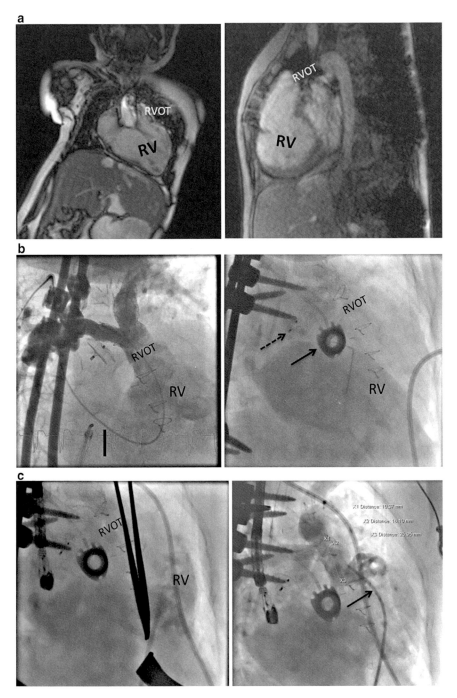

Fig. 22.2 Pre-procedure planning for hybrid procedure in a patient with multiple comorbidities including severe kyphoscoliosis, chronic respiratory failure, multiple previous operations, and transcatheter interventions, presenting with right heart failure. The patient had bilateral femoral

d

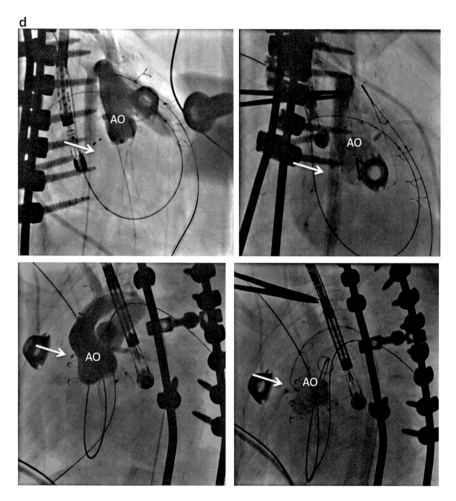

Fig. 22.2 (continued) venous occlusion and a left SVC to the coronary sinus; thus, only the right SVC was available for access. The planned intervention was double-balloon flower-blossom technique for Melody valve implantation. Importantly, all the routine steps as performed during transcatheter placement need to be followed. (**a**) Frontal and lateral MRI images showing the massively enlarged right ventricle and the site for potential perventricular puncture (surgical access site). (**b**) Previous angiography in RAO projection and similar fluoroscopic view on the day of the procedure further help to plan surgical access site. Solid arrow points to infusa-port and dashed arrow points to an atrial septal defect occluder device. (**c**) Fluoroscopic images show the introducer placed from the surface of the right ventricle and the alignment of the introducer with the right ventricular outflow tract. An angiogram is performed through the right ventricle introducer. (**d**) To test for coronary compression prior to placing the larger introducer in the right ventricle, the double-balloon technique was used. The first balloon angioplasty catheter was placed from the right internal jugular vein and centered across the right pulmonary artery stent, and the other was centered across the left pulmonary artery stent via the ventricular introducer (8Fr introducer). RAO and LAO views showing compression of the right coronary artery with the balloons inflated, and the patent right coronary artery without the balloons inflated

pre-procedural planning also requires detailed assessment of the interventional tools that will be necessary, including guidewires, introducers, catheters, bare-metal stents, etc. The right ventricular outflow tract should be well defined in order to help determine the optimal site for surgical access. It is important to maximize the real estate available for unsheathing of the balloon-expandable pulmonary valve and the trajectory necessary for proper alignment of the delivery system to the right ventricular outflow tract. This will require evaluation of prior advanced imaging studies or angiograms. If none of these are available, a pre-procedural right ventricular angiogram to create a road map is a must prior to preparing the surgical site. As mentioned before, complete documentation of occluded vessels is critical, especially if these become necessary for bailout cardiopulmonary support. Finally, space mapping should be done to maximize the space around the table with all of the potential equipment needs in an environment different than the standard catheterization laboratory or operating room.

Standard cardiac catheterization techniques are routinely utilized; however, a number of factors need to be remembered. The interventionist is routinely accustomed to working with long catheters and guidewires, with a significant length of these within the patient. The typical introducer, when well seated, resides almost entirely within the vessel. The muscle memory that is developed during standard catheterization needs to be modified. For example, with the perventricular approach, most of the introducers are outside the patient and on the field. The support provided by the long wires and introducers is no longer available, and the beating heart creates high potential for the introducer to move out and cause significant bleeding if careful attention is not given to the access site. The real estate available for manipulation of the delivery systems is similarly different. All these minor, yet important, factors need to be newly learnt and constitute the learning curve. Very frequently, the hybrid suite has only a single plane system, and even when a biplane system is available, the ability for angulation can be limited by the setup.

Femoral arterial and, if necessary, venous access is obtained to perform hemodynamic assessment as well as to perform aortic root or coronary artery angiography when testing for coronary compression. Once the optimal surgical site is chosen, the patient is heparinized and the surgical team places a standard side arm introducer/ sheath. The interventionist then performs hemodynamic assessment. A right ventricular angiogram is performed to serve as a road map. A standard balloon-tipped end-hole catheter is advanced into the right or left pulmonary artery. The existing introducer is then upsized to the necessary dimensions after sequentially dilating the access site. Careful attention is directed frequently to the access site to avoid inadvertent dislodgement of the introducer by the beating heart. Next, the right ventricular outflow tract is prepared with balloon angioplasty as needed, coronary artery compression is ruled out, and if necessary the right ventricular outflow tract is balloon sized. A balloon-expandable bare-metal stent is then placed in the right ventricular outflow tract, taking care to avoid the contractile portion. Finally, the balloon-expandable pulmonary valve is deployed in the usual fashion, taking care to avoid jailing of the branch pulmonary arteries. This is especially important in smaller children where the length of the outflow can be quite short. After valve deployment, standard hemodynamic assessment and angiography are performed. At the discretion of the hybrid team, intracardiac or transesophageal echocardiography is performed. At this point, the surgical team once again takes over and controls the access site and completes the surgical aspects of wound closure and placement of a drain.

At the present time, standard catheterization and interventional tools are utilized for these procedures. As mentioned above, if the hybrid suite is not the usual cardiac catheterization laboratory, then preplanning requires careful attention to the availability of usual supplies. We have found that an additional team member should be readily available to serve as a runner in the event additional supplies are necessary. Optimal position of standard operating room equipment should be determined. Once the ideal setup is identified, it is useful to write down the setup and photo document for future use. Innovative solutions for equipment limitations such as modification of introducers and catheters as well as the balloon-expandable valve may be necessary.

The major technical challenges are described above but are worth reiterating. Especially when starting a new hybrid program, remember that none of the team members have worked together in unison before. There are inevitable "cultural clashes" for how things are done and the role of each team member. Pre-procedural planning and closed-loop communication is critical to the success of the program. Careful preplanning will help minimize the "unknown." In fact, for the first few times, the entire team should discuss each step of the procedure in sequence. It is also worthwhile to record the events for the early procedures and document aspects that went well and opportunities for improvement. A post-procedural debriefing is a good idea. All the usual assessments, including that for coronary compression, must be performed. A willingness to modify standard catheterization and interventional tools is a must. The beating heart creates a unique situation in terms of the introducer. Although the surgical team is quite familiar with this environment, the interventional team manipulating the introducer needs to be fully cognizant of the tendency of the beating heart to milk out the introducer/sheath, which can result in significant bleeding. The access site should be carefully chosen since it can significantly alter the ease with which the procedure can be performed. If a full sternotomy is performed, it can affect the adequacy of coronary evaluation, and hence careful attention and a high index of suspicion should be maintained for potential coronary compression when the chest is closed.

Although there are several advantages to the hybrid approach, the intermediate and long-term outcomes still need to be studied and monitored. For example, the relatively large introducers placed via the right ventricle may serve as an arrhythmia substrate. Also, since patient size is no longer a limitation, the outcome of this particular patient population will need to be studied before routinely proceeding with hybrid pulmonary valve replacement. It should be remembered that it is still unknown whether earlier pulmonary valve replacement translates to long-term improvement in outcomes.

There are several attributes of a successful hybrid pulmonary valve replacement program. As described above, a hybrid procedure is a collaborative effort between the surgical and interventional teams. Complete trust, a good working relationship, and collaboration throughout all aspects of the procedure from pre-procedural planning to post-procedural debriefing are the key toward good outcomes. It should be remembered that the collaboration is between all the members of the surgical and interventional team, and not only the physicians. Ideally, a hybrid cardiac catheterization suite is available for performing such procedures. Finally, when new procedures are introduced, it is worthwhile to have discussions with other teams that have successfully performed the procedure and will help avoid relearning the lessons that the other team has already learned. Other team members that should be involved with the planning include the cardiac anesthesiologist as well as the imaging cardiologist. A close, working relationship with the device manufacturer will also be beneficial because most of the field specialists have extensive experience and have often observed multiple procedures at multiple institutions.

Summary

The role of pulmonary valve replacement for the insufficient and/or obstructed pulmonary valve has been established. The population of patient that will benefit from a competent pulmonary valve is constantly changing and growing. The accumulating evidence suggests that although the optimal timing of pulmonary valve replacement is not yet defined, there is a point at which the recovery of right heart function may no longer be possible. In the next years, we will be able to more clearly define this optimal timing. In the modern era, we now have two primary approaches to pulmonary valve replacement: open surgical replacement and percutaneous transcatheter valve replacement. We have now embarked on a new era of hybrid pulmonary valve replacement which represents the epitome of surgical and interventional teamwork to maximize the advantages of each approach, minimize the limitations, and ultimately optimize patient care. Not only is the hybrid approach immediately applicable to patient care but also likely represents the approach for developing new prototypes in animal models and in patients with large native outflow tracts requiring sizable delivery systems. Advances in both valve design and delivery systems will be crucial to the successful delivery of pulmonary valve replacement technology to all patients who need it.

References

1. Hoffman JI, Kaplan S, Liberthson RR. Prevalence of congenital heart disease. Am Heart J. 2004;147:425–39.
2. Oster ME, Lee KA, Honein MA, et al. Temporal trends in survival among infants with critical congenital heart defects. Pediatrics. 2013;131:e1502–1508.
3. Shimazaki Y, Blackstone EH, Kirklin JW. The natural history of isolated congenital pulmonary valve incompetence: surgical implications. Thorac Cardiovasc Surg. 1984;32:257–9.
4. Therrien J, Provost Y, Merchant N, et al. Optimal timing for pulmonary valve replacement in adults after tetralogy of Fallot repair. Am J Cardiol. 2005;95:779–82.

5. Geva T. Indications and timing of pulmonary valve replacement after tetralogy of Fallot repair. Semin Thorac Cardiovasc Surg Pediatr Card Surg Annu. 2006;9:11–22.
6. Lee C, Kim YM, Lee C, et al. Outcomes of pulmonary valve replacement in 170 patients with chronic pulmonary regurgitation after relief of right ventricular outflow tract obstruction: implications for optimal timing of pulmonary valve replacement. J Am Coll Cardiol. 2012;60:1005–14.
7. Geva T. Indications for pulmonary valve replacement in repaired tetralogy of Fallot: The quest continues. Circulation. 2013;128:1855–7.
8. Chen XJ, Smith PB, Jaggers J, et al. Bioprosthetic pulmonary valve replacement: contemporary analysis of a large, single-center series of 170 cases. J Thorac Cardiovasc Surg. 2013;146:1461–6.
9. Jacobs JP, Mavroudis C, Quintessenza JA, et al. Reoperations for pediatric and congenital heart disease: an analysis of the Society of Thoracic Surgeons (STS) congenital heart surgery database. Semin Thorac Cardiovasc Surg Pedriatr Card Surg Annu. 2014;17:2–8.
10. Bonhoeffer P, Boudjemline Y, Saliba Z, et al. Percutaneous replacement of pulmonary valve in a right-ventricle to pulmonary-artery prosthetic conduit with valve dysfunction. Lancet. 2000; 356:1402–5.
11. Cheatham JP, Hellenbrand WE, Zahn EM, et al. Clinical and hemodynamic outcomes up to 7 years after transcatheter pulmonary valve replacement in the US Melody valve investigational. Circulation. 2015;131(22):1960–70.
12. Zahn EM, Hellenbrand WE, Lock JE, et al. Implantation of the melody transcatheter pulmonary valve in patients with a dysfunctional right ventricular outflow tract conduit: early results from the U.S. clinical trial. J Am Coll Cardiol. 2009;54:1722–9.
13. McElhinney DB, Hellenbrand WE, Zahn EM, et al. Short- and medium-term outcomes after transcatheter pulmonary valve placement in the expanded multicenter U.S. melody valve trial. Circulation. 2010;122:507–16.
14. Bacha EA, Marshall AC, McElhinney DB, et al. Expanding the hybrid concept in congenital heart surgery. Semin Thorac Cardiovasc Surg Pediatr Card Surg Annu. 2007;10:146–150.
15. Berman DP, McElhinney DB, Vincent JA, et al. Feasibility and short-term outcomes of percutaneous transcatheter pulmonary valve replacement in small (<30 kg) children with dysfunctional right ventricular outflow tract conduits. Circ Cardiovasc Interv. 2014;7:142–8.
16. Simpson KE, Huddleston CB, Foerster S, et al. Successful subxiphoid hybrid approach for placement of a melody percutaneous pulmonary valve. Catheter Cardiovasc Interv. 2011;78:108–11.
17. Cubeddu RJ, Hijazi ZM. Bailout perventricular pulmonary valve implantation following failed percutaneous attempt using the Edwards Sapien transcatheter heart valve. Catheter Cardiovasc Interv. 2011;77:276–80.
18. Berman DP, Burke R, Zahn EM. Use of a novel hybrid approach to salvage an attempted transcatheter pulmonary valve implant. Pediatr Cardiol. 2012;33:839–42.
19. Travelli FC, Herrington CS, Ing FF. A novel hybrid technique for transcatheter pulmonary valve implantation within a dilated native right ventricular outflow tract. J Thorac Cardiovasc Surg. 2014;148:e145–146.
20. Wilhelm C, Swinning J, Sisk M, et al. Melody valve implantation using a double-balloon "flower-blossom" technique. Congenital Cardiology Today. 2014;12(8).
21. Zhang B, Chen X, Xu TY, et al. Transcatheter pulmonary valve replacement by hybrid approach using a novel polymeric prosthetic heart valve: proof of concept in sheep. PLoS One. 2014;13:9.
22. Marianeschi SM, Santoro F, Ribera E, et al. Pulmonary valve implantation with the new Shelhigh Injectable Stented Pulmonic Valve. Ann Thorac Surg. 2008;86:1466–71.
23. Berdat PA, Carrel T. Off-pump pulmonary valve replacement with the new Shelhigh Injectable Stented Pulmonic Valve. J Thorac Cardiovasc Surg. 2006;131:1192–3.

Chapter 23
Anatomic Considerations for Tricuspid Valve Interventions

Emily Downs and Gorav Ailawadi

Introduction

The tricuspid valve is one of the most challenging valves to address due to high mortality with surgical treatment. Thus, percutaneous approaches may be appealing. However, the tricuspid valve lacks commercially available options for transcatheter approaches. Available transcatheter valves have been successfully used for valve-in-valve tricuspid applications, and several potential repair and replacement techniques are being developed. Tricuspid pathologies often accompany and follow the progression of left-sided lesions, and open surgical techniques have likewise followed the developments in mitral valve surgery. In reality, the tricuspid valve is anatomically and physiologically unique and careful attention to the specific characteristics of this valve is imperative to the safe development of catheter-based tricuspid therapies.

Overview of Tricuspid Valve Anatomy

The tricuspid valve serves as the atrioventricular valve of the right heart. It exists in a relatively low-pressure system, and its function and pathology are similar to that of the mitral valve but with several unique features.

E. Downs, MD • G. Ailawadi, MD (✉)
Section of Adult Cardiac Surgery, Department of Surgery, University of Virginia,
PO Box 800679, Charlottesville, VA 22908, USA
e-mail: ead6m@virginia.edu

© Springer Science+Business Media New York 2016
G. Ailawadi, I.L. Kron (eds.), *Catheter Based Valve and Aortic Surgery*,
DOI 10.1007/978-1-4939-3432-4_23

Annulus

The annulus of the tricuspid valve is relatively indistinct compared to what is observed in the other cardiac valves. It is in continuity with the right atrium, right ventricle, interventricular septum, and leaflets at different points along the circumference of the valve. The annulus is not planar in shape, and in fact its geometry varies with the cardiac cycle due to dynamic movements of the neighboring structures. The antero-septal and posteroseptal commissures are located toward the apex, while the annulus along the anterior leaflet adjacent to the aortic valve is oriented higher (more atrial), following the right ventricular outflow tract. During diastole the overall shape of the annulus is essentially circular, and during systole the valve shape becomes oval due to the bulging of the septum toward the right ventricle and the contraction of the right ventricle free wall. This dynamic activity of the annulus during the cardiac cycle is integral to proper closure of the leaflets, and annular dilation results in and increasingly planar, circular shape of the valve with leaflet tethering and improper valve closure [1, 2]. The geometry and physiology of the annulus must be considered when planning tricuspid procedures to ensure the desired effect is achieved.

Leaflets

The tricuspid valve, as its name implies, includes three distinct leaflets: anterior, posterior, and septal, with smaller commissural leaflets. The leaflets of the tricuspid valve are rather thin and delicate, especially when compared to the left-sided atrioventricular valve (mitral). The anterior leaflet is the largest and is semicircular in shape. Its broad coaptation surface provides adequate valve closure in the face of changing right ventricular filling volume. The posterior leaflet is of intermediate size with 2–3 scallop subdivisions. The septal leaflet is smaller than the posterior leaflet and its excursion is more limited than the anterior and posterior leaflets at baseline.

Papillary Muscles and Chordae Tendineae

The subvalvular apparatus is comprised of three groups of papillary muscles (anterior, posterior, and septal) and chordae tendineae extending from the papillary muscles to the leaflets. The anterior papillary muscle is found near the apex and is usually dominant in the group. The posterior group is composed on one or two muscle heads and implants on the posterior ventricular wall, while the septal group includes several small muscles on the septum. The papillary muscles contract during systole to prevent leaflet prolapse, and relaxation in diastole aids in active opening of the valve. The chordae are attached at three levels along the leaflets' length: the free margin (primary), ventricular side at mid-leaflet (secondary), and at the base (basal or tertiary). The primary chordae are attached at intervals of no less than 3 mm (in general), preventing prolapse of the free margin of the leaflet [1].

Anatomic Relationships of the Tricuspid Valve to Neighboring Structures

There are several structures in close proximity to the tricuspid valve, pertinent to the planning and execution of catheter-based interventions. These include the conduction system, the aortic root, the right coronary artery, and the membranous septum.

Conduction System

One of the feared complications of tricuspid valve intervention is damage to the conduction system, as the location of conduction tissue must be imagined and anticipated but cannot be visualized directly. The triangle of Koch provides a useful "map" of anticipated conduction system tissue using right atrial and tricuspid valve landmarks. The triangle is delineated by the ostium of the coronary sinus, the annulus at the septal leaflet attachment, and the tendon of Todaro (a fibrous extension of the Eustachian valve proceeding medially; see Fig. 23.1). The bundle of His proceeds across the tricuspid valve annulus near the anteroseptal commissure, represented by the apex of the triangle of Koch. Within the triangle lies the atrioventricular node. Current "open" tricuspid rings are designed to avoid the need for placement of anchoring stitches near conduction tissues [1].

Aortic Root

The medial aspect of the anterior leaflet annulus is adjacent to the aortic root at the right coronary/noncoronary commissure. It is possible to infringe on the aortic sinuses during placement of sutures in the region of the tricuspid's anteroseptal commissure. The other important consideration with respect to the proximity of the aortic root is the dynamic movement of the root toward the tricuspid valve with systole. This motion plays a role in adequate closure of the tricuspid valve [1].

Right Coronary Artery

The right coronary artery (RCA) travels anteriorly from its sinus, following the path of the tricuspid annulus at the anterior and posterior leaflets along the right ventricular free wall. The RCA is typically several millimeters from the tricuspid annulus, and

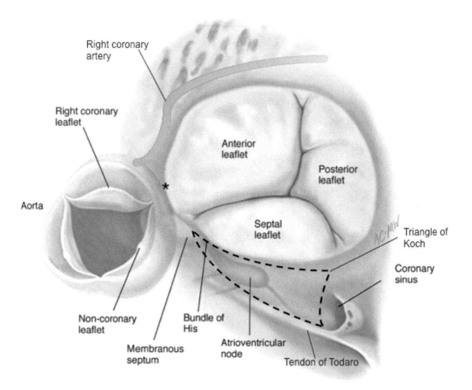

Fig. 23.1 Anatomy of the tricuspid valve and relationships to surrounding structures. Reprinted from Carpentier's Reconstructive Valve Surgery, Tricuspid Valve: Surgical Anatomy and Physiology, page 178, Copyright (2010), with permission from Elsevier

injuries are uncommon during open surgical approaches [2]. However, with the pursuit of interventional approaches, proximity to the RCA is important when considering placement of catheter-based anchoring devices or planning stented prostheses with the potential for compression of the coronary artery or its companion coronary vein.

Membranous Septum

The septal leaflet of the tricuspid valve attaches, as its name implies, directly to the membranous septum. This part of the annulus is most resistant to dilation in functional tricuspid regurgitation due to the stability of the septal structures. Additionally, it is important to recognize that the bundle of His traverses the septal leaflet annular attachment and then follows the membranous septum prior to branching into ventricular bundles [1]. The proximity of the membranous septum to the tricuspid valve is important when considering the pathology of tricuspid annular dilation and potential modes of percutaneously correcting resulting functional regurgitation.

Overview of Tricuspid Valvular Pathologies

Tricuspid valve disease is broadly categorized as organic (related to defects of the valve structures themselves) or functional (related to annular dilation or ventricular dysfunction with normal valve structures). The underlying etiology of tricuspid disease plays a large role in determining which valves may be amenable to percutaneous intervention and in planning catheter-based strategies.

Organic Tricuspid Disease

This category encompasses diseases and disorders which result in damage to the tricuspid leaflets or subvalvular apparatus. A growing etiology is infective endocarditis, which has increased in incidence with intravenous drug use and is also seen in patients with indwelling central venous access devices. Rheumatic fever remains a major cause of tricuspid disease in the developing world with stenosis or insufficiency. Rheumatic tricuspid involvement virtually always accompanies rheumatic disease of the mitral valve or mitral and aortic valve together. Tricuspid damage is observed in a portion of heart transplant patients due to trauma to the subvalvular apparatus during right ventricular myocardial biopsies. Permanent pacemaker or implantable cardioverter defibrillator leads may also cause iatrogenic injury to the valve. Degenerative myxomatous changes are a recognized cause of tricuspid disease, accompanying mitral valve disease. Less common causes of organic tricuspid disease are carcinoid syndrome, medication-related fibrotic valve disease (due to appetite suppressants), lupus, and mediastinal fibrosis [2].

Functional Tricuspid Disease

The majority of tricuspid dysfunction falls into the "functional" category, without lesions of the tricuspid valve itself. Mitral valve disease causes a substantial burden of tricuspid insufficiency. While tricuspid disease is likely to improve after addressing mitral valve disease, Song et al. demonstrated that older age, female gender, rheumatic etiology, and atrial fibrillation were all predictors of late development of TR after left-sided valve surgery [3]. Pulmonary hypertension and right ventricular dysfunction are two other major primary disorders causing secondary tricuspid insufficiency. The tricuspid valve is particularly sensitive to pressure and volume overload conditions of the right ventricle due to the lack of a firm fibrous annulus and the ease of dilation of the anterior and posterior annular regions which are linked to the right ventricular free wall. The compliance of the right ventricle makes tricuspid valvular assessment a challenge, as the degree of functional regurgitation can vary greatly with changes in preload and afterload of the right ventricle [4]. Transthoracic echocardiography provides the optimal assessment of tricuspid regurgitation while the patient is awake and alert, while transesophageal echocardiography can provide additional anatomic information at the time of surgery. The generally accepted annular dilation sizes of >40 mm on echocardiography or >70 mm intraoperatively are indications for tricuspid annuloplasty for functional disease when concomitant left-sided valve surgery is planned [2]. Several authors have suggested that annular dilation is a progressive process and that annular measurement is a better indication than degree of regurgitation when deciding whether to address the valve during left-sided valvular surgery [5]. As interventional approaches are developed, timing of intervention will likely be contingent on symptoms, extent of annular dilation, and correcting the functional disorder prior to irreversible right ventricular dysfunction.

Case Example and Discussion of Tricuspid Anatomic Implications for Interventional Approaches

Case Example: Valve-in-Valve with Melody® Prosthesis

Our group has previously reported the use of a Melody® transcatheter balloon-expandable valve in an 84-year-old female patient with prior sternotomy for coronary artery bypass grafting and bioprosthetic tricuspid valve placement. The bioprosthesis had degenerated, resulting in severe tricuspid regurgitation and stenosis and symptomatic edema and fatigue. Conservative medical management had failed, and while the patient had good functional status, her predicted mortality risk with repeat open operation was 9 %. Decision was made to proceed with a percutaneous transjugular approach with the Melody® valve. The valve was deployed with a 22 mm balloon within the existing 23 mm inner diameter bioprosthesis, and a 25 mm balloon was used to further expand the valve and ensure proper seating. Intraoperative transesophageal echocardiography demonstrated improvement in the gradient across the tricuspid valve, from 15 mmHg pre-procedure to 5 mmHg post-procedure. The patient did well and experienced improvement in symptoms at 3-month and 9-month follow-up [6] (Fig 23.2).

A series by Roberts et al. has previously demonstrated a multicenter experience with placement of Melody® prostheses within tricuspid position bioprosthetic valves or RA to RV valved conduits. The authors identified 15 patients at 8 centers, with 10 patients having a bioprosthetic tricuspid valve in place. The etiologies requiring initial tricuspid procedure encompassed both acquired (infective endocarditis, rheumatic) and congenital causes. Approaches included femoral, right internal jugular, and left internal jugular vein. The authors listed complications including one case of complete heart block requiring permanent pacemaker, one case of endocarditis, and one mortality in a patient who had multisystem organ failure prior to the transcatheter valve placement [7]. This series demonstrates one application of transcatheter technology for the tricuspid valve which, while off-label, introduces the possibility of additional innovations (Table 23.1).

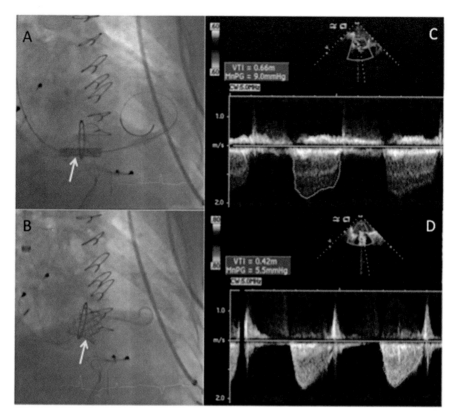

Fig. 23.2 Valve-in-valve prosthesis for treatment of degenerated bioprosthetic tricuspid valve. The transcatheter valve is depicted positioned within the degenerated valve before (**a**) and after (**b**) balloon expansion (transcatheter valve indicated with arrows). The pre-procedure tricuspid gradient by transesophageal echocardiography is shown in (**c**), with the post-deployment gradient improvement in panel (**d**)

Table 23.1 Etiologies of tricuspid valve disease

Organic *indicates presence of discrete valvular or myocardial lesions, and the TR cannot be reversed* [2, 4]	**Functional** *indicates grossly normal valve structures without identifiable lesions; TR can potentially be reversed if right ventricular preload and afterload are adjusted* [2, 4]
Causes include:	Causes include:
• Congenital malformations	• Mitral valve disease
• Rheumatic disease	• Pulmonary hypertension
• Lupus erythematosus	• Dilated cardiomyopathy
• Myxomatous disease	• Ischemic cardiomyopathy
• Endocarditis	
• Trauma (repeated biopsies or endocardial leads)	
• Tumor	
• Carcinoid valve	
• Radiation therapy	

Stented Tricuspid Prosthesis Within Native Tricuspid Valve

The major constraints preventing placement of stented prostheses in the native tricuspid annulus are (1) the lack of a firm fibrous annulus and (2) the dynamic movement of the annulus and surrounding myocardium during the cardiac cycle. Animal studies have demonstrated initial feasibility of using a nitinol stent with bovine pericardial leaflets as a percutaneously delivered valve in a sheep model; the sheep, however, did not have annular dilation or other pathology similar to human tricuspid diseases. The authors describe successful placement in 8 of 10 sheep, with early mortalities due to arrhythmias or stent malpositioning, and survival past 6 months in the successfully recovered animals [8]. While there are several challenges in attempting to deliver a catheter-based stented bioprosthesis in the tricuspid position, high-risk or inoperable patients may benefit from the availability of such an option in the future.

Percutaneous Annuloplasty

Early development efforts for percutaneous mitral annuloplasty utilized the coronary sinus as an anatomic structure in which to place an annuloplasty ring. The tricuspid valve has no analogous preexisting route for placement of percutaneous annuloplasty. Development is ongoing with placement of percutaneous annular anchors and adjustable band support, as well as percutaneous annular modification/plication; this technology will be discussed separately. The main considerations when developing or using such techniques are the major structures surrounding the tricuspid valve: the conduction system and aortic root at the septal and anteroseptal regions, right coronary artery along the anterior and posterior annulus, and the coronary sinus ostium near the posteroseptal commissure. Moreover, as the tricuspid annulus is not a distinct fibrous structure, securing and downsizing or plicating the annulus may not provide a secure repair.

Edge-to-Edge Repair

The technology of percutaneous edge-to-edge mitral valve repair, MitraClip, is now commercially available. Challenges to employing a similar technique include the added complexity of the tricuspid's three leaflets as opposed to the mitral's two and the importance of the tricuspid valve's annular dilation which may make edge-to-edge repair inadequate in some cases. A case example of use of the MitraClip device for tricuspid repair has been reported in a patient with congenitally corrected transposition of the great arteries. Franzen et al. present the case of previously undiagnosed congenitally corrected transposition of the great arteries in a 62-year-old woman with congestive heart failure and NYHA class III symptoms. Evaluation demonstrated that the systemic ventricle was dilated and trabeculated, consistent with right ventricular morphology, with a tricuspid atrioventricular valve. The anatomic tricuspid valve demonstrated significant regurgitation, and when the patient declined open-heart surgery, she was offered MitraClip placement. The procedure necessitated three attempts at positioning and repositioning the clip until it adequately addressed the major regurgitant jet between the anterior and septal leaflets. The procedure was successful with minimal tricuspid regurgitation on 3-month follow-up as well as improvement in symptoms to NYHA class I [9]. This case demonstrates that the MitraClip technology could address tricuspid regurgitation with proper identification of the location of the regurgitant jet but would require adjustments in deployment strategy specific to the right-sided structures. Anecdotally, the authors have attempted select cases of transcatheter tricuspid repair using the MitraClip system with suboptimal efficacy (data not published). Of note, one of the greatest challenges is that imaging of the tricuspid valve still lags behind the mitral valve. Thus, real-time assessment of leaflet insertion is limited.

Conclusions

The tricuspid valve has lagged behind the left-sided valves in knowledge of its dysfunction and in approaches to its repair. Open surgical techniques have largely evolved from mitral valve surgery, but the tricuspid valve's unique anatomy and physiology demand tailored solutions when developing percutaneous therapies. The easily distensible and dynamically shaped annulus, delicate leaflet tissue and annulus, and important neighboring structures all warrant consideration when contemplating percutaneous approaches. Since many patients with tricuspid disease have accompanying left-sided valve disease or prior left-sided valve surgery, the applications of transcatheter tricuspid interventions are appealing. As such, catheter-based tricuspid therapies will give clinicians and patients a broader range of options to more comprehensively address valve disease.

References

1. Carpentier A, Adams DH, Filsoufi F. Surgical anatomy and physiology. In: Carpentier A, Adams DH, Filsoufi F (eds.). Carpentier's reconstructive valve surgery: from valve analysis to valve reconstruction. Elsevier; 2010. pp. 175–182.
2. Duran CMG. Surgical treatment of the tricuspid valve. In: Selke F, del Nido PJ, Swanson SJ (eds.). Sabiston and spencer surgery of the chest. 8th ed. Elsevier; 2010. pp. 241–1257.
3. Song H, Kim M-J, Chung CH, et al. Factors associated with development of late significant tricuspid regurgitation after successful left-sided valve surgery. Heart. 2009;95:931–6.
4. Carpentier A, Adams DH, Filsoufi F. Pathophysiology, preoperative valve analysis, and surgical indications. In: Carpentier A, Adams DH, Filsoufi F (eds.). Carpentier's reconstructive valve surgery: from valve analysis to valve reconstruction. Elsevier; 2010. pp. 183–191.

5. Bianchi G, Solinas M, Bevilacqua S, Glauber M. Which patient undergoing mitral valve surgery should also have the tricuspid repair? Interact Cardiovasc Thorac Surg. 2009;9(2009):1009–20.
6. Bhamidipati CM, Scott Lim D, Ragosta M, Ailawadi G. Percutaneous transjugular implantation of MELODY® valve into tricuspid bioprosthesis. J Card Surg. 2013;28:391–3.
7. Roberts PA, Boudjemline Y, Cheatham JP, et al. Percutaneous tricuspid valve replacement in congenital and acquired heart disease. J Am Coll Cardiol. 2011;58(2):118–22.
8. Bai Y, Zong GJ, Wang HR, et al. An integrated pericardial valved stent special for percutaneous tricuspid implantation: an animal feasibility study. J Surg Res. 2010;160(2):215–21.
9. Franzen O, Von Samson P, Dodge-khatami A, Geffert G, Baldus S. Percutaneous edge-to-edge repair of tricuspid regurgitation in congenitally corrected transposition of the great arteries. Congenit Heart Dis. 2011;6:57–9.

Chapter 24
Percutaneous Mitral and Tricuspid Annuloplasty

Maurizio Taramasso and Francesco Maisano

Percutaneous Mitral Annuloplasty

Percutaneous mitral valve therapies have been emerging as an alternative option for high-risk patients. Multiple technologies and diversified approaches are today under clinical study or in development [1]. They can be categorized based on the anatomical and pathophysiological addressed target: leaflet and chordal repair procedures, indirect and direct annuloplasty, and LV remodeling devices.

Surgical Mitral Annuloplasty

Mitral annuloplasty is widely performed during conventional mitral surgery. The rationale is to restore the normal ratio between the leaflet surface area and the annular area and to improve leaflet coaptation. Moreover, mitral annuloplasty prevents progressive annular dilatation and consequent recurrent mitral regurgitation after surgery [2–4]. From a mechanical standpoint, the stress forces acting on the valve leaflet are decreased after annuloplasty [5, 6], protecting from suture dehiscence and leaflet tissue tears.

Suture annuloplasty is very rarely performed nowadays, while implantation of a prosthetic mitral ring is the gold standard surgical technique today for mitral annuloplasty [7–10]. Different shaped mitral rings have been developed for different etiologies of MR [11, 12], and the choice of the device usually depends on the preference and experience of the surgeon (complete or incomplete, rigid, semirigid, or flexible).

M. Taramasso, MD (✉) • F. Maisano, MD
Department of Cardiovascular Surgery, University Hospital of Zurich,
Raemistrasse, 100, Zurich 8091, Switzerland
e-mail: Maurizio.Taramasso@usz.ch; Francesco.Maisano@usz.ch

© Springer Science+Business Media New York 2016
G. Ailawadi, I.L. Kron (eds.), *Catheter Based Valve and Aortic Surgery*,
DOI 10.1007/978-1-4939-3432-4_24

In the context of degenerative mitral regurgitation (DMR), where mitral leaflets are intrinsically diseased, surgical annuloplasty is usually performed in association with other repair techniques, to reinforce the leaflet repair and to fix the mural portion of the ring to the fibrous skeleton of the heart. This adjunct has been shown to reduce MR recurrence due to further annular dilatation [4].

On the contrary, in functional MR (FMR), isolated undersized annuloplasty (2 sizes smaller than the size measured) is effectively performed as stand-alone procedure, and it is associated with satisfactory results, when proper patient selection is carried out [13–18]. The rationale of undersized annuloplasty in FMR is to force leaflet coaptation, by reducing the septolateral diameter of the mitral annulus, balancing the coaptation defect due to leaflet tethering [19]. However, durability is a major concern of undersized annuloplasty in FMR, with an overall recurrence of significant MR ranging from 10 to 30 % at 1 year, largely depending on preoperative patient selection [13, 14, 20–24].

The Clinical Need of a Reliable Transcatheter Mitral Annuloplasty

The lack of reliable transcatheter annuloplasty devices effectively limits the patient population for transcatheter mitral interventions. Transcatheter annuloplasty may both improve outcomes and expand therapeutic options. From a theoretical point of view, when annuloplasty devices become available, the operator will be able to combine different leaflet and annular transcatheter repair, and percutaneous mitral repair techniques may potentially become a true alternative to surgery even in standard-risk patients.

Transcatheter edge-to-edge repair with the MitraClip system (Abbott Vascular Inc., Menlo, USA) is today the most advanced technology available for clinical use, with a proven safety and efficacy profile in selected patients with both FMR and DMR [25–27]. Most patients treated with MitraClip are high-risk or inoperable patients. Improvements of symptoms and quality of life as well as MR reduction have been observed in the majority of the cases, but about 20 % of patients have still residual MR after the procedure, often due to the concomitant annular dilatation, which is not sufficiently addressed by MitraClip alone [25, 28].

Moreover, the absence of mitral annuloplasty is a major concern regarding durability of MitraClip, as surgical experience clearly showed that long-term results of surgical edge to edge in absence of annuloplasty are suboptimal [29], and this aspect is of crucial importance if the aim of transcatheter mitral treatments is the expansion of the indication toward a lower risk population.

The absence of transcatheter annuloplasty devices is also limiting the global number of patients with symptomatic MR who could benefit from a less invasive transcatheter treatment: up to 1/3 of patients screened for MitraClip are not eligible due to anatomical limitations, including annular dilatation [30], suggesting that there is a clinical need for a different transcatheter mitral repair approach to address annular dilatation.

The Clinical Role of Transcatheter Mitral Annuloplasty

The precise clinical role of transcatheter mitral annuloplasty is still not yet well established, since it is a new therapeutic approach and clinical results are still limited. However, based on the preliminary results of the different technologies and on the lessons learned from surgery, it is possible to try to extrapolate what the clinical role of this therapy will be.

In DMR patients, annuloplasty has to be considered as an adjunctive therapy in combination with leaflet repair. The results obtained with the MitraClip system in DMR could certainly benefit from the association of an annuloplasty to achieve better acute results and improve repair durability, as it is the case in conventional surgery.

In FMR patients, annuloplasty might represent a stand-alone procedure. Therefore, it will be extremely important to identify the ideal candidate who could most benefit from annuloplasty. Patients with predominant annular dilatation and limited valve tethering could be ideal candidates for annuloplasty alone, while in presence of predominant leaflet tethering, MitraClip could still represent the more appropriate therapy. Combination of different technologies may represent a better option in selected FMR patients: surgical literature reported improved repair durability with the association of the edge to edge to the annuloplasty in patients with FMR and advanced tethering [17].

The clinical introduction of transcatheter mitral technologies could promote the adoption of an "early indication" approach. When patients are treated with advanced mitral disease, outcomes become poor and transcatheter mitral procedures may be unable to modify the clinical course of the disease and may not influence prognosis [31–33]. The impact of transcatheter interventions will be much more effective when executed early in the clinical course of the disease. Only a very safe transcatheter procedure can justify an "early indication" approach. In fact, when considering an early indication, beyond efficacy, safety plays a dominant role. Transcatheter direct annuloplasty may represent the ideal procedure that could be used a safe first-line therapy in FMR patients. Considering an early indication approach, if comparable efficacy will be proven, direct annuloplasty may present some advantages compared to MitraClip: possibility of valve-in-ring implantation does not preclude the option of surgical repair.

Description of the Different Annuloplasty Devices and Preliminary Results

One of the most appealing features of the transcatheter mitral annuloplasty is that this approach preserves the native valve anatomy, differently from the majority of the leaflet repair techniques, keeping the option for future valve treatment open. Different catheter-based devices have made use of the coronary sinus to achieve indirect annuloplasty, whereas other devices achieve direct annuloplasty.

Indirect Annuloplasty

The indirect annuloplasty approach is based on the anatomical proximity of the coronary sinus (CS) to the posterior mitral annulus. The CS encircles about two thirds of the mitral annulus and can be used as a route to push the posterior annulus toward the anterior, reducing the septolateral diameter and forcing leaflet coaptation. The cannulation of the CS is simple and safe, and the procedure can be done without general anesthesia and TEE guidance. Therefore, this approach is particularly appealing since it is technically not demanding.

Early attempts to remodel the mitral annulus with coronary sinus devices have not been satisfactory [34–36], mainly due to suboptimal efficacy and the risk of delayed complications (including coronary occlusion) [34, 37, 38].

The Carillon Mitral Contour System (Cardiac Dimension, Inc., Kirkland, Washington) is the only technology still using this approach and received CE mark approval in 2011. The TITAN trial (Transcatheter Implantation of Carillon Mitral Annuloplasty Device) evaluated the clinical impact of Carillon Mitral in HF patients where it is commercially available in Europe with at least moderate FMR. The results of the trial showed a significant reduction in FMR grade with a reduction in LV diastolic and systolic volumes, compared to a control group composed of non-implanted patients. In addition, functional and performance status markedly improved for the implanted patients. Late results showed that CS annuloplasty was associated with delayed reverse LV remodeling and clinical improvement up to 24 months even in acute "nonresponders" [39]. The REDUCE FMR randomized trial will compare the Carillon device to optimal medical therapy in 120 heart failure patients with FMR. The first patient was enrolled in June 2015.

Although clinical benefits have been observed, this approach has a restricted applicability in the real world, mainly due to its limited efficacy (due to the fact that CS and mitral annulus are not coplanar) and to the risk of coronary artery compression and device dislocation. The major concern regarding the long-term outcomes of CS approach is the absence of a solid surgical background.

Direct Annuloplasty

Since it closely reproduces the conventional surgical approach, direct mitral valve annuloplasty is so far the most promising approach for transcatheter mitral valve annuloplasty. Different technologies are under clinical and preclinical investigation (Fig. 24.1).

The Mitralign System

The Mitralign system (Mitralign, Inc., Tewksbury, USA) is designed to perform selective plication in the posterior mitral annulus (in the P1 and P3 annular segments), by deploying couples of transannular pledgets, which are delivered from the

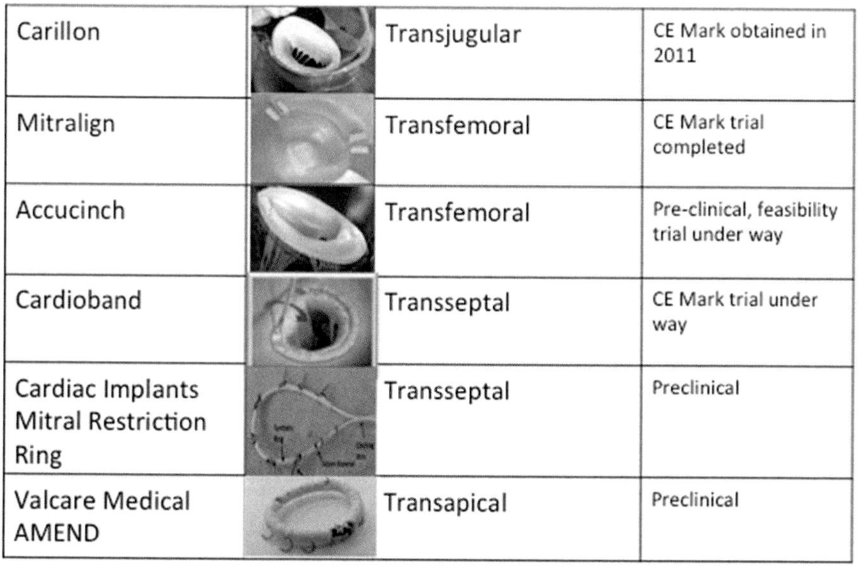

Carillon		Transjugular	CE Mark obtained in 2011
Mitralign		Transfemoral	CE Mark trial completed
Accucinch		Transfemoral	Pre-clinical, feasibility trial under way
Cardioband		Transseptal	CE Mark trial under way
Cardiac Implants Mitral Restriction Ring		Transseptal	Preclinical
Valcare Medical AMEND		Transapical	Preclinical

Fig. 24.1 Transcatheter mitral annuloplasty devices

femoral artery through a retrograde approach from the left ventricle through the mitral annulus [40]. The procedure is performed under transesophageal echocardiography and fluoroscopic guidance. The result of the CE mark trial has been recently reported in 51 high-risk patients with FMR (mean ejection fraction 32 %). No intra-procedural deaths or conversion to emergent open surgery was observed. A thirty-day mortality was 7.8 % (4/51 patients); a 6-month survival was 88 % with an 80 % of freedom from valve intervention. Significant improvement in MR severity and in LV dimension was reported at 6 months, as well as improvement in walking distance (Schofer J. Mitralign procedure and results of the CE Mark Trial. Chicago, TVT 2015). CE mark approval is expected in 2015.

The Accucinch System

The Accucinch system (Guided Delivery Systems, Inc., Santa Clara, USA) is another direct annuloplasty device using the retrograde transventricular approach. A series of anchors are implanted in the subannular space, beneath the MV in the base of the LV. This space is in direct contiguity with the annulus and it is relatively free from chordae. The anchors are connected by a nitinol wire in which tethering the cord under echo guidance cinches the basal LV and mitral annulus. A peculiar aspect of the Accucinch system is that it also causes remodeling of the basal portion of the LV, thereby promoting papillary muscle approximation. Limited clinical data are available. The feasibility and the safety of the device have been shown in 18 patients: among them, 5 were converted to surgery and no 30-day deaths occurred.

In the 4 most recent patients of this small series, there was a 40 % reduction of MR (quantified as regurgitant volume and effective regurgitant area) as well as clinical improvement for the patient (Kleber F. Basal Ventriculoplasty: Guided Delivery Systems: Accucinch® Design Iterations and Clinical Results. San Francisco, TCT 2013). No further clinical updates have been reported thus far.

The Valtech Cardioband

The Valtech Cardioband (ValtechCardio, Inc., Or Yehuda, Israel) is the closest transcatheter device to a surgical ring [41]. It is delivered from a transseptal approach, and the implant is performed on the atrial side of the mitral annulus. An incomplete adjustable surgical-like sutureless Dacron band with multiple anchor elements is secured along the posterior mitral annulus from commissure to commissure, under echo and fluoroscopic guidance, using multiple anchor elements. The interaction with the cardiac function and the hemodynamic impact are minimal. After the implantation, Cardioband length may be shortened on the beating heart, under echo guidance, to improve leaflet coaptation and reduce MR. The CE mark trial is currently enrolling high-risk patients with FMR. Initial clinical experience is promising, confirming the feasibility and safety of Cardioband. Preliminary data from the CE mark trial in 40 symptomatic patients with FMR have been recently reported; the Cardioband implant was associated with significant septolateral annular dimension reduction (20 % in average) and increased leaflet coaptation surface (Vahanian A. Cardioband: Procedure; Insights from CT planning, and CE Mark Trial Results. Chicago, TVT 2015). Acute significant MR reduction was achieved in more than 95 % of the patients and 85 % of the patients had MR $\leq 2+$ at 6 months. A thirty-day mortality was 5 % (2/40 patients), with a very low incidence of major adverse events, suggesting the procedure is safe even in high-risk patients. Six months after the implantation, 80 % of the patients were in NYHA functional classes I–II. Improvements in quality of life and in performance status were accordingly reported. The results reported with the Cardioband device are of particular value because MR reduction has been assessed by an independent Core-Lab.

Cardiac Implants Mitral Restriction Ring

Cardiac Implants Mitral Restriction Ring (Cardiac Implant Solutions LLC, USA) is another direct annuloplasty device delivered from transseptal route, which is currently under preclinical investigations (35 acute and chronic animal implants so far reported). It allows the implantation of a complete adjustable mitral ring with an internal cinching wire on the atrial annular side by means of multiple anchor elements. The implantable actuator is designed to enable noninvasive chronic progressive cinching also at follow-up, following the completion of tissue healing. In case of MR recurrence, the complete mitral ring may serve as retention mechanism for a transcatheter valve-in-ring implantation. Feasibility has been reported in animal models (Kuck KH. Progressive Mitral Ring Annuloplasty and Mitral Valve Replacement. Based on Single Shot Percutaneous Implantation of Complete Circumferential Ring. San Francisco, TCT 2014).

The Valcare Medical AMEND

The Valcare Medical AMEND (Valcare Medical, Israel) is a complete, semirigid, D-shaped mitral ring, which is implanted on the atrial side of the mitral annulus by means of 12 anchors, through transapical access. Acute animal study on 40 adult pigs showed feasibility of the procedure, with a 20–25 % reduction of the septolateral annular dimension after the implantation. This device can potentially serve as a platform for future valve-in-ring implantation (Meerkin D. AMEND. The Mitral Solution from Valcare. Paris, EuroPCR 2015).

Other Annular Repair Techniques

Beyond indirect CS annuloplasty and direct annuloplasty, other methods have been attempted to remodel the mitral annulus, including external compression of atrioventricular groove [42], implant of cinching devices [43], and application of RF or US energy sources to shrink the annular collagen [44, 45]. Reproducibility, efficacy, and safety of these appealing technologies still need to be proved as they are based on completely novel concepts, without a validated and reproducible surgical or preclinical background.

Percutaneous Tricuspid Annuloplasty

Currently, moderate to severe tricuspid regurgitation (TR) affects approximately 1.6 million patients in the USA, of whom only 8000 undergo tricuspid surgery annually (6); thus, there are an extremely large number of untreated patients with significant TR and a large unmet clinical need for patients with severe TR not referred for conventional surgery, mainly due to expected high surgical risk.

Percutaneous procedures may be an attractive alternative to surgery for patients deemed to be high-risk surgical candidates. Whereas over the past few years, the development and clinical use of percutaneous approaches to the aortic valve and valve have been widespread, few data are available about the feasibility and the efficacy of the percutaneous tricuspid valve (TV) treatment. Some of the concepts that have been developed for the percutaneous treatment of MR may be adapted to percutaneous repair of the TV, such as percutaneous annuloplasty. However, anatomical diversity between the two atrioventricular valves makes a direct translation of a mitral into a tricuspid application improbable.

Mechanism of Tricuspid Regurgitation

The etiology underlying TR is functional in more than 90 % of the cases, typically due to RV dilation and dysfunction from left heart disease, as in cases of MV disease. Functional TR (FTR) is invariably associated with tricuspid annular dilatation secondary to right ventricle enlargement. Progressive TV annulus enlargement prevents normal leaflet coaptation, which is the underlying pathophysiology of FTR. Dilatation of the tricuspid annulus occurs mainly in the anterior and posterior annulus, corresponding to the free wall of the right ventricle, while dilation of the septal segment is limited because of its close anatomical relationship with the fibrous skeleton of the heart [46].

The standard surgical treatment of FTR is tricuspid annuloplasty, which can be performed with suture technique or with implantation of a prosthetic ring. The rationale behind tricuspid annuloplasty is to fix the annular dimensions, force leaflet coaptation reducing the anteroseptal diameter of the TV, and counteract further annular dilatation.

Percutaneous Tricuspid Annuloplasty Device and Preliminary Results

The experience with percutaneous tricuspid valve therapies is very preliminary. While different approaches have been tested in preclinical setting, the most promising concept in this field seems to be an annuloplasty concept, since it addresses annular dilatation by reducing the anteroseptal distance.

Different annuloplasty devices are under preclinical and clinical evaluation (Fig. 24.2).

The Millipede system (Millipede, LLC, Ann Arbor, Michigan) involves the placement of a tricuspid annular ring with an attachment system via either minimally invasive surgical or percutaneous methods to restore the native tricuspid annular shape and diameter. It is repositionable and retrievable before deployment. No updated preclinical feasibility or safety data are available.

The abovementioned Mitralign device, originally designed for the treatment of FMR, has recently been used to treat FTR performing a transcatheter bicuspidization of the TV through transvenous jugular approach [47]. A steerable catheter is advanced in the right ventricle across the tricuspid valve and positioned under echocardiographic guidance. An insulated radio-frequency wire is then advanced from the ventricular side of the leaflet and within the annulus, directed toward the right atrium in the desired position in correspondence with the anteroposterior commissure. Once the wire is through the annulus, a pledgeted delivery catheter is advanced over the wire across the annulus. The steps are then repeated on the opposite anatomic site of the posterior commissure. A dedicated plication lock device is used to bring the 2 pledgeted sutures together, plicating the annulus and effectively

Millipede	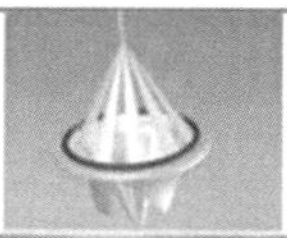	Transjugular	Preclinical
Mitralign	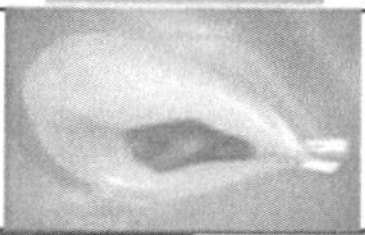	Transjugular	7 compassionate cases performed
Tricinch	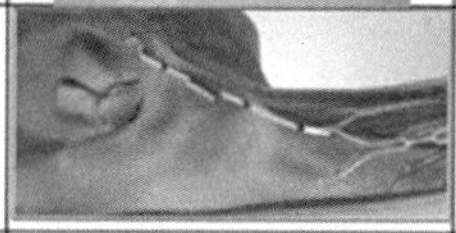	Transfemoral	CE Mark trial under way
TRAIPTA	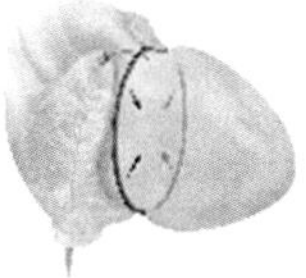	Intrapericardial	Preclinical

Fig. 24.2 Transcatheter tricuspid annuloplasty devices

bicuspidizing the TV. Preliminary results obtained in seven high-risk patients with symptomatic FTR have been reported. Implant was feasible in 5/7 patients with no reported adverse events. Tricuspid annular dimension was observed in all the implanted patients, with an acute reduction of TR in 4/5 patients (Groothuis A. Direct annuloplasty for treatment of tricuspid regurgitation. Paris, EuroPCR 2015).

The TriCinch (4Tech Cardio, Galway, Ireland) is a catheter-based device designed to perform tricuspid annular cinching, in order to reduce anteroseptal annular dimension and reduce TR, improving leaflet coaptation. A steerable catheter is introduced in the femoral vein and delivered to the tricuspid annulus. The tip of the steerable catheter is positioned between the anteroposterior commissure and the mid-anterior annulus. A corkscrew is implanted in the proximity of the midpart of the anterior tricuspid annulus (target zone). Right coronary artery angiography is then performed to exclude coronary injury. Once the corkscrew is secured, the delivery system is retrieved and a self-expandable nitinol stent is introduced over the wire and coupled to the implant. The whole system is then tensioned to reshape the TV promoting annular cinching and to increase the leaflet coaptation, on a beating heart, under echo guidance. Finally, the stent is deployed in the inferior vena cava (IVC) to maintain the tension applied. Multicentre CE mark trial is ongoing (PREVENT trial). Preliminary results obtained in the first three successfully implanted patients showed stable reduction of the septolateral dimension of the tricuspid annulus 6 months after the implantation, with sustained clinical and functional improvement (Maisano F. Fortech Percutaneous Annuloplasty for Tricuspid Regurgitation. Chicago, TVT 2015).

A different approach is used by the TRAIPTA concept (transatrial intrapericardial tricuspid annuloplasty) [48]. Pericardial access is obtained puncturing the right atrial appendage from within, after transfemoral venous access. A circumferential implant, which exerts compressive force over the tricuspid annulus, is delivered along the atrioventricular groove within the pericardial space. Tension on the implant is then adjusted interactively to modify tricuspid annular geometry and reduce therefore TR. The right atrial puncture is then sealed using off-the-shelf nitinol closure devices. The procedure is mainly guided by fluoroscopy. Preclinical experience showed safety of the implant. Significant improvement in leaflet coaptation and reduction of tricuspid valve area and diameters were also observed. The major limitation of this approach is that it requires a free pericardial space. Therefore, it cannot be used in patients with previous heart surgery. This aspect may reduce the adoption of the TRAIPTA device, since patients with late recurrence of FTR after mitral surgery represent a big proportion of the potential candidates for percutaneous TV annuloplasty.

References

1. Maisano F, Alfieri O, Banai S, Buchbinder M, Colombo A, Falk V, Feldman T, Franzen O, Herrmann H, Kar S, Kuck KH, Lutter G, Mack M, Nickenig G, Piazza N, Reisman M, Ruiz CE, Schofer J, Sondergaard L, Stone GW, Taramasso M, Thomas M, Vahanian A, Webb J, Windecker S, Leon MB. The future of transcatheter mitral valve interventions: competitive or complementary role of repair vs. replacement? Eur Heart J. 2015;36(26):1651–9.
2. Gillinov AM, Cosgrove DM, Blackstone EH, Diaz R, Arnold JH, Lytle BW, Smedira NG, Sabik JF, McCarthy PM, Loop FD. Durability of mitral valve repair for degenerative disease. J Thorac Cardiovasc Surg. 1998;116(5):734–43.
3. Flameng W, Herijgers P, Bogaerts K. Recurrence of mitral valve regurgitation after mitral valve repair in degenerative valve disease. Circulation. 2003;107(12):1609–13.
4. Maisano F, La Canna G, Grimaldi A, Vigano G, Blasio A, Mignatti A, Colombo A, Maseri A, Alfieri O. Annular-to-leaflet mismatch and the need for reductive annuloplasty in patients undergoing mitral repair for chronic mitral regurgitation due to mitral valve prolapse. Am J Cardiol. 2007;99(10):1434–9.
5. Kunzelman KS, Reimink MS, Cochran RP. Annular dilatation increases stress in the mitral valve and delays coaptation: a finite element computer model. Cardiovasc Surg. 1997;5(4):427–34.
6. Votta E, Maisano F, Soncini M, Redaelli A, Montevecchi FM, Alfieri O. 3-D computational analysis of the stress distribution on the leaflets after edge-to-edge repair of mitral regurgitation. J Heart Valve Dis. 2002;11(6):810–22.
7. Timek TA, Liang D, Daughters GT, Ingels Jr NB, Miller DC. Effect of semi-rigid or flexible mitral ring annuloplasty on anterior leaflet three-dimensional geometry. J Heart Valve Dis. 2008;17(2):149–54.
8. Jensen MO, Jensen H, Smerup M, Levine RA, Yoganathan AP, Nygaard H, Hasenkam JM, Nielsen SL. Saddle-shaped mitral valve annuloplasty rings experience lower forces compared with flat rings. Circulation. 2008;118(14 Suppl):S250–5.
9. Chong CF. Are rigid annuloplasty rings better than flexible annuloplasty rings in ischemic mitral regurgitation repair: where is the evidence? Ann Thorac Surg. 2009;88(6):2073. author reply 2073–4.
10. Bothe W, Kvitting JP, Stephens EH, Swanson JC, Liang DH, Ingels Jr NB, Miller DC. Effects of different annuloplasty ring types on mitral leaflet tenting area during acute myocardial ischemia. J Thorac Cardiovasc Surg. 2011;141(2):345–53.
11. Maisano F, Redaelli A, Soncini M, Votta E, Arcobasso L, Alfieri O. An annular prosthesis for the treatment of functional mitral regurgitation: finite element model analysis of a dog bone-shaped ring prosthesis. Ann Thorac Surg. 2005;79(4):1268–75.

12. McCarthy PM, McGee EC, Rigolin VH, Zhao Q, Subacius H, Huskin AL, Underwood S, Kane BJ, Mikati I, Gang G, Bonow RO. Initial clinical experience with Myxo-ETlogix mitral valve repair ring. J Thorac Cardiovasc Surg. 2008;136(1):73–81.
13. Magne J, Pibarot P, Dumesnil JG, Senechal M. Continued global left ventricular remodeling is not the sole mechanism responsible for the late recurrence of ischemic mitral regurgitation after restrictive annuloplasty. J Am Soc Echocardiogr. 2009;22(11):1256–64.
14. Braun J, Bax JJ, Versteegh MI, Voigt PG, Holman ER, Klautz RJ, Boersma E, Dion RA. Preoperative left ventricular dimensions predict reverse remodeling following restrictive mitral annuloplasty in ischemic mitral regurgitation. Eur J Cardiothorac Surg. 2005;27(5):847–53.
15. Calafiore AM, Di Mauro M, Gallina S, Di Giammarco G, Iaco AL, Teodori G, Tavarozzi I. Mitral valve surgery for chronic ischemic mitral regurgitation. Ann Thorac Surg. 2004;77(6):1989–97.
16. Lee AP, Acker M, Kubo SH, Bolling SF, Park SW, Bruce CJ, Oh JK. Mechanisms of recurrent functional mitral regurgitation after mitral valve repair in nonischemic dilated cardiomyopathy: importance of distal anterior leaflet tethering. Circulation. 2009;119(19):2606–14.
17. De Bonis M, Lapenna E, La Canna G, Ficarra E, Pagliaro M, Torracca L, Maisano F, Alfieri O. Mitral valve repair for functional mitral regurgitation in end-stage dilated cardiomyopathy: role of the "edge-to-edge" technique. Circulation. 2005;112(9 Suppl):I402–8.
18. Mann DL, Kubo SH, Sabbah HN, Starling RC, Jessup M, Oh JK, Acker MA. Beneficial effects of the CorCap cardiac support device: five-year results from the Acorn Trial. J Thorac Cardiovasc Surg. 2012;143(5):1036–42.
19. Bolling SF, Pagani FD, Deeb GM, Bach DS. Intermediate-term outcome of mitral reconstruction in cardiomyopathy. J Thorac Cardiovasc Surg. 1998;115(2):381–6. discussion 387–8.
20. Tahta SA, Oury JH, Maxwell JM, Hiro SP, Duran CM. Outcome after mitral valve repair for functional ischemic mitral regurgitation. J Heart Valve Dis. 2002;11(1):11–8. discussion 18–9.
21. Ciarka A, Braun J, Delgado V, Versteegh M, Boersma E, Klautz R, Dion R, Bax JJ, Van de Veire N. Predictors of mitral regurgitation recurrence in patients with heart failure undergoing mitral valve annuloplasty. Am J Cardiol. 2010;106(3):395–401.
22. De Bonis M, Lapenna E, Verzini A, La Canna G, Grimaldi A, Torracca L, Maisano F, Alfieri O. Recurrence of mitral regurgitation parallels the absence of left ventricular reverse remodeling after mitral repair in advanced dilated cardiomyopathy. Ann Thorac Surg. 2008;85(3):932–9.
23. Takeda K, Sakaguchi T, Miyagawa S, Shudo Y, Kainuma S, Masai T, Taniguchi K, Sawa Y. The extent of early left ventricular reverse remodelling is related to midterm outcomes after restrictive mitral annuloplasty in patients with non-ischaemic dilated cardiomyopathy and functional mitral regurgitation. Eur J Cardiothorac Sur. 2012;41(3):506–11.
24. Bax JJ, Braun J, Somer ST, Klautz R, Holman ER, Versteegh MI, Boersma E, Schalij MJ, van der Wall EE, Dion RA. Restrictive annuloplasty and coronary revascularization in ischemic mitral regurgitation results in reverse left ventricular remodeling. Circulation. 2004;110(11 Suppl 1):Ii103–8.
25. Maisano F, Franzen O, Baldus S, Schafer U, Hausleiter J, Butter C, Ussia GP, Sievert H, Richardt G, Widder JD, Moccetti T, Schillinger W. Percutaneous mitral valve interventions in the real world: early and 1-year results from the ACCESS-EU, a prospective, multicenter, nonrandomized post-approval study of the MitraClip therapy in Europe. J Am Coll Cardiol. 2013;62(12):1052–61.
26. Glower DD, Kar S, Trento A, Lim DS, Bajwa T, Quesada R, Whitlow PL, Rinaldi MJ, Grayburn P, Mack MJ, Mauri L, McCarthy PM, Feldman T. Percutaneous mitral valve repair for mitral regurgitation in high-risk patients: results of the EVEREST II study. J Am Coll Cardiol. 2014;64(2):172–81.
27. Lim DS, Reynolds MR, Feldman T, Kar S, Herrmann HC, Wang A, Whitlow PL, Gray WA, Grayburn P, Mack MJ, Glower DD. Improved functional status and quality of life in prohibitive surgical risk patients with degenerative mitral regurgitation after transcatheter mitral valve repair. J Am Coll Cardiol. 2014;64(2):182–92.

28. Taramasso M, Denti P, Buzzatti N, De Bonis M, La Canna G, Colombo A, Alfieri O, Maisano F. Mitraclip therapy and surgical mitral repair in patients with moderate to severe left ventricular failure causing functional mitral regurgitation: a single-centre experience. Eur J Cardiothorac Surg. 2012;42(6):920–6.

29. De Bonis M, Lapenna E, Maisano F, Barili F, La Canna G, Buzzatti N, Pappalardo F, Calabrese M, Nisi T, Alfieri O. Long-term results (</=18 years) of the edge-to-edge mitral valve repair without annuloplasty in degenerative mitral regurgitation: implications for the percutaneous approach. Circulation. 2014;130(11 Suppl 1):S19–24.

30. Grayburn PA, Roberts BJ, Aston S, Anwar A, Hebeler Jr RF, Brown DL, Mack MJ. Mechanism and severity of mitral regurgitation by transesophageal echocardiography in patients referred for percutaneous valve repair. Am J Cardiol. 2011;108(6):882–7.

31. Neuss M, Schau T, Schoepp M, Seifert M, Holschermann F, Meyhofer J, Butter C. Patient selection criteria and midterm clinical outcome for MitraClip therapy in patients with severe mitral regurgitation and severe congestive heart failure. Eur J Heart Fail. 2013;15(7):786–95.

32. Taramasso M, Maisano F, Latib A, Denti P, Buzzatti N, Cioni M, La Canna G, Colombo A, Alfieri O. Clinical outcomes of MitraClip for the treatment of functional mitral regurgitation. EuroIntervention; 2014.

33. Taramasso M, Latib A, Denti P, Candreva A, Buzzatti N, Giannini F, La Canna G, Colombo A, Alfieri O, Maisano F. Acute kidney injury following MitraClip implantation in high risk patients: incidence, predictive factors and prognostic value. Int J Cardiol. 2013;169(2):e24–5.

34. Harnek J, Webb JG, Kuck KH, Tschope C, Vahanian A, Buller CE, James SK, Tiefenbacher CP, Stone GW. Transcatheter implantation of the MONARC coronary sinus device for mitral regurgitation: 1-year results from the EVOLUTION phase I study (Clinical Evaluation of the Edwards Lifesciences Percutaneous Mitral Annuloplasty System for the Treatment of Mitral Regurgitation). J Am Coll Cardiol Intv. 2011;4(1):115–22.

35. Schofer J, Siminiak T, Haude M, Herrman JP, Vainer J, Wu JC, Levy WC, Mauri L, Feldman T, Kwong RY, Kaye DM, Duffy SJ, Tubler T, Degen H, Brandt MC, Van Bibber R, Goldberg S, Reuter DG, Hoppe UC. Percutaneous mitral annuloplasty for functional mitral regurgitation: results of the CARILLON Mitral Annuloplasty Device European Union Study. Circulation. 2009;120(4):326–33.

36. Dubreuil O, Basmadjian A, Ducharme A, Thibault B, Crepeau J, Lam JY, Bilodeau L. Percutaneous mitral valve annuloplasty for ischemic mitral regurgitation: first in man experience with a temporary implant. Catheter Cardiovasc Interv. 2007;69(7):1053–61.

37. Machaalany J, St-Pierre A, Senechal M, Larose E, Philippon F, Abdelaal E, Charbonneau E, Dagenais F, Trahan S, Bertrand OF. Fatal late migration of viacor percutaneous transvenous mitral annuloplasty device resulting in distal coronary venous perforation. Can J Cardiol. 2013;29(1):130 e1–4.

38. Piazza N, Bonan R. Transcatheter mitral valve repair for functional mitral regurgitation: coronary sinus approach. J Interv Cardiol. 2007;20(6):495–508.

39. Siminiak T, Wu JC, Haude M, Hoppe UC, Sadowski J, Lipiecki J, Fajadet J, Shah AM, Feldman T, Kaye DM, Goldberg SL, Levy WC, Solomon SD, Reuter DG. Treatment of functional mitral regurgitation by percutaneous annuloplasty: results of the TITAN Trial. Eur J Heart Fail. 2012;14(8):931–8.

40. Siminiak T, Dankowski R, Baszko A, Lee C, Firek L, Kalmucki P, Szyszka A, Groothuis A. Percutaneous direct mitral annuloplasty using the Mitralign Bident system: description of the method and a case report. Kardiol Pol. 2013;71(12):1287–92.

41. Maisano F, La Canna G, Latib A, Denti P, Taramasso M, Kuck KH, Colombo A, Alfieri O, Guidotti A, Messika-Zeitoun D, Vahanian A. First-in-man transseptal implantation of a "surgical-like" mitral valve annuloplasty device for functional mitral regurgitation. J Am Coll Cardiol Intv. 2014;7(11):1326–8.

42. Raman J, Jagannathan R, Chandrashekar P, Sugeng L. Can we repair the mitral valve from outside the heart? A novel extra-cardiac approach to functional mitral regurgitation. Heart Lung Circ. 2011;20(3):157–62.

43. Palacios IF, Condado JA, Brandi S, Rodriguez V, Bosch F, Silva G, Low RI, Rogers JH. Safety and feasibility of acute percutaneous septal sinus shortening: first-in-human experience. Catheter Cardiovasc Interv. 2007;69(4):513–8.
44. Heuser RR, Witzel T, Dickens D, Takeda PA. Percutaneous treatment for mitral regurgitation: the QuantumCor system. J Interv Cardiol. 2008;21(2):178–82.
45. Jilaihawi H, Virmani R, Nakagawa H, Ducharme A, Shi YF, Carter-Monroe N, Ladich E, Iyer M, Ikeda A, Asgar A, Bonan R. Mitral annular reduction with subablative therapeutic ultrasound: pre-clinical evaluation of the ReCor device. EuroIntervention. 2010;6(1):54–62.
46. Taramasso M, Vanermen H, Maisano F, Guidotti A, La Canna G, Alfieri O. The growing clinical importance of secondary tricuspid regurgitation. J Am Coll Cardiol. 2012;59(8):703–10.
47. Schofer J, Bijuklic K, Tiburtius C, Hansen L, Groothuis A, Hahn RT. First-in-human transcatheter tricuspid valve repair in a patient with severely regurgitant tricuspid valve. J Am Coll Cardiol. 2015;65(12):1190–5.
48. Rogers T, Ratnayaka K, Sonmez M, Franson DN, Schenke WH, Mazal JR, Kocaturk O, Chen MY, Faranesh AZ, Lederman RJ. Transatrial intrapericardial tricuspid annuloplasty. J Am Coll Cardiol Intv. 2015;8(3):483–91.

Chapter 25
Percutaneous Tricuspid Repair Techniques

Samir R. Kapadia and Mohammad Qasim Raza

Introduction

Tricuspid valve (TV) disease has long been a forerunner in terms of medical and surgical management. It is the 3rd most-commonly performed valve surgery in the USA, trailing behind aortic and mitral [1]. Percutaneous repair techniques for tricuspid regurgitation (TR) are no exception to this sequence. Transcatheter aortic valve replacement (TAVR) is an established practice for aortic valve (AV) disease, and large trials for percutaneous mitral valve (MV) replacement/repair are well underway. Percutaneous tricuspid repair is now slowly but surely making promising developments. The prevalence of moderate-severe TR is about 1.6 million people, even though a mere 0.5 % (less than 8000) of them get treatment (Fig. 25.1) [2, 3]. TR patients are undertreated by a factor of 4 when compared to MR patients of the same grade, despite the fact that it causes significant symptoms [3, 4]. Persistent and progressive TR can result in reduced cardiac output, eventual symptoms of right heart failure, and overall reduced quality of life [4]. About 80 % of TR is functional, i.e., either secondary to left heart disease or in the setting of RV remodeling from volume/pressure overload leading to annular dilation and leaflet tethering [5, 6]. The remaining 10–20 % are primary disorders of the TV as shown in Tables 25.1 and 25.2 [7].

Regardless of the type, the impact of TR on patient prognosis and clinical condition cannot be ignored [8]. Earlier concepts of TR automatically resolving after left heart surgery are not entirely true [8–10] because the tricuspid annulus is not as robust as its mitral counterpart; it tends to not return to its former shape after relief of overload [6]. For this reason, both old and new guidelines recommend concurrent treatment of TR when performing left heart surgery [6, 11]. Dreyfus recommended "prophylactic" tricuspid annuloplasty when patients undergoing left heart repair

S.R. Kapadia, MD, FACC (✉) • M.Q. Raza, MD
Department of Cardiovascular Medicine, Cleveland Clinic Hospital,
9500 Euclid Avenue, Cleveland, OH 44195, USA
e-mail: kapadis@ccf.org; razam3@ccf.org

© Springer Science+Business Media New York 2016
G. Ailawadi, I.L. Kron (eds.), *Catheter Based Valve and Aortic Surgery*,
DOI 10.1007/978-1-4939-3432-4_25

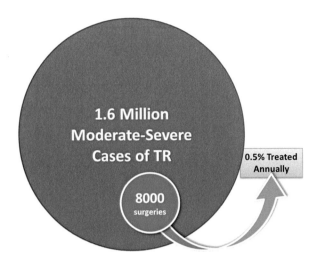

Fig. 25.1 Tricuspid regurgitation patients are vastly undertreated [2, 3]

Table 25.1 Primary causes of tricuspid regurgitation

Organic	Traumatic
Congenital	Blunt chest wall trauma
Ebstein's anomaly	RV endomyocardial biopsy-related trauma
Valve prolapse	RV pacemaker/ICD lead interference
Valve dysplasia/hypoplasia	
Acquired	
Rheumatic disease	
Carcinoid disease	
Drugs (e.g., fenfluramine-phentermine)	
Endomyocardial fibrosis	
Infectious endocarditis	
Radiation exposure	

RV right ventricle, *RH* right heart, *ICD* implantable cardioverter defibrillatory

Table 25.2 Secondary (functional) causes of tricuspid regurgitation

Left-sided heart failure
Mitral stenosis/regurgitation
Right ventricular ischemia
Atrial fibrillation
LTR shunts (e.g., ASD, VSD)
Primary pulmonary disease (e.g., CP, PE, PHTN)
Right atrial myxomas
Hyperthyroidism

LTR left-to-right, *ASD* atrial septal defect, *VSD* ventricular septal defect developed progressive TV dysfunction because their enlarged tricuspid annulus was left uncorrected (Fig. 25.1) [12].

However, not all left heart repairs can be a 100 % successful, nor can the patients be disease-free indefinitely [13, 14]; thus preexisting TR may persist. Indeed, isolated TR is being observed more frequently in spite of normal left heart function after MV annuloplasty or replacement [8]. While ≤1+ TR may not be concerning, ≥2+ TR is associated with significantly worse prognoses as it tends to persist and progress (Fig. 25.2) [7, 8, 10].

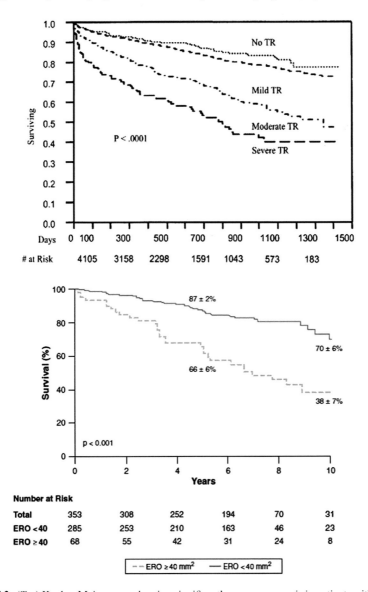

Fig. 25.2 (*Top*) Kaplan-Meier curve showing significantly worse prognosis in patients with moderate and severe TR [7]. (*Bottom*) Kaplan-Meier curve showing low survival in patients with isolate TR and severely increased effective regurgitant orifice (ERO) [15]

The need for percutaneous TV repair is rapidly increasing. Severe TR, whether managed medically or surgically, carries poor prognosis and high risks of postoperative morbidity and mortality [7, 16]. Prohibitively high mortality rates of 35 % and 22 % have been reported for redo TV surgeries or TV surgery concurrent with the aortic/mitral valve, respectively [17, 18]. Thus percutaneous techniques for TR offer an attractive alternative for such high-risk patients who would otherwise have limited chances at survival [19].

Functional Anatomy

The anatomy and pathophysiology of valvular heart disease are deeply inter-twined; one cannot be understood without the other [20]. The tricuspid valve (TV) complex is found somewhat inferiorly and anterolateral to the left side, angulated at about 45° to the sagittal plane [19]. It is a conglomerate of the tricuspid annulus (TA), leaflets, papillary muscles, and associated chordae tendineae, all working synchronously. Valvular dysfunction is a consequence of disruption in this synchrony (Fig. 25.3).

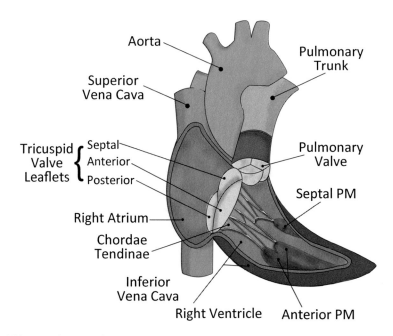

Fig. 25.3 The tricuspid valve with its leaflets, chordae tendinea, and septal muscles

Annulus

Located at the junction of the right atrium (RA) and right ventricle (RV) is the TA. This is not quite the definable fibrous ring of its mitral counterpart, but it is still identifiable [21]. From an atrial perspective, it forms an almost oval structure with a triangular orifice, spanning a diameter of about 40 ± 7 mm and an area of 10 ± 3 cm [2, 21–23]. Anchored along the annulus are three tricuspid leaflets.

The most fibrous part of the annulus is where its relation with the membranous septum and the aortic valve offers increased stability, while several points peripherally only have fibroadipose tissue separating the RA and RV [19, 24]. This precludes the TA from being as robust as the mitral annulus which, in contrast, has much more fibrous tissue support from the right and left fibrous trigones.

From a 3-dimensional perspective, the TA forms a non-planar shape, with two points (anteroposterior) oriented superiorly toward the right atrium and two (mediolateral) oriented inferiorly toward the right ventricular apex. The highest point on the TA is the anteroseptal segment which lies closest to the RV outflow tract and is adjacent to the AV (Fig. 25.4) [25, 26].

In the course of the cardiac cycle, the TA undergoes significant changes in size owing to forces originating from the RA and RV [27, 28]. The end of the p-wave (late diastole) marks the largest annular size, with the smallest observed at mid-systole [25, 28, 29]. This implies that the TA is similar to the mitral annulus in function, i.e., it aids leaflet coaptation during systole and provides a conduit for ventricular filling during diastole.

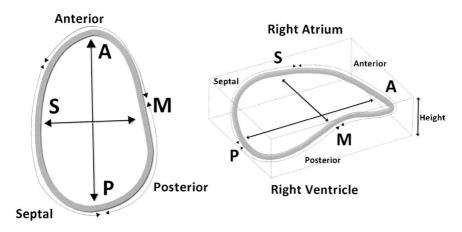

Fig. 25.4 Reconstruction of the tricuspid annulus' non-planar structure. *A* anterior, *P* posterior, *M* medial, *S* septal

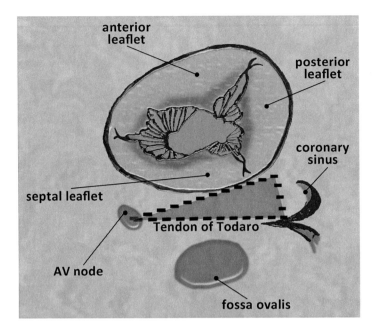

Fig. 25.5 Anatomic associations of the tricuspid valve and the triangle of Koch (*red*)

Tricuspid Leaflets

The tricuspid annulus anchors three leaflets—classically named the anterior, posterior, and septal—that descend into the right ventricle like a curtain [23]. They are of unequal sizes, with the anterior being the largest of the three and also the more mobile [22, 30]. The smallest septal leaflet predominantly arises directly from the septal wall and runs parallel to the interventricular septum, while the posterior leaflet arises from the free wall [22, 23, 31]. The septal leaflet also forms one of the boundaries of the *Triangle of Koch*, an important landmark in the right atrium. The triangle's apex points to the location of the AV node. Other structures contributing to the triangle are the coronary sinus at the base and the tendon of Todaro at the side (Fig. 25.5) [4, 24].

Three commissures, namely, the anteroposterior, anteroseptal, and posteroseptal, produce deep indentations in leaflet tissue creating a roughly triangular orifice [24]. The posterior leaflet forms the base of the orifice, while the rest of the area is occupied by the anterior and septal leaflets [22, 23]. The undersurface of the leaflets is tethered to the right ventricular wall with the assistance of chordae tendinea and papillary muscles.

As with the tricuspid annulus, the mobility of the tricuspid leaflets during the course of the cardiac cycle is a product of different forces acting upon them. The reduction of annular size during systole leads to adequate leaflet coaptation and closure. Similarly, diastolic expansion of the annulus leads to opening of the tricuspid orifice [31, 32].

Papillary Muscles and Chordae Tendinea

Three papillary muscle groups lie beneath the three commissures and support the tricuspid leaflets [23, 30]. When compared to the left heart, their spacing, number, and size may not be as constant [24, 31]. The anterior papillary muscle is the largest, most well-defined of the group and sends chordae to anterior and posterior leaflets along with the anteroposterior commissure. The medial or septal PM arises from the septal band of the crista supraventricularis, and its chordae give support to the anterior and septal leaflets along with the anteroseptal commissure. These chordae may on occasion arise from the septal wall itself. The posterior PM is of inconstant size and shape and arises from the ventricular muscle just beneath the posteroseptal commissure, which is where its chordae insert [19, 23, 32].

The chordae and papillary muscles experience dynamic changes during the cardiac cycle and work in harmony with the rest of the tricuspid valve complex. Chordal lengthening and straightening occurs during systole as papillary muscles undergo a combination of contraction and torsion [32]. The tension in chordae has been found to be vital in maintaining coaptation of leaflets and preventing prolapse [33]. This is followed by relaxation of both structures in diastole.

Mechanisms of Tricuspid Regurgitation

As mentioned earlier, the etiology of tricuspid regurgitation is predominantly secondary or functional, with primary causes accounting for about 10–20 % of the population [6, 7]. Primary causes can be organic or traumatic, such as in the case of Ebstein's anomaly or road traffic accidents leading to blunt chest wall trauma. The regurgitation in these valves is a result of intrinsic valve abnormality that limits adequate leaflet coaptation during systole. One such contributor to primary TR, an ICD/pacemaker wire in the RV, has been subject to considerable debate in the past. Abundant evidence is available both for [34] and against [35] its impact on TR. A recently published study [36] involving around 1600 patients demonstrated that cardiac device implantation was indeed associated with an increase in prevalence of moderate and severe TR. Post-implantation TR was also an independent risk factor for late death ($p \leq 0.05$), hence demonstrating an increased risk of mortality. Multiple mechanisms have been described for this phenomenon [37], such as the device lead causing valve obstruction, annular dilation, leaflet entrapment/laceration, or scarring and fibrosis leading to inadequate closure (Fig. 25.6).

Secondary or functional tricuspid regurgitation occurs in cases where the valve complex itself is intrinsically normal. The most common cause is left-sided heart disease such as mitral regurgitation which leads to rising left atrial pressures that travel back to the right heart via the pulmonary vasculature [39]. It is characterized by RV dilation, distortion of TA shape, tethering of leaflets, and eventual volume overload which all culminate into a vicious and self-perpetuating cycle. This concept is elucidated in Fig. 25.7. A critical point made by many studies regarding TA dilation

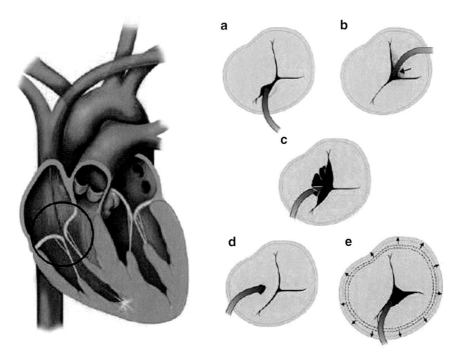

Fig. 25.6 Mechanisms of TR associated with ICD/PPM lead placement: (**a**) leaflet obstruction, (**b**) leaflet scarring, (**c**) lead entrapment, (**d**) valve perforation, and (**e**) annular dilation [38]

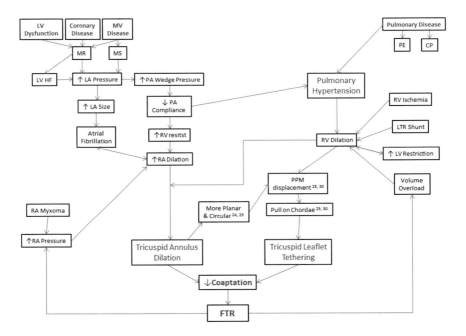

Fig. 25.7 Mechanism of functional tricuspid regurgitation

is that it is asymmetric and more so along the free posterior wall that has least fibrous support tissue [19, 25, 28, 40]. Understanding of the mechanism of secondary TR is a crucial step toward innovation of percutaneous techniques to treat it.

Diagnostic Studies for Tricuspid Valve Disease

Clinical evaluation of severe tricuspid regurgitation is fairly simple considering the most prominent symptoms are those of right heart failure. These may include initial shortness of breath which progresses over time to peripheral edema, cachexia, and ascites. Imaging modalities have enabled the detection of TR in its earlier, more manageable grades.

The non-planar structure of the tricuspid valve precludes it from being completely visualized by imaging methods such as 2D echocardiography. However, 2D TTE (transthoracic echocardiography) combined with color flow Doppler is the current recommendation for assessing cause and severity of TR along with any RV or associated LV dysfunction [6, 41]. These are highly sensitive modalities that allow detection of trivial-mild TR in 80–90 % of patients [31]. The proximity of tricuspid valvular structures to the chest wall may give rise to geometric constraints which may be overcome in some cases with the use of TEE (transesophageal echocardiography) [42, 43]. A comparison between normal and valve pathology (flail) is shown in Figs. 25.8 and 25.9.

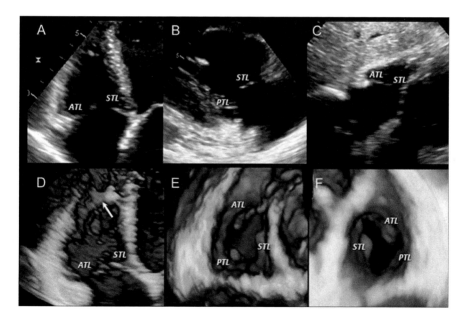

Fig. 25.8 Different echocardiographic views of the heart in 2D (*top*) and 3D (*bottom*): (**a**) apical four-chamber; (**b**) right ventricular inflow; (**c**) subcostal; (**d**) apical four-chamber (with *arrow* pointing to moderator band); (**e**) en face from right ventricle and (**f**) from right atrium. *ATL* anterior tricuspid leaflet, *PTL* posterior tricuspid leaflet, *STL* septal tricuspid leaflet [31]

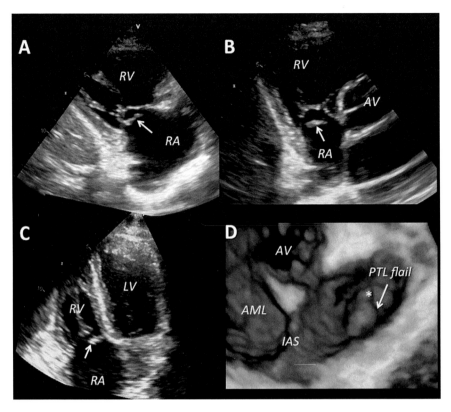

Fig. 25.9 Flail of posterior tricuspid leaflet assessed with different views (*arrows* point at the flail leaflet): (**a**) Parasternal long-axis; (**b**) Parasternal short-axis; (**c**) Apical four-chamber; (**d**) 3D Atrial (or surgical) view; *RA* right atrium, *RV* right ventricle, *AV* aortic valve, *LV* left ventricle, *AML* anterior mitral leaflet, *PTL* posterior tricuspid leaflet, *IAS* interatrial septum

Suboptimal images from 2D methods may require supplementation with more elaborate imaging such as the real-time 3D echocardiogram or the cardiac MR. Both these modalities provide an accurate assessment of RV dysfunction, annular dilation, and leaflet tethering [6, 44].

Invasive imaging and measurements are usually reserved to assess pulmonary artery pressures and pulmonary vascular resistance when there is a discrepancy between TTE, ECG, and physical exam data. These techniques are rarely, if ever, utilized for diagnosis or grading of TR.

Percutaneous Techniques

Historical Perspective

Percutaneous techniques have evolved over the past decade. Some of the earliest animal studies were by Boudjemline et al. [45] who used a disk-based nitinol stent housing a tricuspid valve made of bovine pericardium. A transcatheter approach was used to successfully implant the stent in the tricuspid position in 7 out of 8 ewes. Bai et al. [46] used a unidirectional valve made of porcine pericardium mounted onto a nitinol ring and assembled on a nitinol stent. The stent was percutaneously implanted and successfully reduced TR in 8 out of 10 sheep. Zegdi et al. [47] reported their endovascular valve replacement experience with a self-expanding nitinol stent bearing a porcine aortic valve. The valved stent was repositionable owing to the compression or relaxation mechanism of the stent.

Greenberg et al. [43] pioneered one of the first-in-human transcatheter valve implantation for tricuspid valve disease. Commercially available materials were used to construct a novel device at the Cleveland Clinic. It was placed in the inferior vena cava first for compassionate use in a patient with severe biventricular failure and radiation-induced heart disease, to prevent organ damage from elevated right-sided pressures. The patient experienced significant symptomatic improvement, and thereafter it was implanted into the SVC as well, with the patient continuing to improve on follow-up.

Current Developments

There have been many breakthroughs in the percutaneous management of MV disease over the past 5 years, systematically targeting components of the mitral valve complex. To name a few, the MitraClip™ (Abbott Laboratories, Abbott Park, Illinois) for leaflet repair, the Cardioband™ (Valtech Cardio Ltd, Or-Yehuda, Israel) for annular repair, and the BACE [48] device for external wall remodeling.

Unfortunately, significant differences exist between the atrioventricular junctions of the right and left heart and the same devices cannot be used to treat TR. For instance, the MV enjoys a convenient approach from the coronary sinus which is utilized by percutaneous annuloplasty devices like the Carillon™ device (Cardiac Dimensions, Kirkland, WA). In contrast, lying adjacent to the TV are the AV node, CS ostium, and other structures that must not be compressed or blocked. The design and approach of percutaneous devices are further limited due to potential for creating device-associated TR due to leaflet entrapment and annular dilation [37].

Nonetheless, novel percutaneous devices and techniques for TR in different developmental stages are arising and are discussed in Table 25.3.

Table 25.3 Percutaneous techniques in managing tricuspid valve disease

Technique	Developmental phase
Orthotopic TC valve-in-valve implantation	Human case reports/case series
Heterotopic TC valve implantation	Human case reports
Bicaval valve implantation	FIH procedure performed
TC valve implantation at native valve	FIH procedure performed
The tricuspid valve occluder device (CCF, Cleveland, OH)	Animal studies
The TRAIPTA device (National Institutes of Health, Bethesda, MD)	Animal studies
The Mitralign device (Mitralign Inc., Boston, MA)	FIH procedure performed
The TriCinch device (4Tech Inc., Waltham, MA)	Human trial (PREVENT) ongoing

TC transcatheter, *TRAIPTA* transatrial intrapericardial tricuspid annuloplasty, *FIH* first-in-human, *CCF* Cleveland Clinic Foundation

Transcatheter Tricuspid Valve-in-Valve Implantation

As mentioned earlier, primary surgical repair for tricuspid disease carries high rates of postoperative mortality and morbidity. Additionally, patients with failure of previously placed prostheses in the tricuspid position that require a redo procedure are also significantly high-risk. Transcatheter valve-in-valve (ViV) procedures are emerging as an attractive field for failed prosthetic valves [49]. While reducing the surgical burden, they also avoid removal of failing bioprosthesis, a maneuver that carries significant risk of damaging surrounding cardiac structures [50]. This technique has been well-established for aortic, pulmonary, and mitral positions [51]. As far as employing it for the tricuspid position is concerned, data at present are scarce and limited to mostly case reports or a few case series [52, 53]. The core concept, pioneered by Boudjemline et al. [45] through animal studies, is essentially unchanged (Fig. 25.10).

Transcatheter ViV technique can be technically challenging as it involves factoring in of several details once a patient has been deemed inoperable:

The Type, Size, and Radiological Positioning of the Previously Placed Prosthetic Valve

The internal and external diameters and positioning of the failed bioprosthesis are a crucial starting point for the ViV technique, impacting the kind of valve that will eventually be used. Tricuspid prostheses are known to develop TS, TR, or a combination of disease [51]. In cases of TS, balloon sizing may be necessary to ascertain the best valve size to use along with the optimal position for placing the valve [54].

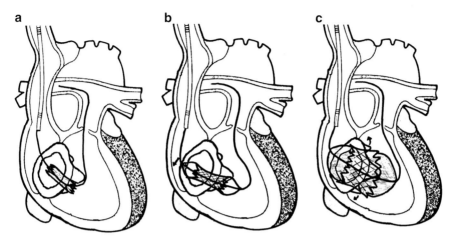

Fig. 25.10 Schematic illustrations showing (**a**) a stiff wire in the right pulmonary artery and a SAPIEN valve advanced into a tricuspid prosthesis; (**b**) partial inflation of the balloon and wire readjustment; (**c**) full inflation of the balloon to place the valve in its final position [50]

Access Route Selection

After the first-in-human percutaneous tricuspid ViV implantation experience by Van Garsse et al. [55] using the right internal jugular vein, many other approaches have also been explored. These include the more familiar but potentially more challenging transfemoral [38, 56], transatrial, and transapical [57]. All of these have been shown to have more or less equal benefit [52], as long as the choice is made keeping in consideration individual patient needs and the expertise of the operator. Our own ViV implantation experience with one patient involved an initial transjugular route which resulted in the slow migration of the valve toward the ventricle [38]. A decision to place a second valve was made using the transfemoral approach for fear of completely dislodging the first valve if the transjugular approach was again used. The procedure was successful with the valve being stable in its position and no paravalvular leak.

Valve Selection

So far there are two stented valves that have been studied for use in tricuspid ViV procedures: the Melody® (Medtronic, Inc., Minneapolis, MN) and the SAPIEN (Edwards Lifesciences Corp., Irvine, CA).

As cited earlier, the first-in-human ViV implantation in the tricuspid position was performed using an Edwards SAPIEN valve. Since then, reports demonstrating the use of both the Melody [58, 59] and Edwards SAPIEN [60, 61] valves have been documented. Not unlike the various implantation approaches, these valves offer no superiority of one over the other [52, 53, 62] and have both been used with considerable success. They do however have differences in their inherent design which can serve as a guide when making the most appropriate selection for patients.

The Edwards SAPIEN is a balloon-expandable valve with a metal stent frame housing bovine pericardium. It is shorter in length than the Melody and goes up to an expanded external diameter of 29 mm [51, 58]. In contrast, the Melody is made of bovine jugular venous valve tissue mounted on to a platinum-iridium stent scaffold, delivered using a balloon-in-balloon system [51]. It is longer but goes up to a maximum diameter of 22 mm [52].

The Edwards SAPIEN has the ability to go to larger diameters and thus may cater to an increasing number of patients, but the small length of the stent may make positioning a challenge, along with an increased risk of embolization [49]. On the other hand, while Melody is limited by its maximum diameter, it was designed to be used in the pulmonary circulation, and its balloon-in-balloon delivery system may facilitate repositioning at the time of implantation [51]. The longer length also facilitates better coaxial alignments and allows coverage of the entire prosthetic valve [54].

With no long-term trials projecting one valve's superiority over the other, and evidence based on case series [52, 53], it can be concluded that these valves are best used when complementing each other.

Presenting

Presenting, as the name suggests, is placing a bare-metal stent in the tricuspid position as a means of creating a radiologically visible "landing zone" for when the valve is introduced [49, 51]. It also provides radial strength and reduces the risk of valve fracture in the case of some valves. This risk may be avoidable in most cases when the valve is being place within the frame of a prosthesis [59]. Other reports have mentioned that presenting is not always necessary [60, 62]; hence a decision must be made on a case-to-case basis.

Pacing

One of the final aspects to consider is rapid pacing, which is when a pacemaker wire, placed in the left ventricle or coronary sinus, is used during balloon inflation. Reports have shown that this is not always necessary, but the Edwards SAPIEN valve may require pacing for adequate positioning [55, 56, 62]. One report described that due to the patient's low pressure system, slow heart rate, and minimal cardiac motion, the decision to not pace outweighed any potential benefits [61].

Transcatheter tricuspid valve-in-valve (TCTVIV) is a growing field, providing therapy to patients of all age groups with favorable outcomes. However complications such as endocarditis, heart block, and on occasion death have been reported [49, 52, 53]. On an average, many the patients receiving ViV implantation are young, with few comorbidities. As long-term follow-up data accumulate, the durability of this procedure can be assessed [63].

TCTVIV Implantation in Native Tricuspid Valve

TCTVIV implantation is becoming a reliable alternative for patients with failed prostheses, but very little progress has been made in implanting a valved stent over the native TV. To date, the first-in-human report of such a procedure is by Kefer et al. [64]. The case is of a 47-year-old female with multiple valve repairs and replacements, including three tricuspid repairs, none of which resulted in the placement of a prosthetic ring or valve. Hence the procedure bore several challenges including the absence of radiological landmarks, a rigid anchor site, and difficulty in annulus measurement. Prestenting was done to create a landing zone where an Edwards SAPIEN valve was eventually deployed. Owing to a paravalvular leak, a second SAPIEN valve was then implanted to achieve optimal reduction of both stenosis and regurgitation. The clinical and echocardiographic follow-up of this patient at 5 months has been good.

This experience may be the foundation for future tricuspid counterparts of mitral valve replacements such as the Edwards FORTIS® and Neovasc TIARA® (Neovasc Inc., Richmond, BC).

Heterotopic Transcatheter Valve Implantation

Davidson et al. [65] first proposed transcatheter valve implantation in the central venous system, a technique known as *heterotopic* valve implantation. This is in contrast to the previous discussion about TCTVIV, which is a form of *orthotopic* valve implantation (i.e., at the tricuspid position). Placement of self-expanding valves into the SVC and IVC reduces regurgitation of blood in the central venous system, thereby protecting distal organs from the damaging effects of right-sided heart failure. The first animal model where this approach was utilized showed favorable results. TR was created artificially in thirteen sheep and cardiac output (CO) went down from a baseline of 5.15 L/min to about 3.0. Post-procedure on acute examination of 9 sheep, an increase of CO to 4.2±0.84 L/min was noted. Chronic follow-up of 4 animals showed no decrease in hemodynamic parameters [66].

After demonstrating feasibility in an animal model, the first-in-human procedure was performed on a compassionate basis for a 79-year-old female with severe functional TR [67]. Initial presentation was with symptoms of right-sided heart failure including peripheral edema, ascites, and New York Heart Association stage-IV dyspnea. Her significant comorbidities and earlier open-heart surgeries precluded her from reoperation. A self-expanding percutaneous heart valve was custom-made to be placed into the IVC such that the upper segment protruded into the RA and the lower segment could be anchored into the IVC. The diameter was tailored to the dimensions of the anticipated landing zone using a CT angiogram. The valve was implanted via a transfemoral approach under fluoroscopic and echocardiographic guidance. Post-procedure the patient showed almost immediate hemodynamic improvement including IVC pressure going down from 29/19 mmHg to 19/12 mmHg. Within 8 weeks of follow-up, NYHA class went from IV to III, and valve function remained consistent.

Bicaval Valve-in-Valve Implantation

Following caval valve implantation (CAVI) for TR in the IVC, the bicaval first-in-human procedure was performed on an octogenarian female with a similar case presentation, including severe functional TR and NYHA stage-IV symptoms [68]. Right heart catheterization revealed elevated pressures in the IVC, SVC, and RA. Two self-expanding custom-made percutaneous stents were simultaneously implanted into the SVC and then the IVC via the transfemoral route. Post-procedural hemodynamics showed decrease in IVC and SVC pressures from 28/19 mmHg to 16/14 mmHg and 27/14 mmHg to 21/13 mmHg, respectively. CO increased from 3.9 to 4.2 L/min. More strikingly however, there was pronounced improvement in the patient's heart failure symptoms. NYHA class went from IV to II–III and overall improvement in physical capacity. At 12-month follow-up, the patient remained in NYHA class II and had no clinical signs of right heart failure. The valve showed sustained functioning and continued improvement in hemodynamics.

The Tricuspid Valve Occluder Device

The tricuspid valve occluder (Cleveland Clinic Foundation, Cleveland, OH) is a novel device for the treatment of functional regurgitation of the tricuspid valve (Fig. 25.11). It is positioned across the enlarged TV orifice where it acts as a bridge between

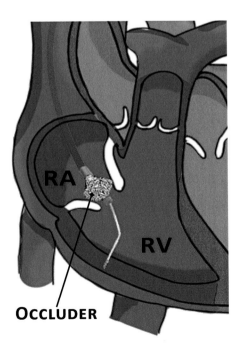

Fig. 25.11 Tricuspid valve occluder device increasing surface area for coaptation between tricuspid leaflets

leaflets. It provides leaflets an additional surface to coapt with and, in doing so, also reduces the regurgitant orifice. The device enters the TV orifice through the transjugular route while the proximal end lies subcutaneous, similar to a pacemaker wire. The degree of occlusion is adjustable by manipulating controls at the proximal end.

The device is currently undergoing animal studies. Severe TR (4+) was created manually in 2 swine and the device was successfully implanted via the transjugular approach. Postoperative reduction of TR to moderate (4+ to 2+) was achieved after which the animals were sacrificed.

The Trans-Atrial Intrapericardial Tricuspid Annuloplasty Device (TRAIPTA)

The TRAIPTA (National Institutes of Health, Bethesda, MD) is another novel device for treating functional TR via an indirect annuloplasty (Fig. 25.12) [69]. The rationale is similar to that of the CARILLON® device (Cardiac Dimensions, Kirkland, WA) for treating functional MR. The device takes a transfemoral route and then punctures through the right atrial appendage, allowing it to enter pericardial space. The device encircles the heart in the atrioventricular groove within the pericardial space and is then tightened to modify the geometry of the tricuspid annulus. So far, this is the first extracardiac structural intervention achieving a degree of tricuspid annuloplasty comparable to surgical techniques.

Currently, the device is in the preclinical phase. Fifteen swine with functional TR underwent successful extracardiac tricuspid annuloplasty resulting in a 53 % increase in tricuspid leaflet coaptation length ($p \leq 0.001$) and reduction in annular area by 59 % ($p \leq 0.001$). Small pericardial effusions were noticed immediately post-procedure but had resolved on follow-up.

Fig. 25.12 The transatrial intrapericardial tricuspid annuloplasty (TRAIPTA) device for extracardiac annuloplasty [69]

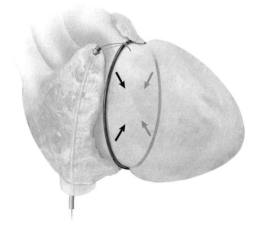

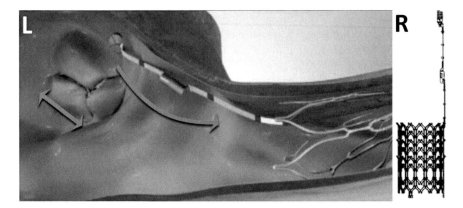

Fig. 25.13 The TriCinch device (R), decreasing septo-lateral dimension of the TV and fixated with a stent in the IVC (L)

The 4Tech TriCinch

The TriCinch device (4Tech Inc., Waltham, MA) is a percutaneous variant of a clinically proven surgical tricuspid repair technique. The Kay repair [70] remodels the tricuspid valve on a commissural level, converting it from tricuspid to bicuspid, and also reduces annular size (Fig. 25.13). Using a venous transfemoral access, the device is guided through a 24Fr sheath under fluoroscopic and echocardiographic guidance. A fixation element is implanted into the anterior annulus between the anteroposterior commissure and the mid-anterior annulus, where it acts as an anchor. The attached system is tensioned under echocardiographic guidance to reshape the TV and increase leaflet coaptation length. Finally a stent is deployed in the IVC to fixate the cinch. Initial safety and feasibility studies with 31 adult swine showed 100 % successful device implantation with favorable results: a 30 % reduction in septo-lateral dimensions (35.5 ± 6 mm to 24.6 ± 5 mm) and a 70 % increase in tricuspid coaptation length (4.55 ± 0.7 mm to 7.78 ± 1.3 mm).

The PREVENT trial is the first-in-human trial on this novel technique, working out of 3 different sites with a targeted total of 24 patients. The first successful human implant was in a 72-year-old female with severe (4+) TR, enlarged annulus, and increased anteroseptal coaptation gap. Post-implant, the TR was decreased to moderate (2+) and coaptation length increased from none to 5 mm. The patient continues to show clinical improvement at 1-month follow-up.

The Mitralign System

The Mitralign System for functional TR (Mitralign Inc., Boston, MA) aims to more directly mimic the aforementioned surgical Kay bicuspidization procedure. A wire delivery catheter is advanced through the transjugular route and across the tricuspid valve (Fig. 25.14).

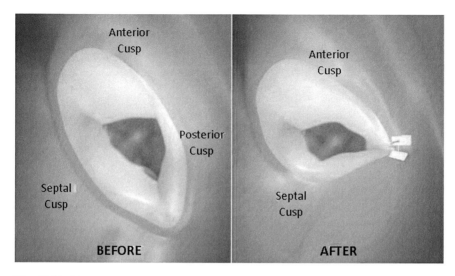

Fig. 25.14 The tricuspid valve, before and after bicuspidization procedure with the Mitralign device

Two pledgets functioning as anchors are placed at the posteroanterior and septo-anterior commissures and then cinched together. This essentially obliterates the posterior leaflet, leaving behind a functional bicuspid valve with a septal and anterior cusp.

Animal studies showed favorable results and the first-in-human procedure was reported recently. The patient was an 89-year-old female with recurrent cardiac decompensation due to severe TR and signs and symptoms of severe RV dysfunction. Her clinical state precluded her from surgery, and the decision to proceed with percutaneous management was made. Pledget placement and plication was successful and postoperative hemodynamics revealed decrease in RA pressure (22 mmHg to 9 mmHg) and increase in LV stroke volume (42 ml to 72 ml).

Conclusion

The tricuspid is no longer the "forgotten" valve that it once was. The development of novel percutaneous techniques in the management of tricuspid valve diseases has been on the rise for the past decade. This is primarily because interventional cardiology is intimately associated with advances in technology, allowing it to evolve rapidly. As the TAVR and MitraClip procedures for aortic and mitral valve become more commonplace, the impact of TR on these is becoming more prominent. This has led to a further growth in interest in developing techniques to manage the disease for a cohort of patients that is already deemed too frail to receive invasive procedures. Nonetheless managing tricuspid regurgitation percutaneously remains a challenging task owing to the valve's location, anatomy, and the overall environment of the right heart. The novel techniques that have been developed so far are in their infancy but are gaining momentum. Their efficacy will increase over time with the learning curve, and additional training and skill sets may be needed to achieve the best results. At this moment, it would be judicious to say that all the steps are in the right direction and that the percutaneous management of TR may become a concurrent procedure while treating other valves.

References

1. Kilic A, Saha-Chaudhuri P, Rankin JS, Conte JV. Trends and outcomes of tricuspid valve surgery in north america: an analysis of more than 50,000 patients from the society of thoracic surgeons database. Ann Thorac Surg. 2013;96:1546–52. discussion 1552.
2. Singh JP, Evans JC, Levy D, Larson MG, Freed LA, Fuller DL, Lehman B, Benjamin EJ. Prevalence and clinical determinants of mitral, tricuspid, and aortic regurgitation (the Framingham heart study). Am J Cardiol. 1999;83:897–902.
3. Stuge O, Liddicoat J. Emerging opportunities for cardiac surgeons within structural heart disease. J Thorac Cardiovasc Surg. 2006;132:1258–61.
4. Rogers JH, Bolling SF. The tricuspid valve: current perspective and evolving management of tricuspid regurgitation. Circulation. 2009;119:2718–25.
5. Chan KM, Zakkar M, Amirak E, Punjabi PP. Tricuspid valve disease: pathophysiology and optimal management. Prog Cardiovasc Dis. 2009;51:482–6.
6. Nishimura RA, Otto CM, Bonow RO, Carabello BA, Erwin III JP, Guyton RA, O'Gara PT, Ruiz CE, Skubas NJ, Sorajja P, Sundt III TM, Thomas JD. 2014 aha/acc guideline for the management of patients with valvular heart disease: executive summary: a report of the american college of cardiology/american heart association task force on practice guidelines. J Am Coll Cardiol. 2014;63:2438–88.
7. Nath J, Foster E, Heidenreich PA. Impact of tricuspid regurgitation on long-term survival. J Am Coll Cardiol. 2004;43:405–9.
8. Antunes MJ, Barlow JB. Management of tricuspid valve regurgitation. Heart. 2007;93: 271–6.
9. Braunwald NS, Ross Jr J, Morrow AG. Conservative management of tricuspid regurgitation in patients undergoing mitral valve replacement. Circulation. 1967;35:I63–9.
10. Goldstone AB, Howard JL, Cohen JE, MacArthur Jr JW, Atluri P, Kirkpatrick JN, Woo YJ. Natural history of coexistent tricuspid regurgitation in patients with degenerative mitral valve disease: implications for future guidelines. J Thorac Cardiovasc Surg. 2014;148:2802–9.
11. Bonow RO, Carabello BA, Kanu C, de Leon Jr AC, Faxon DP, Freed MD, Gaasch WH, Lytle BW, Nishimura RA, O'Gara PT, O'Rourke RA, Otto CM, Shah PM, Shanewise JS, Smith Jr SC, Jacobs AK, Adams CD, Anderson JL, Antman EM, Fuster V, Halperin JL, Hiratzka LF, Hunt SA, Nishimura R, Page RL, Riegel B. Acc/aha 2006 guidelines for the management of patients with valvular heart disease: a report of the american college of cardiology/american heart association task force on practice guidelines (writing committee to revise the 1998 guidelines for the management of patients with valvular heart disease): developed in collaboration with the society of cardiovascular anesthesiologists: endorsed by the society for cardiovascular angiography and interventions and the society of thoracic surgeons. Circulation. 2006;114:e84–231.
12. Dreyfus GD, Corbi PJ, Chan KM, Bahrami T. Secondary tricuspid regurgitation or dilatation: which should be the criteria for surgical repair? Ann Thorac Surg. 2005;79:127–32.
13. Fedak PW, McCarthy PM, Bonow RO. Evolving concepts and technologies in mitral valve repair. Circulation. 2008;117:963–74.

14. Flameng W, Herijgers P, Bogaerts K. Recurrence of mitral valve regurgitation after mitral valve repair in degenerative valve disease. Circulation. 2003;107:1609–13.
15. Topilsky Y, Nkomo VT, Vatury O, Michelena HI, Letourneau T, Suri RM, Pislaru S, Park S, Mahoney DW, Biner S, Enriquez-Sarano M. Clinical outcome of isolated tricuspid regurgitation. JACC Cardiovasc Imaging. 2014;7:1185–94.
16. King RM, Schaff HV, Danielson GK, Gersh BJ, Orszulak TA, Piehler JM, Puga FJ, Pluth JR. Surgery for tricuspid regurgitation late after mitral valve replacement. Circulation. 1984;70:I193–7.
17. Bernal JM, Morales D, Revuelta C, Llorca J, Gutierrez-Morlote J, Revuelta JM. Reoperations after tricuspid valve repair. J Thorac Cardiovasc Surg. 2005;130:498–503.
18. Filsoufi F, Salzberg SP, Abascal V, Adams DH. Surgical management of functional tricuspid regurgitation with a new remodeling annuloplasty ring. Mt Sinai J Med. 2006;73:874–9.
19. Agarwal S, Tuzcu EM, Rodriguez ER, Tan CD, Rodriguez LL, Kapadia SR. Interventional cardiology perspective of functional tricuspid regurgitation. Circ Cardiovasc Interv. 2009;2:565–73.
20. Virmani R. The tricuspid valve. Mayo Clin Proc. 1988;63:943–6.
21. Taramasso M, Vanermen H, Maisano F, Guidotti A, La Canna G, Alfieri O. The growing clinical importance of secondary tricuspid regurgitation. J Am Coll Cardiol. 2012;59:703–10.
22. Anwar AM, Geleijnse ML, Soliman OI, McGhie JS, Frowijn R, Nemes A, van den Bosch AE, Galema TW, Ten Cate FJ. Assessment of normal tricuspid valve anatomy in adults by real-time three-dimensional echocardiography. Int J Cardiovasc Imaging. 2007;23:717–24.
23. Silver MD, Lam JH, Ranganathan N, Wigle ED. Morphology of the human tricuspid valve. Circulation. 1971;43:333–48.
24. Calafiore AM, Bartoloni G, Al Amri H, Iaco AL, Abukhudair W, Lanzaro BI, Di Mauro M. Functional tricuspid regurgitation and the right ventricle: What we do not know is more than we know. Expert Rev Cardiovasc Ther. 2012;10:1351–66.
25. Fukuda S, Saracino G, Matsumura Y, Daimon M, Tran H, Greenberg NL, Hozumi T, Yoshikawa J, Thomas JD, Shiota T. Three-dimensional geometry of the tricuspid annulus in healthy subjects and in patients with functional tricuspid regurgitation: a real-time, 3-dimensional echocardiographic study. Circulation. 2006;114:I492–8.
26. Ton-Nu TT, Levine RA, Handschumacher MD, Dorer DJ, Yosefy C, Fan D, Hua L, Jiang L, Hung J. Geometric determinants of functional tricuspid regurgitation: insights from 3-dimensional echocardiography. Circulation. 2006;114:143–9.
27. Miglioranza MH, Mihaila S, Muraru D, Cucchini U, Iliceto S, Badano LP. Dynamic changes in tricuspid annular diameter measurement in relation to the echocardiographic view and timing during the cardiac cycle. J Am Soc Echocardiogr. 2014.
28. Tei C, Pilgrim JP, Shah PM, Ormiston JA, Wong M. The tricuspid valve annulus: study of size and motion in normal subjects and in patients with tricuspid regurgitation. Circulation. 1982;66:665–71.
29. Tsakiris AG, Mair DD, Seki S, Titus JL, Wood EH. Motion of the tricuspid valve annulus in anesthetized intact dogs. Circ Res. 1975;36:43–8.
30. Badano LP, Agricola E, Perez de Isla L, Gianfagna P, Zamorano JL. Evaluation of the tricuspid valve morphology and function by transthoracic real-time three-dimensional echocardiography. Eur J Echocardiogr. 2009;10:477–84.
31. Badano LP, Muraru D, Enriquez-Sarano M. Assessment of functional tricuspid regurgitation. Eur Heart J. 2013;34:1875–85.
32. Fawzy H, Fukamachi K, Mazer CD, Harrington A, Latter D, Bonneau D, Errett L. Complete mapping of the tricuspid valve apparatus using three-dimensional sonomicrometry. J Thorac Cardiovasc Surg. 2011;141:1037–43.
33. He Z, Jowers C. A novel method to measure mitral valve chordal tension. J Biomech Eng. 2009;131:014501.
34. Kim JB, Spevack DM, Tunick PA, Bullinga JR, Kronzon I, Chinitz LA, Reynolds HR. The effect of transvenous pacemaker and implantable cardioverter defibrillator lead placement on tricuspid valve function: an observational study. J Am Soc Echocardiogr. 2008;21:284–7.

35. Kucukarslan N, Kirilmaz A, Ulusoy E, Yokusoglu M, Gramatnikovski N, Ozal E, Tatar H. Tricuspid insufficiency does not increase early after permanent implantation of pacemaker leads. J Card Surg. 2006;21:391–4.
36. Al-Bawardy R, Krishnaswamy A, Rajeswaran J, Bhargava M, Wazni O, Wilkoff B, Tuzcu EM, Martin D, Thomas J, Blackstone E, Kapadia S. Tricuspid regurgitation and implantable devices. Pacing Clin Electrophysiol. 2015;38(2):259–66.
37. Al-Bawardy R, Krishnaswamy A, Bhargava M, Dunn J, Wazni O, Tuzcu EM, Stewart W, Kapadia SR. Tricuspid regurgitation in patients with pacemakers and implantable cardiac defibrillators: a comprehensive review. Clin Cardiol. 2013;36:249–54.
38. Mick SL, Kapadia S, Tuzcu M, Svensson LG. Transcatheter valve-in-valve tricuspid valve replacement via internal jugular and femoral approaches. J Thorac Cardiovasc Surg. 2014;147:e64–5.
39. Navia JL, Nowicki ER, Blackstone EH, Brozzi NA, Nento DE, Atik FA, Rajeswaran J, Gillinov AM, Svensson LG, Lytle BW. Surgical management of secondary tricuspid valve regurgitation: annulus, commissure, or leaflet procedure? J Thorac Cardiovasc Surg. 2010;139:1473–82. e1475.
40. Spinner EM, Shannon P, Buice D, Jimenez JH, Veledar E, Del Nido PJ, Adams DH, Yoganathan AP. In vitro characterization of the mechanisms responsible for functional tricuspid regurgitation. Circulation. 2011;124:920–9.
41. Lancellotti P, Moura L, Pierard LA, Agricola E, Popescu BA, Tribouilloy C, Hagendorff A, Monin JL, Badano L, Zamorano JL. European association of echocardiography recommendations for the assessment of valvular regurgitation. Part 2: Mitral and tricuspid regurgitation (native valve disease). Eur J Echocardiogr. 2010;11:307–32.
42. Meluzin J, Spinarova L, Hude P, Krejci J, Kincl V, Panovsky R, Dusek L. Prognostic importance of various echocardiographic right ventricular functional parameters in patients with symptomatic heart failure. J Am Soc Echocardiogr. 2005;18:435–44.
43. Navia JL, Al-Ruzzeh S. Percutaneous valve technology: present and future. Hauppauge, NY: Nova Science; 2012.
44. De Castro S, Cavarretta E, Milan A, Caselli S, Di Angelantonio E, Vizza Carmine D, Lucchetti D, Patel A, Kuvin J, Pandian NG. Usefulness of tricuspid annular velocity in identifying global RV dysfunction in patients with primary pulmonary hypertension: a comparison with 3D echo-derived right ventricular ejection fraction. Echocardiography. 2008;25:289–93.
45. Boudjemline Y, Agnoletti G, Bonnet D, Behr L, Borenstein N, Sidi D, Bonhoeffer P. Steps toward the percutaneous replacement of atrioventricular valves an experimental study. J Am Coll Cardiol. 2005;46:360–5.
46. Bai Y, Zong GJ, Wang HR, Jiang HB, Wang H, Wu H, Zhao XX, Qin YW. An integrated pericardial valved stent special for percutaneous tricuspid implantation: an animal feasibility study. J Surg Res. 2010;160:215–21.
47. Zegdi R, Khabbaz Z, Borenstein N, Fabiani JN. A repositionable valved stent for endovascular treatment of deteriorated bioprostheses. J Am Coll Cardiol. 2006;48:1365–8.
48. Raman J, Jagannathan R, Chandrashekar P, Sugeng L. Can we repair the mitral valve from outside the heart? A novel extra-cardiac approach to functional mitral regurgitation. Heart Lung Circ. 2011;20:157–62.
49. Godart F, Baruteau AE, Petit J, Riou JY, Sassolas F, Lusson JR, Fraisse A, Boudjemline Y. Transcatheter tricuspid valve implantation: a multicentre french study. Arch Cardiovasc Dis. 2014;107:583–91.
50. Cerillo AG, Chiaramonti F, Murzi M, Bevilacqua S, Cerone E, Palmieri C, Del Sarto P, Mariani M, Berti S, Glauber M. Transcatheter valve in valve implantation for failed mitral and tricuspid bioprosthesis. Catheter Cardiovasc Interv. 2011;78:987–95.
51. Gurvitch R, Cheung A, Ye J, Wood DA, Willson AB, Toggweiler S, Binder R, Webb JG. Transcatheter valve-in-valve implantation for failed surgical bioprosthetic valves. J Am Coll Cardiol. 2011;58:2196–209.
52. Roberts PA, Boudjemline Y, Cheatham JP, Eicken A, Ewert P, McElhinney DB, Hill SL, Berger F, Khan D, Schranz D, Hess J, Ezekowitz MD, Celermajer D, Zahn E. Percutaneous tricuspid valve replacement in congenital and acquired heart disease. J Am Coll Cardiol. 2011;58:117–22.

53. Tzifa A, Momenah T, Al Sahari A, Al Khalaf K, Papagiannis J, Qureshi SA. Transcatheter valve-in-valve implantation in the tricuspid position. EuroIntervention. 2014;10:995–9.
54. Cullen MW, Cabalka AK, Alli OO, Pislaru SV, Sorajja P, Nkomo VT, Malouf JF, Cetta F, Hagler DJ, Rihal CS. Transvenous, antegrade melody valve-in-valve implantation for bioprosthetic mitral and tricuspid valve dysfunction: a case series in children and adults. JACC Cardiovasc Interv. 2013;6:598–605.
55. Van Garsse LA, Ter Bekke RM, van Ommen VG. Percutaneous transcatheter valve-in-valve implantation in stenosed tricuspid valve bioprosthesis. Circulation. 2011;123:e219–21.
56. Calvert PA, Himbert D, Brochet E, Radu C, Iung B, Hvass U, Darondel JM, Depoix JP, Nataf P, Vahanian A. Transfemoral implantation of an Edwards SAPIEN valve in a tricuspid bioprosthesis without fluoroscopic landmarks. EuroIntervention. 2012;7:1336–9.
57. Gaia DF, Palma JH, de Souza JA, Buffolo E. Tricuspid transcatheter valve-in-valve: an alternative for high-risk patients. Eur J Cardiothorac Surg. 2012;41:696–8.
58. Bhamidipati CM, Scott Lim D, Ragosta M, Ailawadi G. Percutaneous transjugular implantation of melody(r) valve into tricuspid bioprosthesis. J Card Surg. 2013;28:391–3.
59. Riede FT, Dahnert I. Implantation of a melody valve in tricuspid position. Catheter Cardiovasc Interv. 2012;80:474–6.
60. Kenny D, Hijazi ZM, Walsh KP. Transcatheter tricuspid valve replacement with the Edwards SAPIEN valve. Catheter Cardiovasc Interv. 2011;78:267–70.
61. Mortazavi A, Reul RM, Cannizzaro L, Dougherty KG. Transvenous transcatheter valve-in-valve implantation after bioprosthetic tricuspid valve failure. Tex Heart Inst J. 2014;41:507–10.
62. Raval J, Nagaraja V, Eslick GD, Denniss AR. Transcatheter valve-in-valve implantation: a systematic review of literature. Heart Lung Circ. 2014;23:1020–8.
63. Bapat V, Asrress KN. Transcatheter valve-in-valve implantation for failing prosthetic valves. EuroIntervention. 2014;10:900–2.
64. Kefer J, Sluysmans T, Vanoverschelde JL. Transcatheter SAPIEN valve implantation in a native tricuspid valve after failed surgical repair. Catheter Cardiovasc Interv. 2014;83:841–5.
65. Davidson MJ, White JK, Baim DS. Percutaneous therapies for valvular heart disease. Cardiovasc Pathol. 2006;15:123–9.
66. Lauten A, Figulla HR, Willich C, Laube A, Rademacher W, Schubert H, Bischoff S, Ferrari M. Percutaneous caval stent valve implantation: investigation of an interventional approach for treatment of tricuspid regurgitation. Eur Heart J. 2010;31:1274–81.
67. Lauten A, Ferrari M, Hekmat K, Pfeifer R, Dannberg G, Ragoschke-Schumm A, Figulla HR. Heterotopic transcatheter tricuspid valve implantation: first-in-man application of a novel approach to tricuspid regurgitation. Eur Heart J. 2011;32:1207–13.
68. Lauten A, Doenst T, Hamadanchi A, Franz M, Figulla HR. Percutaneous bicaval valve implantation for transcatheter treatment of tricuspid regurgitation: clinical observations and 12-month follow-up. Circ Cardiovasc Interv. 2014;7:268–72.
69. Rogers T, Ratnayaka K, Sonmez M, Franson DN, Schenke WH, Mazal JR, Kocaturk O, Chen MY, Faranesh AZ, Lederman RJ. Transatrial intrapericardial tricuspid annuloplasty. JACC Cardiovasc Interv. 2015;8:483–491
70. Ghanta RK, Chen R, Narayanasamy N, McGurk S, Lipsitz S, Chen FY, Cohn LH. Suture bicuspidization of the tricuspid valve versus ring annuloplasty for repair of functional tricuspid regurgitation: midterm results of 237 consecutive patients. J Thorac Cardiovasc Surg. 2007;133:117–26.

Index

A

Adjustable Annuloplasty Ring, 211
Adverse left ventricular remodeling, 251–254
  cardiac function and survival
    CABG, 251
    RESTORE group, 251
    STICH trial, 251
  cellular/pharmacologic therapies, 252
  cellular-based therapies, 251
  endoventricular circular patch plasty, 250
  myocardial infarction, 249
  PARACHUTE ventricular partitioning
    device, 252
  partitioning device
    echocardiography and imaging, 254
    PARACHUTE IV trial, 254
    percutaneous, 252–253
    success rate, 254
  percutaneous partitioning device
    PARACHUTE VPD device, 252
    static chamber, 252
  pharmacologic interventions, 250
  right anterior oblique angiographic
    image, 253
  surgical procedures, 250
  wall stress, 250
ALCAPA. *See* Anomalous left coronary artery
  from the pulmonary artery
  (ALCAPA)
Angiograms, 39, 41
Annuloplasty devices, 308–311
  direct annuloplasty
    accucinch system, 309–310
    mitral restriction ring, 310, 311
    mitralign system, 308, 309

Valcare, 311
  valtech cardioband, 310
Anomalous left coronary artery from the
  pulmonary artery (ALCAPA), 7
Aortic insufficiency, 3
Aortic regurgitation, 42
Aortic root, 1, 3
  rupture, 25
Aortic stenosis (AS), 3, 7, 8, 38, 45
  severe, 11
  symptomatic, 65
Aortic valve, 1–3, 5–8, 10
  anatomic variants
    ALCAPA, 7
    anomalous coronary arteries, 7
    bicuspid aortic valves, 7
  anatomy
    aortic annulus, 5
    aortic root, 3
    commissure, leaflet, 5, 6
    coronary ostia, 3
    leaflets, 3, 5
    left atrium, left ventricle, and aortic root, 2
    sinotubular junction (STJ), 1, 3
  imaging
    CMRI, 8
    leaflet calcification, 10
    TTE, 8
Aortic valve annulus, 35
Aortic valve replacement (AVR), 77, 78, 87, 168
  Direct Flow Medical valve, 59
  transcatheter (*see* Transcatheter aortic
    valve replacement (TAVR))
Arrhythmia, 267
AVR. *See* Aortic valve replacement (AVR)

Printed in the United States
By Bookmasters